FOURTH INTERNATIONAL SYMPOSIUM ON BOVINE LEUKOSIS

CURRENT TOPICS IN VETERINARY MEDICINE AND ANIMAL SCIENCE

VOLUME 15

FOURTH INTERNATIONAL SYMPOSIUM ON BOVINE LEUKOSIS

Other titles in this series

Volume 1
Control of Reproduction in the Cow
edited by J.M. Sreenan

Volume 2
Patterns of Growth and Development in Cattle
edited by H. de Boer and J. Martin

Volume 3
Respiratory Diseases in Cattle
edited by W.B. Martin

Volume 4
Calving Problems and Early Viability of the Calf
edited by B. Hoffmann, I.L. Mason and J. Schmidt

Volume 5
The Future of Beef Production in the European Community
edited by J.C. Bowman and P. Susmel

Volume 6
Diseases of Cattle in the Tropics: Economic and Zoonotic Relevance
edited by M. Ristic and I. McIntyre

Volume 7
Control of Reproductive Functions in Domestic Animals
edited by W. Jöchle and D.R. Lamond

Volume 8
The Laying Hen and its Environment
edited by R. Moss

Volume 9
Epidemiology and Control of Nematodiasis in Cattle
edited by P. Nansen, R.J. Jørgensen and E.J.L. Soulsby

Volume 10
The Problem of Dark-Cutting in Beef
edited by D.E. Hood and P.V. Tarrant

Volume 11
The Welfare of Pigs
edited by W. Sybesma

Volume 12
The Mucosal Immune System
edited by F.J. Bourne

Volume 13
Laboratory Diagnosis in Neonatal Calf and Pig Diarrhoea
edited by P.W. de Leeuw and P.A.M. Guinée

Volume 14
Advances in the Control of Theileriosis
edited by A.D. Irvin, M.P. Cunningham and A.S. Young

Series ISBN: 90-247-2429-5

FOURTH INTERNATIONAL SYMPOSIUM ON BOVINE LEUKOSIS

A Seminar in the EEC Programme of Coordination of Research on Animal Pathology organised by O.C. Straub and G. Gentile, and held in Bologna, 5-7 November 1980

Sponsored by the Commission of the European Communities, Directorate-General for Agriculture, Coordination of Agricultural Research

edited by

O.C. STRAUB
Bundesforschungsanstalt für
Viruskrankheiten der Tiere
Tübingen, B.R. Deutschland

1982

SPRINGER-SCIENCE+BUSINESS MEDIA, B.V.

Distributors

for the United States and Canada
Kluwer Boston, Inc.
190 Old Derby Street
Hingham, MA 02043
USA

for all other countries
Kluwer Academic Publishers Group
Distribution Center
P.O. Box 322
3300 AH Dordrecht
The Netherlands

Library of Congress Cataloging in Publication Data

International Symposium on Bovine Leukosis (4th :
1980 : Bologna, Italy)
Fourth International Symposium on Bovine Leukosis

(Current topics in veterinary medicine and animal science ; v. 15)
1. Bovine leukosis--Congresses. I. Straub, O. C. (Otto Christian), 1930- II. Commission of the European Communities. Directorate-General for Agriculture. Coordination of Agricultural Research. III. Title. IV. Series. [DNLM: 1. Cattle diseases--Congresses. 2. Leukemia--Veterinary--Congresses. 3. Retroviridae--Congresses. W1 CU822B v.15 / SF 967.L4 I61 1980f]
SF967.L4I57 1980 636.2'089699419 81-18951
ISBN 978-94-011-8391-8 AACR2

ISBN 978-94-011-8391-8 ISBN 978-94-011-9090-9 (eBook)
DOI 10.1007/978-94-011-9090-9

Publication arranged by
Commission of the European Communities,
Directorate-General Information Market and Innovation

EUR 7445 EN

Manuscript Preparation by
Janssen Services, 33a High Street, Chislehurst, Kent BR7 5AE, UK

PREFACE

The series of international symposia on Enzootic Bovine Leukosis (EBL) sponsored by the Commission of the European Communities, began in 1975 in Copenhagen. This latest symposium, the third, was held in Bologna, 5-7 November 1980. If we compare the two proceedings it is quite evident how much progress has been achieved in EBL research during these few years. Whereas in 1975 there were still discussions on the characterisation and importance of the various identified antigens and the antibodies against them, we now have evidence of base sequence variations of the bovine leukosis provirus derived from cattle in different continents, due to the world-wide cooperation on the subject. Disease control was still largely based on haematology, whereas now some countries are completely free, or on the verge of becoming completely free, of the disease following the introduction of serological methods of diagnosis.

EBL research appears to me to be an excellent example of the production of new fundamental research and its transfer to the applied disciplines of veterinary sciences. I must emphasise that this progress would not have been achieved if the CEC had not sponsored a number of projects and the meetings.

I should like to thank the CEC for this continued sponsorship, Prof. Dr. Gentile, whose invaluable assistance helped to ensure the quality of the symposium and Janssen Services for their work in preparing the proceedings and assistance with the editing of the papers and discussion.

Tübingen, June 1981

Otto Christian Straub

CONTENTS

SESSION I

Chairmen : G. Gentile and O.C. Straub

OPENING REMARKS

G. Gentile
Clinica Medica Veterinaria, Viale Q. Filopante 5,
I-40126 Bologna.

We convene today as a result of the proposal, put forward during the previous meeting held in Brussels on 1st June, 1979, that the IVth International Symposium on bovine leukosis should be held in Bologna. At that time I welcomed the suggestion that I should act as the local organiser, and today it is my duty and pleasure to welcome you at the start of this Symposium.

I should like to express my sincere appreciation of the effort and commitment that each of you, in his own way, has dedicated to the study of bovine leukosis and which have produced innumerable results, as can be seen in the various papers which have been produced at previous meetings. These meetings were begun in 1975, under the auspices of the European Economic Community, to whom we are very grateful for the interest and sensitivity with which it encourages all efforts directed towards improving the health and production potential of the animal population. We are particularly grateful for its financial contribution which enables us to meet here today.

I should also like to thank those corporations and businesses which have contributed towards the organisation of this Symposium.

In the knowledge that this meeting will enrich many personal friendships and revitalise our common theme of research, allow me to extend to you my most cordial greetings, and in addition those of our Chancellor, who will be glad to receive us in person in his office during intervals in the conference today and tomorrow. Please accept also greetings from my colleagues in the Faculty of Veterinary Medicine of the University of Bologna which is our host during the next few days.

O.C. Straub (ed.), Fourth International Symposium on Bovine Leukosis

I should now like to wish you good luck in your work, which is very worthwhile. As we know, in the past few years bovine leukosis has become increasingly widespread and today it presents an ever-increasing risk to cattle. In addition to countries with a history of infection, we are now witnessing an ever-increasing rate of bovine leukosis in countries which were previously unaffected. In fact, modern methods of investigation have revealed the presence of infected animals in countries which, until recently, were thought to be leukosis free.

In view of the growing proportions of this problem, we must recognise the need for a multidisciplinary approach to its theoretical and practical aspects, both of which are to be developed in the course of the scientific programme of this Symposium. During the next three days we will share the results of our research and deepen our knowledge in a free exchange of ideas and opinions. In the final analysis this last point represents the ultimate goal of any scientific encounter, a goal which will certainly be achieved during the next few days due to the exceptional competence of the participants to whom Bologna is proud to play host.

With that assurance, let us begin our work in the hope that the scientific success of the Symposium may overshadow any inevitable organisational deficiencies.

Finally, I should like to thank you for participating. I am aware that your unquestioned scientific authority in the field of bovine leukosis lends great prestige to this Symposium. I should also like to extend a special greeting to those participants from nations which do not belong to the European Economic Community, as well as to our non-European colleagues, whose participation is particularly valued, emphasising as it does the validity of the scientific programme which has been promoted, since 1975, by the Commission of the European Communities.

INTRODUCTORY LECTURE

THE EVOLUTION AND DIMINUTION OF BOVINE LEUKOSIS

O.C. Straub
Federal Research Institute for Animal Virus Diseases, D-7400 Tübingen, Federal Republic of Germany.

It was during the nineteenth century when veterinarians found that leukaemia and tumours occurred in some herds of cattle but not in others. Almost one century passed before it was generally accepted that the 'Bovine Leukosis Virus' (BLV), a member of the oncovirinae subgroup of the retroviridae, was the aetiological agent of the disease. This most important result of 'Enzootic Bovine Leukosis' (EBL) research has led first to the development of a number of serological methods - among other problems to be discussed at this meeting - enabling us to determine whether or not an animal is free of specific antibodies, and secondly to the development of methods for the detection of BLV or BLV antigen in a host.

This knowledge has, however, not solved the question concerning the development or disappearance of clinical EBL symptoms, such as lymphocytosis and/or tumours. It is still largely a matter of speculation as to how the virus is spread other than by the general routes named 'vertical' or 'horizontal' transmission. Vertical transmission is conceived to occur during the prenatal period, horizontal transmission during the postnatal period. The horizontal, i.e. postnatal, spread is thought to occur via colostrum and/or milk, by vectors, semen, saliva or by mechanical (artificial) means such as the bleeding needle. The results of all experiments have not led to any conclusion as to why one seropositive animal can act as a transmitter and others not. It is also still a matter of speculation as to why one animal develops lymphocytosis and/or tumours after an infection with BLV and others do not. Furthermore, it remains unknown why under natural conditions one gets only approximately 60% of the cattle population infected, and under experimental

O.C. Straub (ed.), Fourth International Symposium on Bovine Leukosis

conditions 100%. If bovine leukosis was transmitted like any other infectious disease, we would certainly have all the answers available by now. Because it is not so, I would like to present my personal ideas on the subject based only on my own experience.

In a BLV infected herd of cattle there may be different types of cattle, such as:

1) cattle free of BLV and BLV-specific antibodies, non-susceptible under natural conditions;

2) cattle free of BLV and BLV-specific antibodies but susceptible under natural conditions;

3) horizontally infected cattle which are non-contagious for neighbouring cattle;

4) horizontally infected and stressed cattle which are at times contagious for neighbouring animals and foetuses. Some of them may develop clinical symptoms;

5) vertically infected cattle which are contagious for neighbouring cattle and foetuses. They are prone to develop a lymphocytosis and/or tumours;

6) lymphocytic cattle with or without tumours which may be highly contagious for neighbouring cattle and foetuses.

Cattle of groups 1 and 2 and also of group 3, are of no importance because they never spread the virus and may be detected as the only positive animal in a herd even at an advanced age. In the routine immunodiffusion test (IDT) animals of that category (group 3) have only a gp antibody titre. Their offspring acquire high antibody titres which render them non-susceptible for the first few months of life. If separated from the dam within the first three months they remain serologically negative after the disappearance of the colostral antibodies. In contrast, offspring from the cattle of groups 1 and 2 may be susceptible immediately after birth. However, it is necessary for them to come into close contact with positive cattle. A distance of 2 or more metres prevents transmission, if biological vectors can be excluded. This fact may also explain why leukosis will not necessarily be spread by animals on pasture, if they belong to group 3.

Animals that contact the agent before or at a period of stress appear to be of considerable importance. In contrast to group 3 just mentioned, they become contagious at times and may easily transmit the agent vertically. A certain percentage of them even develops clinical signs of the disease. Whether or not the foetus will form antibodies prenatally depends on the stage of its growth. If a period of stress is followed by non-stressful periods, later calves might be born without the presence of antibodies and attain temporary protection through the dam's colostrum. Vertically infected cattle (group 5) appear to be the most dangerous ones. The antigen is not readily detectable in all of them at birth, but some of them show the presence of antibodies prior to the ingestion of colostrum. The colostral antibodies seem to persist somewhat longer than in the virus free animals. Either they disappear gradually and the animals stay seronegative in the IDT or an increase is noted after 5 - 7 months. Those that have become negative may remain in that stage for as long as 2 - 3 years, after which period they again develop antibodies and may become contagious. It is then very easy to detect antigen in the peripheral blood leukocytes. Animals of that kind are disastrous at times for herds participating in an eradication programme. If an animal is pregnant at that time the virus may easily pass to the foetus again. Such animals often develop a lymphocytosis at a later age, which might be followed by tumour formation.

Cattle of group 6 (lymphocytic with or without tumours) are considered to be frequently contagious for neighbouring animals and foetuses. In the IDT they usually show the presence of antibodies against the gp and p24 antigens; in some cases the concentration of p24 antibodies may even exceed that of gp antibodies. Calves born to them may harbour the virus at birth and will carry it continuously in the peripheral blood leukocytes.

A very high percentage of those animals will come down with lymphocytosis and tumours. They represent the typical lymphosarcomas.

As you can see, it will take many generations of infected cattle before the stage is reached where the annual losses may be as high as 10 to 20%. A situation such as this existed during the late forties to fifties in many cattle herds in the east and middle of Europe. It was the time when the leukosis keys emerged.

Many people consider the early sanitation measures as completely unsuccessful and wrong. I disagree. There is plenty of evidence that the incidence of cases with lymphocytosis and tumours decreased. We can explain this now. By those measures we caught a high number of those animals which spread the disease and caused the tumour cases by vertical transmission. Let me mention an example: a herd of about 150 head was haematologically checked for many years and the positive cattle eliminated. The incidence of tumour development and lymphocytosis went down to 0% and remained at that level for 7 years until serology was introduced. It was then found that 7.5% of the cattle were seropositive. This percentage increased to 30% during the following years. At the same time no lymphocytosis was detected during the routine check-ups, only individual elevated lymphocyte counts were determined during the course of the research programme. It would most likely have taken another few years until the first case of lymphocytosis occurred and later on tumours would have been found again. Here the evolution of the disease was stopped by the introduction of the serological method and we have now reached a diminution of EBL in the country due to the systematic testing and elimination of seropositive animals from the herds.

If I am right, it is possible to explain why the disease obviously spread much faster during recent decades than during earlier ones. In the old days cattle were not sold and transported as much as they are nowadays - from herd to herd, from fair to fair, from country to country, from continent to continent. Usually, those animals are the best ones, the high producers which are already continuously stressed. If the stress of transportation is then added, those animals are easily infected and incapable of handling the infection. They become the best propagators of BLV.

With this in mind it is also possible to explain why some authors point to the importance of vertical transmission, which is certainly true as far as later clinical symptoms are concerned, and others refer to horizontal transmission as the most important one; this is also true as far as seroconversion is concerned. It just depends on what stage of evolution or diminution a herd is in at the time a research programme is conducted.

SESSION II

BLV Studies

Chairmen : Y. Becker and O.-R. Kaaden

INTRODUCTORY REMARKS

Y. Becker
Department of Molecular Virology, Hebrew University,
Hadassah Medical School, P.O. Box 1172, Jerusalem, Israel.

Having looked at the programme of the meeting, and having attended all the previous meetings in this series of international symposia, it seems to me to be very clear that research in this field is now progressing well. During the last few years, there were problems that were of great interest to us but on which opinions differed - for example, on the correct molecular weight of a certain glycoprotein, the structure of the virus, and so on. Most of these issues have now been settled and agreed upon, and the research is now moving on to the major questions of why this is a cancerous virus, why does the virus sometimes spread so rapidly from one animal to another, what actually controls the expression of the virus, and is the virus a leukosis or tumour-forming agent? In this meeting, I think the situation regarding what we now know and what we do not know will become clearer.

I would like to draw your attention to one point which is becoming apparent from research on retroviruses, and which is not mentioned here, namely the question of what is the gene structure of a retrovirus that causes a tumour. From studies done by many workers, among them D. Baltimore, it is becoming clear that we are not dealing with interaction between viral genes alone but with an interaction between viral and cellular genes which function together to cause cancer. Although the meeting is on bovine leukosis virus, I think it is proper to introduce the concept that we have to consider cellular genes that might be involved in the processes leading to cancer. One of the papers in the next session, by Dr. Lévy, actually deals with this concept; a special group of genes will be described, and their function in relation to the oncogenic genes of the virus. However, when we look at the structure of leukomogenic viruses, we see that the viruses undergo a marked change. They

O.C. Straub (ed.), Fourth International Symposium on Bovine Leukosis

differ from the original virus in the sense that they do not have all the viral genes: instead of some of the viral genes, they have cellular genes. In fact, we are dealing here with two classes of viruses - one is a real virus that has all the genes required by a retrovirus and the other is a defective virus which has lost a few of the viral genes but has acquired instead cellular genes and thus forms a new subclass of this virus. The next paper, from Dr. Burny's laboratory, will develop this idea further.

Since one of the major problems that we will be considering is that of cancer, we must contemplate the question of the virus hiding itself away, namely becoming latent, and forming an endogenous virus that does not express any genes and therefore does not lead to the formation of antibodies. All of a sudden, a process of reactivation can occur, and an animal which was, by all criteria, absolutely virus negative can develop an infection and release infectious virus. This must be taken into consideration when we talk about removing the virus from the environment and having virus-free herds at least in the EC member states, as is being planned. In addition to studies on the epidemiology of the virus, I think we should also investigate the possibility that the bovine leukosis virus might become an endogenous virus that can be reactivated. After or during reactivation, there may be an interaction with cellular genes, leading to the formation of a transforming virus. Such investigations would add to our understanding of what constitutes a leukomogenic virus, in addition to understanding leukomogenic virus function in the transformation of a cell and the development of a tumour.

BASE SEQUENCE VARIATIONS IN THE BOVINE LEUKAEMIA PROVIRUS

D. Couez(1), M. Mammerickx(2), C. Olson(3), M. Onuma(4), A-L. Parodi(5), M.J. Van der Maaten(6), A. Burny(1)(7) and R. Kettmann(1)(7).

(1) University of Brussels, Belgium; (2) Institute for Veterinary Research, Uccle, Belgium; (3) University of Wisconsin, Madison, USA; (4) Hokkaido University, Japan; (5) National Veterinary School, Maisons-Alfort, France; (6) National Animal Diseases Center, Ames, USA; (7) Faculty of Agronomy, Gembloux, Belgium.

ABSTRACT

Restriction endonuclease analysis was performed in order to compare the integrated BLV provirus in affected tissues of animals from distant geographic origins (Belgium, France, Japan, USA). Seven BLV genetic mutants were discovered during this short survey performed on 17 BLV infected animals with either persistent lymphocytosis or lymphosarcoma. Most of the variations were probably due to point mutations rather than deletions or insertions. One deleted mutant, lacking about 4 830 (out of 10 000) base pairs at the 5' end of the proviral genome was identified in a tumour from Japan.

O.C. Straub (ed.), Fourth International Symposium on Bovine Leukosis

INTRODUCTION

Bovine leukaemia virus (BLV), an exogenous retrovirus of cattle (Kettmann et al., 1976) is the pathogenic agent of enzootic bovine leukosis (EBL) (see Burny et al., 1980, for a review). The target cell is the B lymphocyte (Muscoplat et al., 1974). BLV infection may induce perisistent lymphocytosis (PL) (characterised by an increased number of apparently normal B lymphocytes in the peripheral blood of the infected animal) and, in a latter stage, lymphnode tumours.

Proviral copies were found to be integrated at many sites in the genomes of a fraction of the leukocytes of animals with PL, but at only one or very few sites in the genomes of a larger fraction of leukocytes or tumour cells of animals with lymphosarcoma (Kettmann et al., 1980a). Since two BLV genetic mutants were detected in the Belgian cattle population (Kettmann et al., 1980b) we wanted to extend the study of BLV proviral genetic stability. This should be very useful for analysing the organisation of exogenous bovine leukaemia virus sequences in bovine cells of outbred cattle populations.

DNAs from buffy coat cells or tumours were digested by bacterial restriction endonucleases and submitted to electrophoresis in agarose gels. After transfer to cellulose nitrate paper, the DNA fragments were annealed to a specific BLV cDNA probe labelled with ^{32}P (Southern, 1975). Genomic DNA fragments containing viral information appear as individual bands, sometimes as smears after autoradiographic development.

In this report, we show that BLV provirus heterogeneity in bovine cell DNA often includes point mutations but sometimes large deletions.

MATERIALS AND METHODS

Cells and tissues

Bovine tissues and cells were collected from 17 animals

with EBL. Three animals (nos 2586, 928 and 65) were in PL and 14 (nos 15, 950, 79-2, 3168, 3261, 3202, 3156, 56, 53, 46, 119, 1347, 1351, 1345) with lymphosarcoma. Leukocytes from animals in PL, tumours from lymphosarcomatous cases and the thymus of a normal calf were used as sources of DNA.

BLV was produced by the BLV infected-foetal lamb kidney (FLK) cells established by Van der Maaten and Miller (1976).

Cellular DNA extraction

This was performed with SDS and phenol-chloroform essentially as described by Kay et al., 1952. The molecular weights of all DNA preparations were found to be higher than 20×10^6 as estimated by 0.5% agarose gel electrophoresis using λ DNA and λ EcoRI digest as molecular weight markers.

Restriction endonuclease digestions

All restriction enzymes, but one, used in this study were purchased from New England Biolabs; EcoRI enzyme was a Boehringer product. About 20 μg of DNA were digested for 2 h in 20 μl of appropriate buffer with an excess of restriction endonuclease. The extent of digestion was usually monitored by including a marker DNA of known cleavage pattern in the digestion mixture.

Gel electrophoresis

Restriction enzyme digests were added directly to horizontal slab agarose (SIGMA) gels. The electrophoresis apparatus was purchased from Bethesda Research Laboratory Inc. (Rockville, MD). We prepared 0.4 cm thick slab gels of 0.8% agarose. Restriction fragments of λ DNA and ØX 174 DNA were used as size standards. The length estimate of restriction fragments is probably accurate to ± 80 nucleotides.

Blotting

After electrophoresis, DNA fragments were denatured and transferred from agarose gels to sheets of 0.45 μm cellulose nitrate (Millipore, Bedford, Mass.) in 3M NaCl pH 11 (Meunier et al., 1979). After rinsing in 3 x SSC, the filter was dried in air and baked at 80°C for 3 h.

Viral RNA and cDNA synthesis

BLV production and purification, viral RNA extraction and purification were carried out as previously described (Ghysdael et al., 1979). In brief, poly A^+ RNAs present in each viral particle were prepared from 60 - 70S viral RNA by heat denaturation and chromatography on oligo (dT)-cellulose. Sedimentation of that poly A^+ RNA on a denaturing sucrose gradient showed that about 25 to 30% of the molecules were full-length 38S, the other molecules having lengths ranging from about 12S to 38S. BLV (^{32}P) cDNA (4.2×10^8 cpm/μg) was synthesised as previously described (Kettmann et al., 1980).

Hybridisation

Baked, blotted nitrocellulose filters were wet in 3 x SSC (SSC = 0.15M NaCl plus 0.015M sodium citrate) and pre-hybridised in a plastic box with 40 ml of a mixture containing 3 x SSC, 10 x Denhardt medium (Denhardt, 1966), 0.1% SDS and 100 μg of denatured calf thymus DNA per ml. The (^{32}P) cDNA probe (about 5×10^6 cpm/ml) was separately prehybridised in the same mixture except that denatured calf thymus DNA was present at a concentration of 2 mg/ml to avoid ribosomal contaminants. After an overnight incubation at 65°C, the filters were removed from their prehybridisation mixture and then hybridised with mixing, for 24 h with the prehybridised (^{32}P) cDNA probe. Filters were washed for about 1 h at 65°C in several changes of 3 x SSC. This was repeated with 0.3 x SSC for 30 min. Dried filters were exposed at -70°C to preflashed KODAK X-Omat-R films in presence of Siemens 'special' intensifying screens for 1 - 3 days.

RESULTS

We have recently established a restriction map of the

linear unintegrated proviral DNA of BLV produced by the BLV infected FLK cells established by Van der Maaten and Miller (1976) (Kettmann et al. manuscript submitted). That same BLV proviral DNA was taken as a reference for the present study. Figure 1 represents the cleavage sites, on that linear unintegrated DNA, for the bacterial restriction endonucleases used in this investigation.

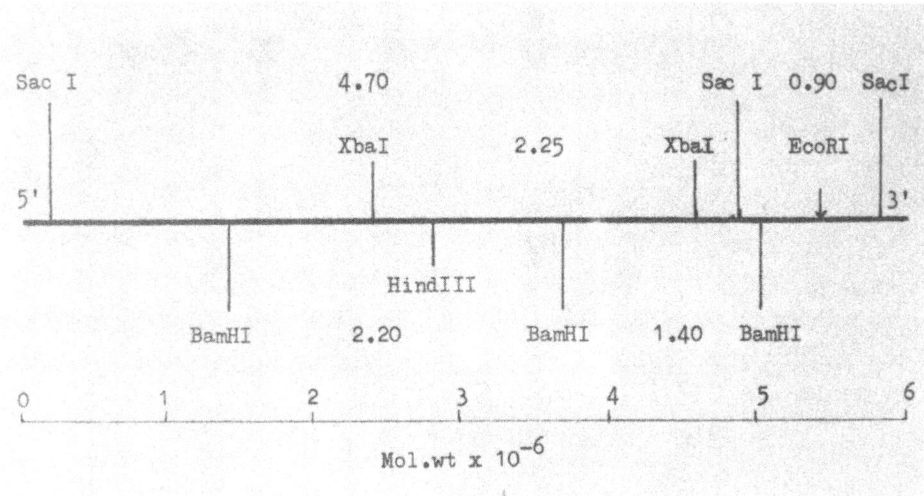

Fig. 1. Restriction map of bovine leukaemia virus (BLV-FLK isolate) unintegrated viral DNA.

Total cellular DNAs from circulating leukocytes from animals in PL or from lymphosarcoma were digested with the endonucleases shown in Figure 1 and analysed according to Southern (1975).

The results obtained when BLV (^{32}P) cDNA was annealed to EcoRI restriction fragments of circulating leukocytes or tumour DNAs from various animals are shown in Figure 2. The electrophoretic pattern of BLV-positive DNA fragments from animals 2586, 928 and 65, in PL, appeared as a continuum of hybridisation from MW = 5×10^6 up to MW = 12×10^6. These data indicated and confirmed (Kettmann et al., 1979, 1980 a, b) that many sites in the bovine genome could accommodate the BLV provirus. However, they did not allow to detect the presence of an EcoRI restriction site.

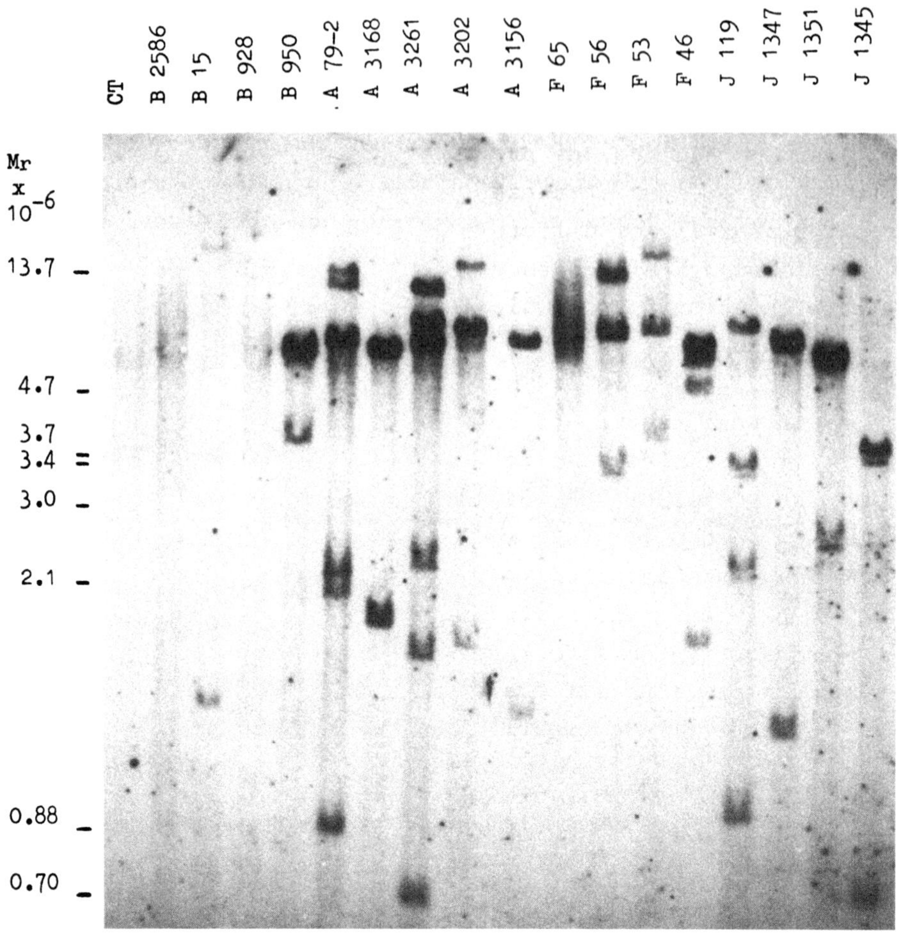

Fig. 2. Hybridisation patterns of BLV (^{32}P) cDNA on DNA restriction fragments from circulating leukocytes of animals in PL or from lymphosarcoma. Twenty micrograms of each DNA were exhaustively digested by <u>EcoRI</u> and electrophoresed on a 0.8% agarose gel. The DNA fragments were blotted and hybridised as described in Materials and Methods. Autoradiography was for 72 h.

In contrast, the EcoRI digests of lymphosarcoma DNAs (15, 950, 79-2, 3168, 3261, 3202, 3156, 56, 53, 46, 1347, 1351) exhibited one to three viral positive fragments of MW above 5×10^6 with respectively one to three smaller viral positive fragments of MW between 0.70×10^6 and 4.80×10^6 (some of these fragments were too weak to be seen on the autoradiogram as reproduced). Our interpretation of these data is that:

1. one EcoRI site was present in all proviruses detected;

2. one to three BLV proviral copies were integrated per haploid genome.

However, we cannot rule out the possibility that one to three clones, each containing one provirus copy located at a different site, were present in these tumours. A comparative restriction analysis of different tumours of the same animal where several proviral copies were detected should help to solve this question. EcoRI digest of tumour 119 showed one hybridisation band of MW = 8.0×10^6 and three bands between 0.80×10^6 and 3.00×10^6. This result strongly suggests the presence, in that tumour, of one complete provirus and one deleted one. More interesting was the result encountered with EcoRI digest of tumour DNA 1345 where two hybridisation bands of 3.20×10^6 and 0.70×10^6 were observed. The sum of the MW of these fragments amounted to 3.90×10^6. Considering that the linear unintegrated provirus has a MW = 6.0×10^6 (Kettmann et al., manuscript submitted) these data very probably indicated that the only provirus integrated in tumour 1345 was deleted. That conclusion will be clearly confirmed by SacI digestion (Figure 4).

XbaI digest of linear unintegrated BLV DNA induced by BLV produced by the BLV infected FLK cells generated one internal fragment of 2.25×10^6 (Figure 1). XbaI digests of all American tumour DNAs (79-2, 3168, 3261, 3202, 3156) as well as French tumour DNA 56 and circulating leukocyte DNA from animal 65, in PL, showed the same 2.25×10^6 viral internal fragment (Figure 3). It should be recalled that, in restriction digests of circulating leukocyte DNA from animals in PL, only viral internal fragments will be visualised as well defined bands because of the polyclonality of the infected cells (Kettmann et al., 1980). It should also be noted that in restriction digests of tumour DNAs containing several proviral copies (i.e. DNA 3261, 79-2), restriction fragments cleaved from within integrated genomes result in intense bands whereas faint bands are produced by provirus end fragments that are attached to diverse host sequences.

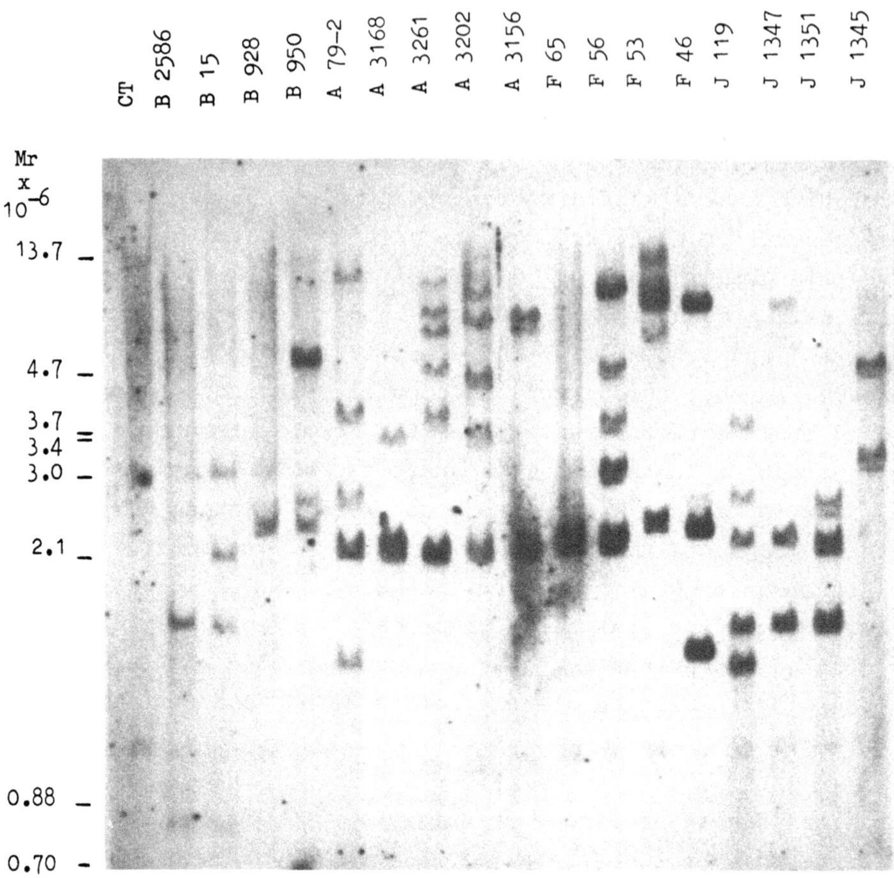

Fig. 3. Hybridisation patterns of BLV (^{32}P) cDNA on DNA restriction fragments from circulating leukocytes from animals in PL or from lymphosarcoma. Twenty micrograms of each DNA were exhaustively digested by XbaI and electrophoresed on a 0.8% agarose gel. The DNA fragments were blotted and hybridised as described in Materials and Methods. Autoradiography was for 72 h.

North Belgian tumour DNA 15 and circulating leukocyte DNA from animal 2586, in PL, showed two proviral internal fragments of 1.75×10^6 and 0.85×10^6 (Figure 3). South Belgian tumour DNA 950 and circulating leukocyte DNA from animal 928, in PL, shared the same viral internal fragment of 2.60×10^6 in common with French tumour DNAs 53 and 56 (Figure 3). Japanese tumour DNAs 119 and 1347 shared in common two viral positive fragments of 2.40×10^6 and 1.75×10^6 (Figure 3). Only one of these fragments might be of proviral internal origin since only three viral positive fragments were detected in DNA 1347 where only one proviral copy was detected (Figure 2). Japanese tumour DNA 1351 shared in common with tumour DNAs 1347 and 119 the 1.75 kb fragment, strongly suggesting its internal position. Japanese tumour DNA 1345 containing one BLV proviral copy (Figure 1) two viral positive fragments of 6.20 x 10^6 and 3.40 x 10^6 implying the existence of one XbaI site in that integrated provirus (Figure 3). This result might well be related to the presence of a deletion in the provirus (Figure 2).

The results obtained after BamHI and HindIII digestions are summarised in Table 1. They also allowed the detection of variations in the integrated BLV genome.

The enzyme SacI cut within terminal sequences at both ends of BLV DNA but also cleaved at another internal site generating two fragments of 4.70 x 10^6 and 0.90 x 10^6 (Figure 1). This enzyme appeared to be a useful tool to detect deleted mutants. Some of the SacI digestions are illustrated in Figure 4. American tumour DNAs 79-2, 3168 and 3261 shared the same two internal fragments of 4.70 x 10^6 and 0.90 x 10^6 in common with those found for the linear unintegrated DNA (Figure 1). The three other bands of 3.10 x 10^6, 2.00 x 10^6 and 1.10 x 10^6 detected in all SacI digests, including the control calf thymus DNA, were due to a contamination of the probe with ribosomal sequences. Belgian tumour DNAs 15 and 950 as well as circulating leukocyte DNAs 2586 and 928 showed only one fragment (5.60 x 10^6) of viral origin. It seems thus very likely that these proviruses had lost the most internal SacI restriction site. Japanese tumour DNA 119 which contained two proviral copies (Figure 2) showed the same 4.70 x 10^6 and 0.90 x 10^6 viral fragments already observed for unintegrated linear DNA (Figure 1). In addition, another fragment of 2.35 x 10^6 was detected. We already knew that one proviral copy was detected (see EcoRi digestion). It seems thus very likely that SacI digestion of the deleted provirus produced the 2.35 x 10^6 fragment (instead of a 4.70 x 10^6 fragment) and probably one 0.90 x 10^6 fragment.

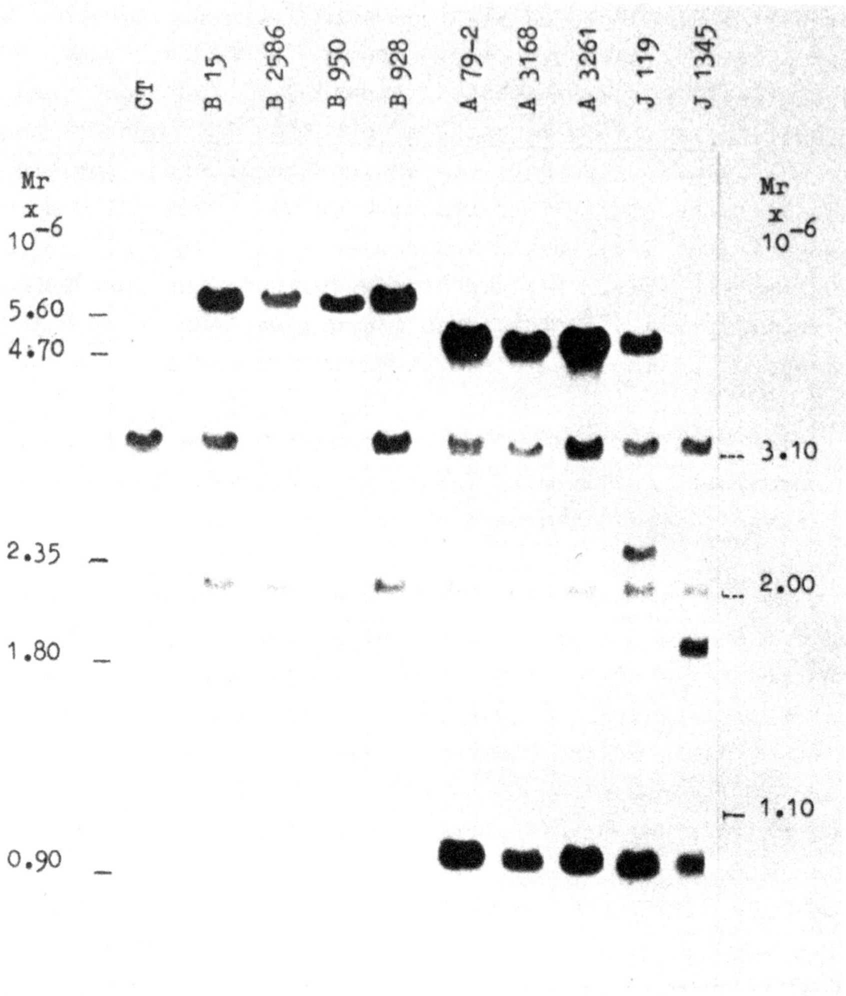

Fig. 4. Hybridisation patterns of BLV (^{32}P) cDNA on DNA restriction fragments from circulating leukocytes from animals in PL or from lymphosarcoma. Twenty micrograms of each DNA were exhaustively digested by SacI and electrophoresed on a 0.8% agarose gel. The DNA fragments were blotted and hybridised as described in Materials and Methods. Autoradiography was for 72 h.

In Japanese tumour DNA 1345, only one deleted provirus was detected (Figure 1). SacI digestion generated two viral fragments of 1.80×10^6 and 0.90×10^6. Our interpretation of that result is that the 4.70×10^6 fragment located at the 5' end of the proviral molecule was deleted of about 2.90×10^6 daltons (4 830 kilobase pairs).

TABLE 1

DIFFERENCES IN CLEAVAGE SITES WITHIN VARIOUS MUTANTS OF INTEGRATED BLV PROVIRUSES.

Variant	Country of origin	Animal number	Number of restriction endonuclease cleavage sites and length of proviral internal fragments in megadaltons (in brackets)				
			EcoRI	XbaI	BamHI	HindIII	SacI
Variant 1 (BLV-FLK)	USA (Wisconsin, Iowa)	79-2, 3168, 3261 3202, 3156	1	2 (2.25)	3 (2.20; 1.40)	1	3 (4.70; 0.90)
Variant 2	Belgium (South) France	928, 950 46, 53	1	2 (2.60)	3 (2.20; 1.47)	0	2 (5.60)
Variant 3	Belgium (North)	2586, 15	1	3 (1.75; 0.85)	3 (2.20; 1.47)	0	2
Variant 4	France	65, 56	1	2 (2.25)	3 (1.40; 0.80)	0	NT
Variant 5	Japan	1347, 119	1	2 (2.40 <u>or</u> 1.75)	3 (2.20; 1.40)	1	3 (4.70; 0.90)
Variant 6	Japan	1351	1	2 (1.75)	1-2 (?)	0	NT
Variant 7	Japan	1345	1	1	0 ?	0 ?	2-3 (0.90 and perhaps 2.35)

NT = not tested.

DISCUSSION

We have analysed integrated BLV proviruses in Southern blots of chromosomal DNA originating either from circulating lymphocytes or from tumour tissue. The unintegrated linear DNA produced by short term infection of permissive cells by BLV from FLK cell line (Van der Maaten and Miller, 1976) was taken as reference and referred to as variant 1 (Table 1). When polyclonal populations of BLV-infected cells are analysed, fragments cleaved from within integrated genomes result in intense bands whereas provirus end fragments attached to diverse hose sequences make up smears of radioactive material in the agarose gels. This is specifically the case when DNA from circulating lymphocytes of animals in PL is examined (Kettmann et al., 1980 a, b). When monoclonal populations of provirus-carrying cells are analysed, all restriction bands are intense. Of course, only those representing internal pieces of proviral DNA serve the purpose of the study reported here. Logically also, the nucleases most useful within the frame of our study are those for which BLV proviruses provide a moderate number of restriction sites. If one restriction site only is present, it can solely be concluded that it is conserved or not (see Table 1, EcoRI and HindIII nucleases). Conversely, enzymes with high frequency of cleavage give rise to complex and uninterpretable profiles. All animals from which material was examined in this report were either in persistent lymphocytosis or with lymphosarcoma. They also showed positive reactions when tested for antibody to BLV envelope glycoprotein gp51 and internal antigen p24.

From the comparison between nucleases EcoRI and HindIII, it comes that the 17 samples analysed do carry one EcoRI site. We favour the idea but have no proof for it yet that we are dealing with the same site, thus located in a crucial region for BLV function. It is indeed remarkable that after EcoRI digestion, all samples (Figure 2) show the presence of a dark high molecular weight band (MW > 5.10^6) together with a faint band of smaller molecular weight. The darkness of the band being correlated with the length of viral information in the fragment, we tend to consider that the unique EcoRI site is highly conserved at the 3' side of the proviral DNA. On the contrary, HindIII site is present in the five samples from North Central USA and in two Japanese cases, which tends to show a much less stringent requirement for this site in BLV function. Moreover, it may be significant to notice that BamHI internal fragments have the same lengths both in the five American and the two Japanese cases 1347 and 119. We incline to believe that the 7 animals considered here were infected by two closely related BLV variants.

A striking feature of this study is the observation that the five field cases of North Central USA harbour a BLV provirus probably identical to variant 1 used by Van der Maaten and Miller to infect FLK cell line. A given variant seems to be conserved when spreading in a given geographical area. An analogous conclusion is reached when considering the four cases analysed in Belgium (North and South) and two French cases. Variants 2 and 3 seem to be closely related, variant 3 exhibiting one supplementary BamHI site. Taken together, these two sets of observations indicate that BLV spread can occur without much genetic drift, a conclusion that fits quite well with the general opinion that BLV spreads horizontally via the cell rather than the virus route through husbandry and veterinary malpractices. Propagation of integrated provirus rather than virus particles possibly avoids replication steps like reverse transcription, integration, etc., where mutations are most likely to occur than during normal DNA duplication.

A next step in these studies will be to locate as precisely as possible the sites of variations. It already appears that mutations do occur at dispersed locations along the proviral genome. We, indeed, noticed modifications at the HindIII site (in the middle of the molecule); at one SacI site (the one that is to the left of the EcoRI site) and we even observed a broad deletion at the 5' end of the provirus. With the exceptions of two large deletions observed, in one of the proviral copies found in DNA 119 and in the unique proviral copy present in DNA 1345, SacI digests did not reveal modifications in the total length of other proviruses, including those found in the majority of leukocytes of animals in PL. Considering the limitations of the technique used, these results exclude large insertions or deletions and allow to postulate the existence of many point mutations. Sequencing data will settle the issue when necessary.

The mechanism by which leukaemia viruses responsible for chronic diseases exert their oncogenic effects is unknown. Expression of 'leuk' genes of viral origin, induction of transcription of downstream genes, etc., have been put forward. Discovery of mutants with very large deletions like case 1345 may help approach the problem. We are currently pursuing this task by characterising the normal and deleted provirus genomes and by studying their infectivity and biological effects on selected target cells.

ACKNOWLEDGEMENTS

This work was supported by the Fonds Cancérologique of the Caisse Générale d'Epargne et de Retraite, Belgium. R.K. is 'Chercheur Qualifié' of the Fonds National Belge de la Recherche Scientifique.

REFERENCES

Burny, A., Bruck, C., Chantrenne, H., Cleuter, Y., Dekegel, J., Ghysdael, J., Kettmann, R., Leclercq, M., Leunen, J., Mammerickx, M. and Portetelle, D., 1980. Bovine leukemia virus: molecular biology and epidemiology. In Viral Oncology (Klein, G., Ed) p. 231, Raven Press, New York.

Denhardt, D.T., 1966. A membrane-filter technique for the detection of complementary DNA. Biochem. Biophys. Res. Commun. 23, 641-646.

Ghysdael, J., Kettmann, R. and Burny, A., 1979. Translation of bovine leukemia virus virion RNAs in heterologous protein-synthesizing systems. J. Virol. 29, 1087-1098.

Kay, E.R.M., Simmons, N.S. and Douce, A.L., 1952. An improved preparation of sodium deoxyribonucleate. J. Am. Chem. Soc. 74, 1724-1726.

Kettmann, R., Cleuter, Y., Mammerickx, M., Meunier-Rotival, M., Bernardi, G., Burny, A. and Chantrenne, H., 1980a. Genomic integration of bovine leukemia provirus: comparison of persistent lymphocytosis with lymph node tumor form of enzootic bovine leukosis. Proc. Natl. Acad. Sci. USA 77, 2577-2581.

Kettmann, R., Marbaix, G., Burny, A., Meunier-Rotival, M., Bernardi, G. and Mammerickx, M., 1980b. Genomic integration of bovine leukemia provirus. Cold Spring Harbor Conferences on Cell Proliferation, vol. 7, pp. 927-941.

Kettmann, R., Meunier-Rotival, M., Cortadas, J., Cuny, G. Ghysdael, J., Mammerickx, M., Burny, A. and Bernardi, G., 1979. Integration of bovine leukemia virus DNA in the bovine genome. Proc. Natl. Acad. Sci. USA, 76, 4822-4826.

Kettmann, R., Portetelle, D., Mammerickx, M., Cleuter, Y., Dekegel, D., Galoux, M., Ghysdael, J., Burny, A. and Chantrenne, H., 1976. Bovine leukemia virus: an exogenous RNA oncogenic virus. Proc. Natl. Acad. Sci. USA 73, 1014-1018.

Meunier-Rotival, M., Cortadas, J., Macaya, G. and Bernardi, G., 1979. Isolation and organization of cell ribosomal DNA. Nucleic Acids Res. 6, 2109-2123.

Muscoplat, C.D., Johnson, D.W., Pomeroy, K.A., Olson, J.M., Larson, V.L., Stevens, J.B. and Sorensen, D.K., 1974. Lymphocyte surface immunoglobulin, frequency in normal and lymphocytotic cattle. Am. J. Vet. Res. 35, 593-595.

Southern, E.M., 1975. Detection of specific sequences among DNA fragments separated by gel electrophoresis. J. Mol. Biol. 98, 503-517.

DISCUSSION

A.A. Ressang *(Netherlands)*

Can you tell us whether it is possible to use this technique for sub-classification of BLV? I presume that the strains you got from Japan, Belgium and France are cross reacting serologically. Will you be able, in the future, to make a sub-classification of BLV or is it simply the case that you will be able to say that one strain is virulent in comparison to the other?

R. Kettman *(Belgium)*

I think that will be very difficult. I mentioned only five enzymes but I have done more and if you use different enzymes it seems that the variation is very important. If you digest with different enzymes you will see a very important variability. I do not say that it is not possible to make a classification but it will be necessary to analyse a lot of samples to be sure of defining, say, 10 classes. The more samples you analyse, the more variants you will find.

Y. Becker *(Israel)*

This is a very important question which ought to be clarified rightaway. We are talking about genes and antigens. What Dr. Ressang referred to is actually antigenic variation. Can you find any variations in the structure of the envelope gene which can be reflected in antigenic variation?

R. Kettman

We have found some variations in the envelope gene region but we have no correlation with the differences in the antigenic properties.

M. Mussgay *(FRG)*

Did you try to take one of these strains from cattle and put it into the sheep?

R. Kettman

The sheep we have in Belgium were infected by Mammerickx but I have not yet checked these DNAs to see whether or not there are variations.

R. Schön *(DDR)*

Just to take Dr. Ressang's question a stage further, is there any evidence from your group or from other workers, that these viruses express any structural variance?

R. Kettman

Not to my knowledge.

R. Mamoun *(France)*

I have another virus from France and there is no difference in the gp by the radioimmunological assay. There is no difference in the gp and in the p24.

O.-R. Kaaden *(FRG)*

Dr. Kettman, as I understood you, you have analysed the integrated form of DNA. Would you expect that the differences in this integrated DNA also relate to antigenic differences, for p24 or the gp antigen, for example?

A. Burny *(Belgium)*

Maybe I can give an opinion on this. We will hear the work of Portetelle later on but I think we can say that the site that is antigenic *in vivo* in infected animals for the envelope glycoprotein which seems to be the region of the virus where most of the variations are, that this site is unique and due to the carbohydrate of the molecule. So, we can imagine that if the mutation occurs at the amino acid to which the carbohydrate side chain is attached, then we can expect to have a variant that would not be detected. But that has not been seen so far to my knowledge.

G.H. Theilen *(USA)*

What you have reported is extremely interesting and intriguing. I have two questions. What you are describing is reminiscent of sarcoma viruses. Dr. Burny has given some explanation on the biochemistry. However, as I recall, leukaemia viruses are fairly stable but the sarcoma viruses, feline, murine and avian, do vary in their integration sites. Are we dealing with a sarcogenic product rather than a leukogenic product? If that is so, something that has concerned me for a number of years since no one has isolated a bovine sarcoma virus, is, are we dealing with a virus that is a combination between what we know of as sarcoma viruses and leukaemia viruses, and here we are dealing with 'one in all' if you like. I am not that much of a geneticist or a biochemist to be able to explain it in your terms but it really intrigues me that we are dealing with a virus that may have the properties of a sarcoma virus.

My second point is this: you did not mention much about the polyclonal and monoclonal aspects of lymphosarcoma or leukosis in the bovine. Is it possible to follow through on some of the hypotheses that we are dealing with many types of cells that are pre-malignant in the persistent lymphocytotic animal but, because the virus is stimulating the immune system continually, an event occurs that causes transformation of one cell. In actual fact, the virus is not causing leukosis; it is only the initiator of the disease. Do you think that happens?

R. Kettman

That could be.

CELL SURFACE ANTIGENS ON SHEEP FIBROBLASTS TRANSFORMED BY BOVINE LEUKAEMIA VIRUS

M. Onuma, S. Watarai, T. Mikami and H. Izawa
Department of Epizootiology, Faculty of Veterinary Medicine, Hokkaido University, Sapporo, 060, Japan

ABSTRACT

When sheep fibroblasts were inoculated with BLV materials from 5'-iodo-2'-deoxyuridine-treated 3178 cells, morphological alteration of cells was observed in a few passages after inoculation. The morphologically altered cells showed such transformed phenotypes as growth in soft agar medium, increased uptake of 2-deoxy-D-glucose and tumorogenicity in athymic nude mice. When the cell surface antigens of transformed sheep were compared with those of FLK cells, the major antigen expressed on the former cells was different from the glycoprotein antigen of BLV expressed on the latter cells. Antibody against the antigen on the transformed sheep cells was found in half of the tested sera from BLV-infected cattle which remained healthy, whereas the same antibody was found in only 1 out of the 23 sera from cattle with lymphosarcoma.

O.C. Straub (ed.), Fourth International Symposium on Bovine Leukosis

INTRODUCTION

Bovine leukosis is enzootic and sporadic. Enzootic bovine leukosis (EBL) is a contagious disease induced by bovine leukaemia virus (BLV). Induction of a neoplastic disease by BLV was confirmed by the evidence that BLV inoculated into sheep and cattle causes lymphosarcoma or leukaemia (Van der Maaten and Miller, 1976). However transformation of sheep and calf cells by BLV *in vitro* is unknown.

In a previous paper, we observed the induction of BLV in cultured cells from calf form lymphosarcoma after treatment with 5'-iodo-2'-deoxyuridine (IdU) and at the same time an alteration of cell morphology (Onuma et al., 1978). This cell line (3178) showed transformed phenotypes. Inoculation of BLV from this cell line into sheep fibroblasts resulted in an alteration of cell morphology. Here we will describe the biological properties of the transformed cell and their cell surface antigens.

MATERIALS AND METHODS

Cell cultures

Virus materials were obtained from IdU-treated 3178 cells. These culture cells expressed only BLV antigen and were negative for known virus particles of bovine origin (Onuma et al., 1978). FLK cells, persistently infected with BLV were provided by Dr. Van Der Maaten.

Inoculation of culture fluids onto fibroblasts

Secondary cultures of fibroblasts originating from 4 different sheep testis were used. Inocula were obtained from culture fluids of the 80th to 100th passage of the 3178 cells. The procedures of the preparation of inocula are described elsewhere (Onuma et al., 1980). Control inocula were prepared from culture fluids from normal sheep embryonic cells by the same procedures.

Soft agar culture

The soft agar medium consisted of Eagle's medium with non-essential amino acid supplemented with 10% Bact tryptose phosphate broth and 15% foetal calf serum plus 0.35% Special Noble Agar (Difco).

Heterotransplantation in athymic nude mice

BALB/c nude mice were used in the examination of tumorogenicity of cells. About 5×10^5 cells were injected subcutaneously into the shoulder regions of 4 to 6 weeks old nude mice.

Uptake of 2-deoxy-D-glucose (2DG)

Labelled sugar uptake was determined by the method of Hatanaka and Hanafusa (1970).

Reference sera

Reference serum V34 was obtained from a sheep experimentally infected with BLV which was from a lymphocyte culture of a natural lymphosarcoma case. Reference serum S28 was obtained from a sheep experimentally infected with BLV which originated from 3178 cells. The CF titres of V34 and S28 were respectively 1 : 2 and 1 : 64 against the purified glycoprotein (gp) antigen of BLV. Detectable antibodies against other known bovine or sheep viruses and those against normal bovine or sheep cells were absent in both sera.

Absorption of sera

Reference S28 serum was absorbed twice with living cells (1×10^8 cells per one ml serum) from FLK or transformed sheep 28 fibroblasts (SF-28). The serum and cell mixture was incubated at $37^{\circ}C$ for 30 min and then centrifuged at 600x g for 10 min. The supernatant was used as absorbed serum. Reference V34 and S28 sera were also absorbed with purified BLV as described previously (Honma et al., 1980).

Membrane fluorescent antibody (MFA) test

An indirect MFA test was performed to detect BLV related membrane antigen on the cell surface of viable cells.

Cytotoxicity tests

The complement-dependent antibody cytotoxicity (CDAC) test was performed to detect cell surface antigen by the trypan-blue dye exclusion method as described previously (Honma et al., 1980).

Detection of BLV antibody

For the detection of BLV antibody in cattle naturally infected with BLV, the complement fixation (CF) test and the immunodiffusion test (gp-ID) using purified gp antigen, were carried out.

RESULTS

Comparison of normal and transformed cells

Table 1 shows the transformed phenotypes in the 3178- and BLV-infected ovine fibroblasts. After IdU treatment, rapid cell proliferation and BLV expression was observed in the 3178 cell line. This cell line could grow in soft agar culture and had tumorogenicity in nude mice. The uptake of the glucose analogue, 2DG in the 3178 cells was 4.1 times higher than that in normal bovine or ovine cells.

When the concentrated culture fluids from the 3178 cells were inoculated into fibroblasts originating from 4 different normal sheep testis, the morphological change from fibroblasts-like to epithelial-like cells and focus formation were observed in cultures after the second to third passages. However, no morphological change was observed in the control cultures. These 4 infected cells showed anchorage independence and grew in nude mice (Table 1). The uptake of 2DG in these infected cultures was 3.0 to 3.5 times higher than that in the control

TABLE 1

COMPARISON OF NORMAL AND TRANSFORMED CELLS

Culture cells	BLV-related antigen detected by			BLV[2] detection	Growth in soft agar medium	Increased rate of uptake of 2-DG	Tumorogenicity in nude mice
	MFA test (%)		CDAC test (CI)[1]				
	V34	S28	S28				
3178	2.7	ND	84.6	+	+	4.1	+
Normal bovine foetal thymus	0	ND	< 10	-	-	1.0	-
Infected sheep fibroblasts							
19	9.2	72.3	92.3	+	+	ND	+
21	7.0	55.4	77.3	+	+	3.0	+
27	4.0	64.4	81.8	+	+	3.5	+
28	7.9	63.6	61.1	+	+	ND	+
Control sheep fibroblasts	0	0	< 10	-	-	1.0	-

1) Cytotoxic index (CI) was calculated by the following formula:

$$CI = \frac{\text{\% viable cells in cell suspension alone - \% viable cells in test samples}}{\text{\% viable cells in cell suspension alone}} \times 100$$

2) BLV was detected by syncytia assay.

ND = Not determined

cultures. When V34 serum was used for the MFA test, 4.0 to 9.2% of the transformed cells were positive for BLV antigen. When S28 serum was used, however, 55.4 to 72.3% of the cells were positive. In the CDAC test about 60 to 90% of the cells were killed by 1 : 2 dilution of S28 serum.

Different cell surface antigens expressed on FLK and SF-28 cells

Table 2 shows the comparison of cell surface antigens expressed on FLK and SF-28 cells by the MFA test. In FLK cells, 68% and 75% of cells were positive with V34 and S28 sera, respectively. Absorption of both sera with purified BLV removed the positive reaction to FLK cells. This result suggested that the major antigens expressed on FLK cells were BLV structural proteins. The expression of BLV antigens on SF-28 cells gradually decreased with passages (7.9% to 0.6%). When S28 serum was used, about 60% of SF-28 cells showed a positive reaction. Absorption of S28 serum with BLV or FLK cells could not remove the positive reaction against SF-28 cells. Absorption experiments in Table 2 clearly showed that the major antigens expressed on SF-28 cells are new antigens which may be different from BLV structural antigens. Similar results were also obtained by the CDAC test (data not shown).

Detection of antibody against SF-28 cells in cattle with and without lymphosarcoma

In order to know the expression of the antibody against SF-28 cells in cattle naturally infected with BLV, 23 sera from cattle with bovine lymphosarcoma and 111 sera from healthy cattle in multiple leukosis herds were tested by the CDAC test (Table 3). In sera from cattle with lymphosarcoma (21 sera were positive for BLV antibody), only 1 out of 21 BLV positive sera had CDAC antibody against SF-28 cells. On the other hand, in sera from cattle in multiple leukosis herds, 26 out of 51 BLV positive and 9 out of 60 BLV negative sera were positive for CDAC antibody against SF-28 cells. In addition, the results of the CDAC test using FLK cells were in good agreement with the results of the CF and gp-ID tests.

TABLE 2

DEMONSTRATION OF CELL SURFACE ANTIGENS ON FLK AND SF-28 CELLS BY MFA TEST

Culture cells	Sera					
	Absorbed V34 with		Absorbed S28 with			
	None	BLV	None	BLV	FLK cells	SF-28 cells
FLK	68[1)]	1.5	75	3.5	0	52.9
SF-28 (p23)[2)]	6.5	0.2	60.3	55.4	45.3	0.5
SF-28 (p107)	0.6	0.3	58.3	56.4	43.4	0.8

1) Percentage of cell surface antigen positive cells

2) p23 : 23rd passage

TABLE 3

DETECTION OF CDAC ANTIBODY AGAINST FLK AND SF-28 CELLS IN CATTLE WITH AND WITHOUT LYMPHOSARCOMA

Status	BLV antibody[1)]	No. of sera tested	CDAC test against FLK cells		CDAC test against SF-28 cells	
			Positive	Negative	Positive	Negative
Lymphosarcoma	Positive	21	21	0	1	20
	Negative	2	0	2	0	2
Healthy[2)]	Positive	51	50	1	26	25
	Negative	60	3	57	9	51

1) Antibody was detected by gp-ID and CF tests

2) Sera were obtained from cattle in multiple leukosis herds

DISCUSSION

IdU-treated 3178 cells and ovine fibroblasts inoculated with BLV from 3178 cells exhibited the characteristics of transformed cells *in vitro:*

1. Anchorage independence
2. Increased uptake of 2-DG
3. Tumorogenicity in athymic nude mice

Since untreated 3178 cells and control ovine fibroblasts did not show the transformed phenotypes after an additional 20 to 30 passages, the transformed phenotypes in these cells may be associated with BLV infection.

Expression of BLV related antigen on the surface of the transformed cells was demonstrated by MFA and CDAC tests using 2 different reference sera. The results of absorption experiments suggested that at least 2 different antigens may express on the surface of transformed ovine fibroblasts; one was a BLV structural antigen and the other was a new antigen. Since this new antigen was antigenically different from BLV structural antigens, it might be associated with transformation such as tumour-associated cell surface antigen.

In a previous paper, we demonstrated that the antibody against SF-28 cells in sera from sheep experimentally infected with BLV remained healthy (Suneya et al., 1981). The same antibody could be detected in half of the sera from cattle which had been naturally infected with BLV but had remained healthy. However, only 1 out of 23 sera from cattle with lymphosarcoma had the antibody. In the feline system, for example, cats inoculated with feline oncornavirus developed rapidly growing tumours, with little or no antibody to feline oncornavirus-associated cell membrane antigen (FOCMA). However, inoculated cats that developed regressor tumours or no tumours had an early response to both FOCMA and high antibody titre (Essex et al., 1975). Since the new antigen detected on the transformed SF-28 cells was not a viral structural protein, it might be the bovine oncornavirus cell membrane antigen (BOCMA) similar to that in the feline system. The results in Table 3 suggest that the humoral response against BOCMA may hinder the progress of the disease.

REFERENCES

Essex, M., Sliski, A., Cotter, S.M., Jakowski, R.M. and Hardy, W.D. Jr., 1975. Immunosurveillance of naturally occurring feline leukemia. Science, 190: 790-792.

Hatanaka, M. and Hanafusa, H., 1970. Analysis of a functional change in membranes in the process of cell transformation by Rouse Sarcoma virus: Alteration in the characteristics of sugar transport. Virology, 41: 647-652.

Honma, T., Onuma, M., Suneya, M., Mikami, T. and Izawa, H., 1980. Cytotoxic antibody in cattle and sheep exposed to bovine leukemia virus. Archiv. Virol., In press.

Onuma, M., Okada, K., Yamazaki, I., Fujinaga, K., Fujimoto Y. and Mikami, T., 1978. Induction of C-type virus in cell lines derived from calf form bovine lymphosarcoma. Microbiol. Immunol., 22: 683-691.

Onuma, M., Watarai, S., Suneya, M., Mikami, T. and Izawa, H., 1980. Induction of transformed phenotypes in sheep fibroblasts by culture fluids from cells persistently infected with bovine leukemia virus. Microbiol. Immunol., In press.

Suneya, M., Onuma, M., Mikami, T. and Izawa, H., 1981. Humoral and cellular immune response to bovine leukemia virus infection in sheep. IV International Symposium on Bovine Leukosis, Bologna, Nov. 5-7, 1980 (this publication).

Van der Maaten, M.J. and Miller, J.M., 1976. Induction of lymphoid tumors in sheep with cell-free preparations of bovine leukemia virus. Bibl. Haemat. 43: 377-379.

DISCUSSION

J.F. Ferrer *(USA)*

Do you know whether the FLK cells are transformed? Have you transplanted them into nude mice?

M. Onuma *(Japan)*

I checked the FLK cells also and this cell line, effector cell, also showed the transformed phenotypes.

J.F. Ferrer

In other words, you have two BLV infected transformed cell cultures which have different cell surface antigens?

M. Onuma

Yes.

A.A. Ressang *(Netherlands)*

To summarise, do you consider the cell surface antigen as equal as those that produce FOCMA in the feline system?

M. Onuma

It is just my speculation because the major antigen expressed on this transformed cell is not a viral structural protein and it may be cross-related to the transformation. So I suppose this new antigen is a BOCMA. In lymphosarcoma cases we seldom find the antibody against this new antigen but in BLV infected cattle that remain healthy, about half of the cattle produce antibody against the new antigen. So this antibody protects the progression of the disease, like FOCMA. But it is just speculation.

MECHANISMS INVOLVED IN BOVINE LEUKAEMIA VIRUS INDUCED EARLY AND LATE POLYKARYOCYTOSIS

B. Guillemain, R. Mamoun and Thérèse Astier
Institut National de la Santé et de la Recherche Médicale, U-117, 229, cours de l'Argonne, 33076 Bordeaux, France.

ABSTRACT

With regard to the length of time which it takes to appear, the phenomenon of syncytia formation induced by BLV has been classified as 'early' or 'late' polykaryocytosis according to Poste (1970). Late polykaryocytosis (4 - 8 days) was observed after infection of normal cells with cell-free infectious BLV. Early polykaryocytosis arose (1 - 24 h) in mixed cultures of BLV-infected cells with indicator cells.

Our results demonstrate that the two phenomena following single-hit kinetics are specific for BLV, but arise from different mechanisms. Late polykaryocytosis requires a virus which is able to infect and replicate, and which results in an active process dependent on the integrity of the viral genome. In contrast, early polykaryocytosis may be considered as a passive process in view of the fact that it does not require any viral metabolic activity.

O.C. Straub (ed.), Fourth International Symposium on Bovine Leukosis

A BOVINE LEUKAEMIA VIRUS PRODUCING CELL LINE OF BOVINE LYMPHOID ORIGIN

R. Mamoun, Thérèse Astier and B. Guillemain
Institut National de la Santé et de la Recherche Médicale, U-117, 229, cours de l'Argonne, 33076 Bordeaux, France.

ABSTRACT

We investigated the possibility of obtaining in vitro established cell lines of lymphoid origin which spontaneously release BLV, from cattle with lymphosarcoma.

One such cell line, termed LB59Ly, is the subject of this report. It is shown that monolayers can easily be derived from bovine leukaemic lymphoid cells and can be maintained permanently without any cell degeneration; such cells produce large amounts of viral particles. These viral particles cannot be distinguished, on the basis of biophysical, biochemical or antigenic properties, from BLV produced by FLK-BLV cells. Furthermore, this report shows that the virus released by LB59Ly cells is infectious for homologous cells and particularly for in vitro derived bovine normal lymphoid cells.

O.C. Straub (ed.), Fourth International Symposium on Bovine Leukosis

SESSION III

Immunology

Chairmen : A. Burny and M. Onuma

IDENTIFICATION AND BIOCHEMICAL CHARACTERISATION OF THE MAJOR HISTOCOMPATIBILITY COMPLEX IN CATTLE

D. Lévy, M. Hoang-Xuan, H. Leveziel, M.T. Zilber,
F. Crespeau and A.L. Parodi

INSERM U 152, Hôpital Cochin, F-75014 Paris
INRA, Jouy-en-Josas,
Ecole Nationale Vétérinaire, F-94704 Maisons-Alfort,
France.

ABSTRACT

Among the animal histocompatibility systems, the major histocompatibility complex of the mouse has been studied in great detail, and has been shown to control different immunological functions and to be involved in the cell mediated killing of virus infected cells. Over the past 10 years, there has been a rapid development of knowledge about HLA, the complex chromosomal region in man homologous to the mouse H-2 system and controlling similar functions to H-2. In addition, very similar chromosomal regions have been described in other species. If a region homologous to HLA exists in cattle, and if it also controls a wide range of functions related to immune responsiveness, then it may well be associated with disease. Lymphocytotoxic sera have been produced in cattle by skin grafting and rendered monospecific by absorption with lymphocytes. The inheritance of the antigen factors detected by these sera in cattle families is consistent with the hypothesis that at least 17 of the factors are inherited in a simple Mendelian fashion. The biochemical characterisation of this BLA region has been done by radioimmunoprecipitation of lymphocyte membrane antigens. The gene product of the BLA genes is a protein that is 45 000 daltons in molecular size and carries a carbohydrate moiety. This 45 000 glycoprotein is non covalently associated with a low molecular weight protein that may resemble the β2-microglobulin.

O.C. Straub (ed.), Fourth International Symposium on Bovine Leukosis

INTRODUCTION

The role of BLV in bovine leukosis seems to be well established. In past years, numerous studies have aimed at establishing the best conditions of diagnosis. A strict correlation between the incidence of the disease and the presence of viral antibodies was found, whatever the method used, and its sensitivity. However, nothing is known about leukaemia susceptibility in cattle. The stimulus for the study of bovine lymphocyte antigens arises particularly from the associations that have been found between H-2 antigens and leukaemia in mice, and between HLA-antigens and disease in man.

GENETIC CONTROL OF VIRUS SUSCEPTIBILITY IN MICE

The discovery that inbred strains of mice differ in their susceptibility to tumour-inducing oncogenic viruses triggered a search for genes specifically involved in the control of viral oncogenesis. In the 1950s, Gross demonstrated that two inbred strains, AKR and C58 mice, develop leukaemia spontaneously and that the disease can be easily transferred to other animals of the same strain by inoculating normal adult mice with cell suspensions from the spleen, lymph nodes and liver of the leukaemic animals. The disease was demonstrated to be due to a virus and to begin in the thymus. Attempts to transfer this Gross virus leukaemia to animals of other inbred strains have resulted in 3 categories being defined with regard to susceptibility or resistance to the disease:

- strains with high incidence of both spontaneous and induced leukaemia: AKR, C58
- strains with a low incidence of spontaneous and a high incidence of induced leukaemia: C3Hf/Bi, C57BR
- strains with a low incidence of both spontaneous and induced leukaemia: C57Bl/6, I/St.

Association between the disease and the H-2 system

(major histocompatibility complex - MHC) was first noted by Boyse. Experimental evidence was provided by Lilly and co-workers (1966) and can be summarised as follows (Klein, 1975):

1. The distribution of susceptibility or resistance to Gross virus among the inbred strains correlates with the distribution of H-2 haplotypes. Thus, all strains carrying $H\text{-}2^k$ or $H\text{-}2^d$ haplotypes are susceptible, and all strains carrying $H\text{-}2^b$ or $H\text{-}2^j$ are resistant.
2. Analysis of segregating F2 or backcross generations revealed a close linkage between susceptibility to Gross virus and the H-2 complex.

Six other murine viruses were also demonstrated to be influenced by the H-2 complex, five RNA viruses (Tennant virus, radiation-induced leukaemia virus, Bittner virus, Friend virus, lymphocytic choriomeningitis virus), and one DNA containing virus (vaccinia virus).

ASSOCIATIONS BETWEEN HLA AND DISEASE

The most striking generalisation to emerge from a survey of HLA and disease associations is that many, if not most, of the HLA and disease associations appear to be due to genes in the HLA-D region. Frequently, a disease was initially reported to be associated with an HLA-A or B locus. Further studies showed that the disease associations were stronger with an HLA-D allele.

Table I classifies some of the major HLA and disease associations with respect to the locus showing the strongest association (McDevitt, 1977). A few diseases, such as ankylosing spondylitis, Reiter's disease and haemochromatosis (not listed) appear to be associated primarily with the HLA-B or -A allele (e.g. haemochromatosis). A number of diseases show a definite association with an HLA-B locus allele, but an even stronger association with an HLA-D locus allele. This category includes multiple sclerosis, Addison's disease, and several others, and exemplifies the most rapidly expanding category of associations. Many of the diseases which are listed in the Table as being associated with the B locus have not yet been tested for association with HLA-D alleles (as indicated with a question-mark). At present, rheumatoid arthritis is the only disease which is associated with an HLA-D allele and shows no association with HLA-A or -B.

TABLE 1

HLA AND DISEASE ASSOCIATIONS

Disease	Locus Association		
	B	B/D	D
Rheumatoid arthritis			x
Ankylosing spondylitis	x		
Reiter's disease	x		
Diabetes mellitus		x	
Addison's disease		x	
Hyperthyroidism		x	
Multiple sclerosis		x	
Myathenia gravis		x	
Gluten-sens, Enteropathy		x	
Dermatitis herpetiformis		x	
Psoriasis	x	?	
Chronic active hepatitis		x	
Sjogren's syndrome		x	

THE BLA SYSTEM

Antisera

The study of bovine lymphocyte antigens was done by using a slightly different approach from previous studies. The aim has been to produce monospecific anti-lymphocyte antisera and so simplify the subsequent genetic analysis. This was done mainly by skin grafting and, in a few cases, by lymphocyte immunisation, followed by repeated absorptions with lymphocytes. Operationally monospecific sera were then used in extensive family material to study the inheritance of the antigens they detected. All immunisations took place between dam-calf pairs, the first significant response was detectable between 10 and 14 days and the peak was reached at 21 days. Sera were tested by cytotoxicity against cells from a panel of different animals. Some appeared to be monospecific without absorption (7/47). The others were absorbed with one of the reacting cells and these absorbed aliquots were tested back on all of the absorbing cells. The reactor patterns obtained enabled an assessment of the number of antigenic factors detected by the serum. The basic definition of sera is given by Table 2. If any one of the positive cells totally absorbs out the serum activity, this serum is considered as monospecific (purity test). If a serum does react with cells from different animals, the number and the characteristics of the antibodies can be determined by the same cross table (Table 3).

TABLE 2

CROSS REACTIONS OF A MONOVALENT ANTISERUM (PURITY TEST) ON 30 TO 40 DIFFERENT CELL SAMPLES

Test on cells no.	Serum absorbed by cells no.						Non absorbed	Antigenic factors present on cells
	1	2	3	4	5	6		
1	-	-	-	-	+	+	+	A
2	-	-	-	-	+	+	+	A
3	-	-	-	-	+	+	+	A
4	-	-	-	-	+	+	+	A
5	-	-	-	-	-	-	-	-
6	-	-	-	-	-	-	-	-

TABLE 3

CROSS REACTION OF A BIVALENT ANTISERUM

Test on cells no.	Serum absorbed by cells no. 1	2	3	4	5	6	Non absorbed	Antigenic factors present on cells
1	-	-	-	+	+	+	+	B -
2	+	-	+	+	+	+	+	B C
3	-	-	-	+	+	+	+	B -
4	+	-	+	-	+	+	+	- C
5	-	-	-	-	-	-	-	- -
6	-	-	-	-	-	-	-	- -

Absorption on cells 1 and 3 defines the anti-C antiserum
Absorption on cell 4 defines the anti-B antiserum

Inheritance of antigens

The family material consisted of groups of half sib families. To study the mode of transmission of a factor present in one bull, only families where the dams were negative and a proportion of the offspring positive were considered. Using these selected families, 18 antigenic factors have been shown to be inherited by approximately 50% of the offspring of bulls. This supports a simple Mendelian mode of inheritance with the presence of the antigen being dominant to its absence. The inheritance of combinations of lymphocyte factors is illustrated in Table 4. A number of pairs of factors appeared to be inherited together, or are in opposition. Thus their segregation is not independent. All information presently available provides strong evidence that these antigens belong to a major histocompatibility complex.

TABLE 4

SEGREGATION OF ANTIGENIC FACTORS IN BULL OFFSPRING

Bull	Antigenic factor	Total	Number of products			
			+/+	-/-	+/-	-/+
Unyka	1;2	41	18	21	O	2
Upsilon	3;4	39	23	15	O	1
	4;5	35	17	14	4	O
Amer	5;6	31	16	15	O	O
Valmin	7;8	11	7	4	O	O
	(7,8);6	10	6	3	1	O
	1;2	8	3	5	O	O
	(6,7,8);(1,2)	9	O	O	6	3
Aureol	(1,2);9	7	O	O	2	5

The 9 factors under study were numbered from 1 to 9

Biochemical characterisation of the BLA

1. Location

The tissue distribution of the BLA has not yet been systematically studied, but it seems reasonable to assume that, as observed in mouse or man, it is present in nearly all tissues. Concerning their sub-cellular distribution, MHC products are situated on the cell surface, even though it is likely that, in some cells and possibly at particular stages in the cell cycle, some antigens may also be located on the internal membrane. The evidence for the location of the BLA antigens on the cell surface comes from studies visualising these antigens at the cell membrane by light microscopy. Additional evidence comes from experiments utilising separated or partially purified membrane fractions.

2. Biochemical properties

Previous studies on the H-2 and HLA systems demonstrated that membrane dissolution with ionic (deoxycholate) or non-ionic (Triton-Nonidet P.40) detergents releases molecules in a native form. We used a similar procedure for characterising the BLA. In all cases, radiolabelled antigen has been used. The cells were incubated prior to solubilisation with amino acid precursors which are then incorporated directly into the MHC proteins, or alternatively, the intact cells were surface-iodinated with lactoperoxidase. The cells were then solubilised with detergent and after an adequate incubation period, the material not sedimented by ultracentrifugation of 100 000 g for 1 hour, was analysed for antigenic activities. The protein was precipitated with an anti-BLA alloantiserum and anti-bovine IgG or protein A from *Staphylococcus aureus*. The precipitate was dissolved in SDS in the presence of 2-mercapto-ethanol and subjected to electrophoresis on an SDS-PAGE. Under these conditions, the samples behave as proteins of a molecular size of 45 000 daltons (Figure 1). The specificity of the reaction is assessed by absorption experiments (Figure 2): pretreatment of the alloreactive antiserum with cold relevant lymphocytes removes totally the activity of the serum for the labelled antigen, whereas non-relevant cells are not effective. On the other hand, the BLA activity is not dependent on any BLV reactivity: serum absorption on purified virus does not remove the anti-BLA reactivity (Figure 3). In some experiments, after cell absorptions which greatly reduce the background, or by using 10 or 12.5% polyacrylamide gels, a protein of approximately 12 000 MW was found, non-covalently associated to the BLA-protein. This is presumably the bovine equivalent of the β 2-microglobulin found in association with both H-2 and HLA antigens. We are still not able to demonstrate the glycoprotein nature of the BLA antigens. However, the labelled BLA binds to lectin columns and the glycoprotein eluted with α-methyl-mannoside is reactive with alloantisera. Double label experiments using tritiated fucose and leucine are now in progress.

3. Model of anchoring to the membrane

Some hypothetical features of the H-2 and HLA complexes are likely to be applied to the BLA. The antigen complex consists of two chains, the glycoprotein and the β-2 micro-

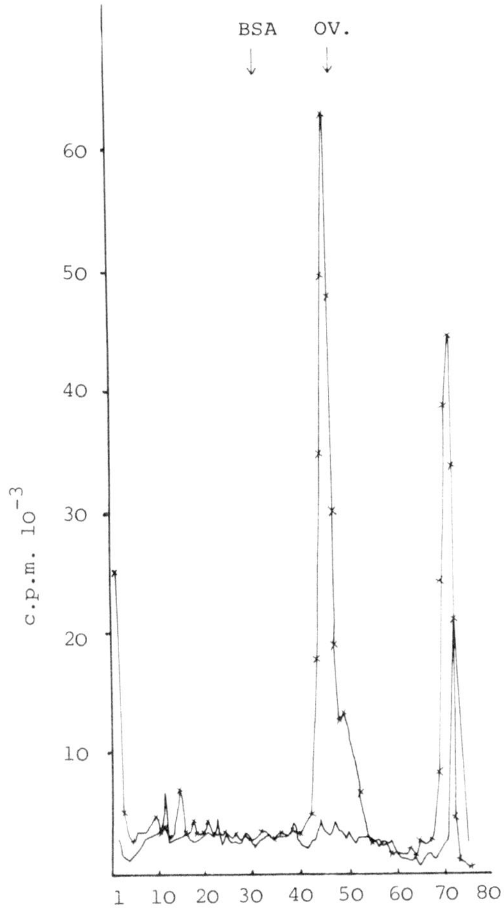

Fig. 1. Precipitation of labelled BLA with a relevant positive serum (x —— x) and a negative serum (· —— ·)

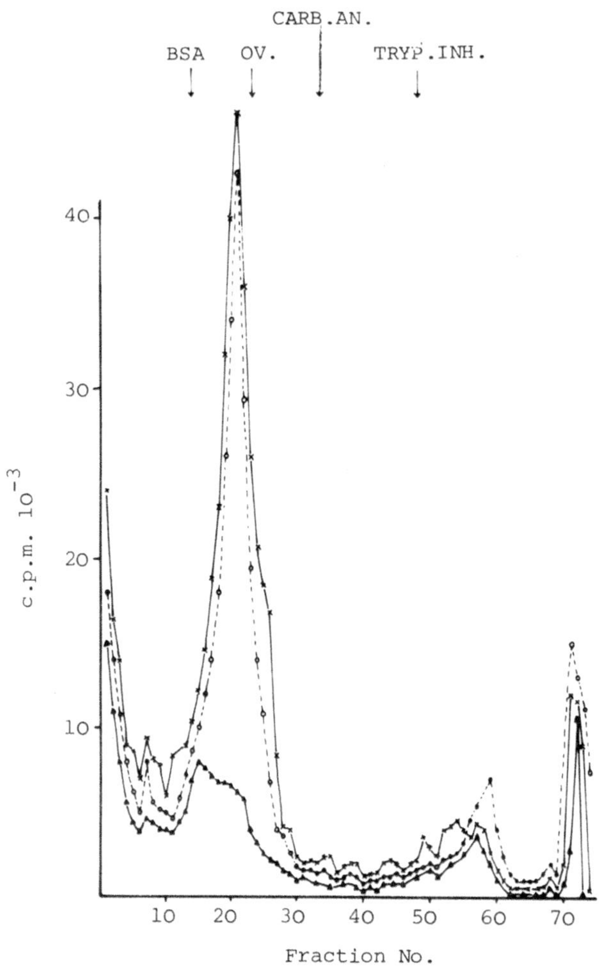

Fig. 2. Precipitation of labelled BLA with a positive antiserum (x —— x) and after absorption on relevant (▲ —— ▲) or irrelevant (o — o) cells

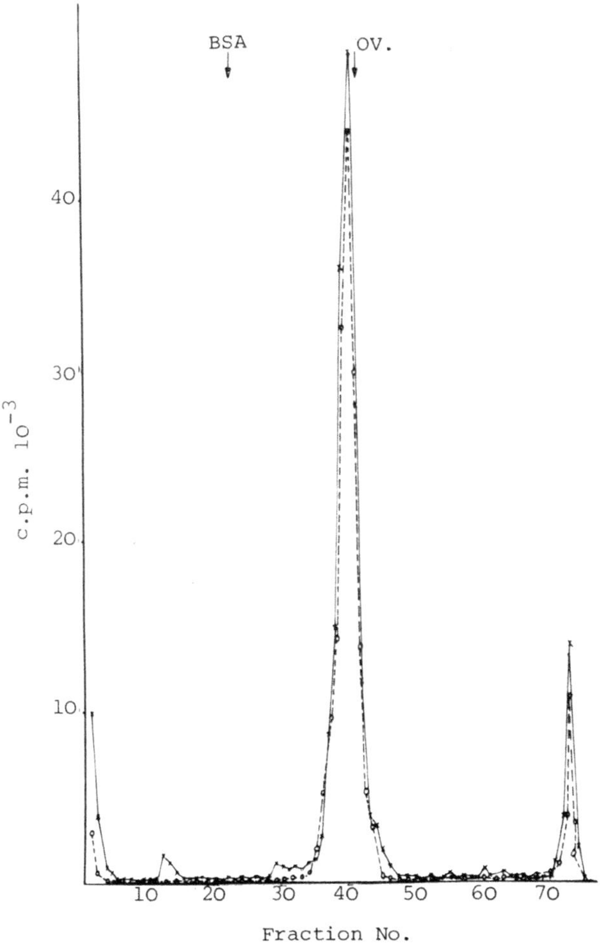

Fig. 3. Precipitation of labelled BLA with a positive antiserum (x —— x) and after absorption on purified BLV (o —— o)

globulin. The glycoprotein has a globular region at the external surface of the lipid bilayer of the membrane. The carbohydrate chain is branched on this external protein. The protein backbone extends through the membrane. The β-2 microglobulin is on the external part of the globular portion. Some data suggest the existence of a tetrameric structure whose structure evokes a relationship with immunoglobulins. In addition, the β-2 microglobulin is partially homologous to the constant region of immunoglobulins.

CONCLUSIONS

The study of infectious diseases has been central to the development of immunology. The humoral aspect of the immune response has been well analysed at the molecular and genetic level. Immunity to extracellular bacteria is mediated by antibodies and complement. Cell mediated immunity is a major factor in the elimination of intracellular parasites (e.g. viruses), but is less well understood. It is however apparent that the major histocompatibility antigens are involved in all T cell interactions with other cells. When a virus enters the organism, there are 3 different levels of control.

1. A genetic control to infection: animals are susceptible or resistant depending on their histocompatibility genes. This may reflect a control in the absorption, penetration or integration of the parasite.

2. The second control is through antibody production: the foreign antigen causes a clonal expansion of specific effector cells or their precursors. In parallel, a pre-committed helper T cell population is expanded and contributes to the differentiation of the activated B cell into a secretory cell. Both B and T helper cells must be compatible in the immune response genes of the MHC to co-operate.

3. The last control is cell mediated. Antigen stimulation in a defined context of major transplantation antigens activates

a pre-committed precursor of cytolytic lymphocytes (P.CTL). A T helper cell, compatible in the immune response region, induces the expansion of these P.CTL by a diffusible factor (TCGF or interleukin-2-IK.2). The differentiated CTL had developed receptors recognising the association of one cellular transplantation antigen and the extracellular parasite. The target, infected or tumoral cell, may be specifically recognised and killed either by CTLs or by specific antibodies and complement. Among a population, some individuals will not have the necessary receptors for a given antigen, and then appear as low responders. Others may have the appropriate receptors and therefore be high responders. The differences in the T cell receptor repertoires are dictated by the Ia genes. K and D molecules provide the effector signal leading to target cell lysis. What is the role of MHC polymorphism? If all individuals carried the same T cell receptors repertoire, they would have the same 'blind spots' and they would all be unresponsive to certain antigens. The end result would be that the entire population would be defenceless against a pathogenic organism. The existence of the species would thus be endangered.

REFERENCES

Gross, L., 1970. Oncogenic viruses, 2nd ed., Pergamon Press, Oxford.

Klein, J., 1975. Biology of the mouse histocompatibility - 2 complex - Springer Verlag, Berlin.

Lilly, F., 1966. The inheritance of susceptibility to the Gross leukemia virus in mice. Genetics 53, 529-539.

McDevitt, H.O., 1977. In: HLA and Disease, J. Dausset and A. Svejgaard, editors, Copenhagen.

DISCUSSION

A.A. Ressang *(Netherlands)*

Congratulations on this work; I think you are one of the first people to investigate the BLA system. I hope that in the near future you will be able to present us with a mapping of the chromosomes. Do you know which chromosome is involved?

D. Lévy *(France)*

We don't know.

IMMUNOLOGICAL REACTIVITY OF THE BOVINE LEUKAEMIA VIRUS GLYCOPROTEIN GP51

D. Portetelle*°, C. Bruck*, Y. Cleuter*, M. Mammerickx+ and A. Burny*°

*Department of Molecular Biology, University of Brussels, B-1640 Rhode St-Genèse

°Faculty of Agronomy, B-5800 Gembloux

+National Institute for Veterinary Research, B-1180 Uccle

Belgium.

ABSTRACT

Natural or experimental infection of cattle, sheep or goats with bovine leukaemia virus (BLV) induces a host humoral antibody response directed against structural protein of the virus. Previous studies have shown that antibodies to envelope glycoprotein gp51 are consistently formed at a higher titre than antibodies to internal p24. Both titres steadily increase from infection to death of the animal in the tumour phase of the disease.

Animals infected by BLV harbour complement-dependent cytotoxic antibodies directed against BLV producing cells which express gp51 at the membrane, whereas serum raised in the rabbit against purified gp51 have no cytotoxic activity.

Digestion of gp51 with a mixture of glycosidases abolished the reactivity of the antigen with sera of infected cattle or sheep. In contrast, the reactivity of gp51 with monospecific rabbit antisera was only slightly modified by the glycosidase treatment. Solid phase radioimmunoassay furthermore showed that the carbohydrate antigenic site is probably unique as opposed to the protein antigenic determinants, which are probably multiple.

In conclusion, a carbohydrate antigenic site, which is probably unique belonging to BLV envelope gp51 is strongly immunogenic for BLV-infected animals.

O.C. Straub (ed.), Fourth International Symposium on Bovine Leukosis

INTRODUCTION

Infection of animals (cattle, sheep, goats, pigs, rabbits etc.) with bovine leukaemia virus (BLV), the aetiological agent of enzootic bovine leukosis, induces a rapid and strong humoral antibody response directed against all structural proteins of the virus (Burny et al., 1980). This humoral reaction does not arrest BLV multiplication in the infected host; surprisingly enough, anti-gp51 antibody titre increases steadily and inexorably until the animal's fatal outcome in the tumour phase of the disease. Failure of the immune system to eliminate an established BLV infection does not prove, however, that adequate vaccination of animals at risk would be unsuccessful. From recent experiments by Mammerickx et al. (1980), we know that passive antibody given to sheep by colostrum feeding prevented BLV take, irrespective of the route of virus administration. The latter observations reinforced our decision to investigate thoroughly the antigenic site of BLV gp51 exposed at the cell membrane of virus producing cells and recognised as target by sera exhibiting strong cytolytic activity towards these cells (Portetelle et al., 1978, 1980).

The series of experiments summarised here showed that cytotoxic antibodies present in BLV infected animals were mostly directed against the carbohydrate part of the gp51 molecule. On the contrary, monospecific immune sera prepared in the rabbit by injection of purified BLV gp51 were directed against determinants of the polypeptide backbone of the antigen.

MATERIALS AND METHODS

Sera 2146 and 2152 were prepared in the rabbit by injection of BLV-infected bovine lymphocytes. Sera 67 and 82 were from cattle in the tumour phase of enzootic bovine leukosis. Serum 3162 was from an animal in persistent lymphocytosis and serum 351628 from an asymptomatic BLV carrier. Rabbit serum 167 was raised by injection of purified BLV gp51.

Foetal lamb kidney (FLK) epithelioid cells chronically infected by and producing BLV were kindly provided by Drs. J.M. Miller and M.J. van der Maaten.

Purification and iodination of virus glycoprotein gp51, liquid phase, solid phase and competition radioimmunoassays, serum cytolytic activity, glycosidase treatment of virus glycoprotein has been described previously (Portetelle et al., 1980).

RESULTS

Complement-dependent antibody-mediated immune cytolysis has previously been shown (Portetelle et al., 1978) to recognise mostly if not solely, gp51 as the target molecular structure. Data presented in Figure 1 illustrate the striking difference between natural sera (serum 67 x——x, serum 351628 ●——●) and rabbit serum 167 (⊙——⊙) prepared against purified gp51.

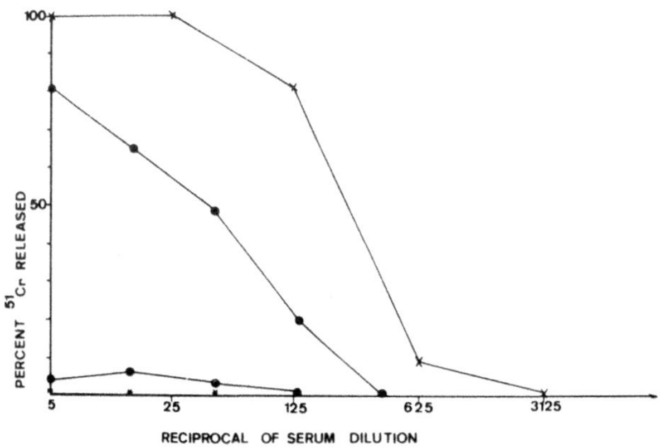

Figure 1. Susceptibility of FLK-BLV cells to lysis by bovine serum 67 (x-x), bovine serum 351628 (●-●), normal bovine serum (*-*) and rabbit serum 167 (⊙-⊙).

^{51}Cr labelled FLK-BLV cells were incubated with dilutions of the serum to be tested and with a 1:8 final dilution of rabbit complement.

To confirm that cytolytic and non-cytolytic antibodies recognised separate sites on the gp51 molecule, a competition radioimmunoassay was performed (Figure 2) between bovine serum 67 and rabbit sera 2146.

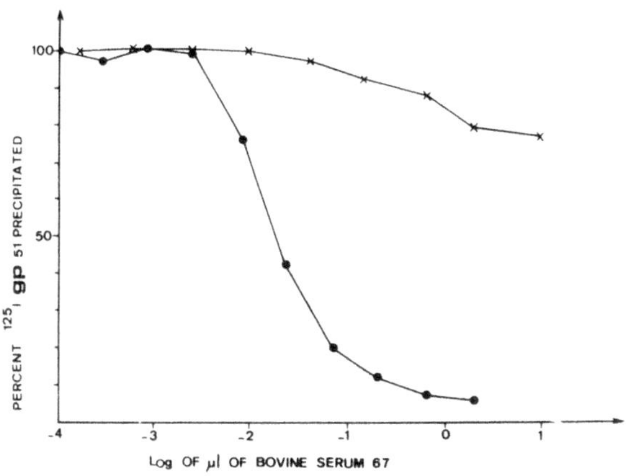

Figure 2. Competition by bovine serum 67 of the immune precipitation of ^{125}I gp51 by rabbit sera 167 (x-x) and 2146 (●-●).

Labelled antigen (0.5 ng) and a limiting rabbit antibody diltution (1/40 000 for serum 167; 1/75 000 for serum 2146) were incubated with increasing amounts of bovine serum 67. After a 72 h incubation, antirabbit Ig-coated cellulose was added to adsorb immune complexes involving rabbit antibody. Pelleted and washed immunosorbent was counted in a γ counter.

Advantage was also taken of a solid phase radioimmunoassay. The results obtained indicated that (Figure 3):

- natural sera and rabbit serum 167 reacted with different antigenic regions of gp51;

- the antigenic site recognised by natural sera was most probably unique.

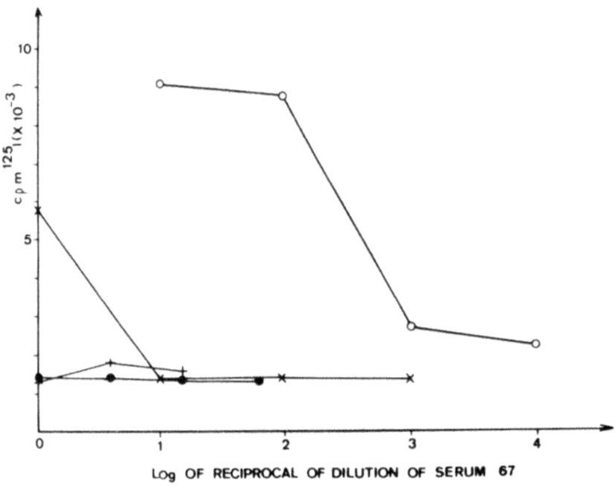

Figure 3. Solid phase radioimmunoassay. Reagents were added to the wells in the following order:

- Ig82-gp51-serum 67-^{125}I gp51 (x-x)
- Ig82-gp51-normal bovine serum-^{125}I gp51 (●-●)
- Ig rabbit 167-gp51-serum 67-^{125}I gp51 (O-O)
- Ig rabbit 167-gp51-normal bovine serum-^{125}I gp51 (+ - +).

At each step, an excess reagent was added, incubation was performed and non adsorbed excess protein was washed away. After completion of the last step, the wells were separately counted in a γ counter.

Importance of the carbohydrate moiety of gp51 was finally assessed by glycosidase treatment of ^{125}I-labelled antigen followed by addition of a variety of antisera. Sera 2152, 3162 and 67 behaved similarly: removal of the carbohydrate moiety of the antigen resulted in almost complete loss of reactivity with the three sera. The behaviour of serum 167 was strikingly different. Glycosidase digestion lowered maximal precipitability of gp51 by only 20%. Consequently, apparent antibody titre was also slightly lowered (Figure 4).

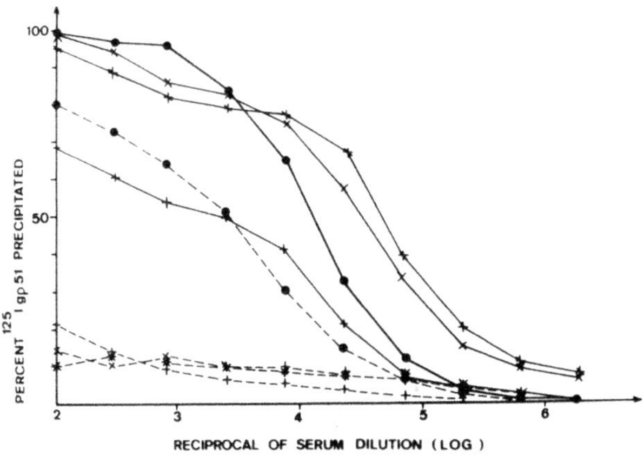

Fig. 4. Effect of glycosidase digestion of ^{125}I gp51 on direct radioimmunoassay with sera of different origins. Precipitation curves obtained with sera from rabbit 167 (●-●), cow 3162 (x-x), cow 67 (*-*) and rabbit 2152 (+ - +) are taken as controls. The precipitation curves obtained with the same sera after glycosidase treatment of the antigen are depicted as interrupted lines.

That the polypeptide backbone of gp51 was the target for serum 167 reactivity was later demonstrated by protease treatment of the antigen (data not shown). Finally, SDS-PAGE analysis of native and glycosidase-treated BLV gp51 showed that the enzyme treatment reduced the apparent molecular weight from 51 000 to about 30 000 (Portetelle et al., 1980).

CONCLUSION

In conclusion, a carbohydrate antigenic site, which is probably unique, belonging to BLV envelope gp51 is strongly immunogenic for naturally infected animals or for rabbits injected with BLV lymphocytes. On the contrary, when purified gp51 is used as immunogen, it induces synthesis of antibodies directed to the protein skeleton of the glycoprotein antigen.

From a very practical point of view, it follows that purified BLV gp51 should not be used as a vaccinal preparation against BLV infection.

Results very similar to those reported here have been obtained by Schmerr et al., 1980.

REFERENCES

Burny, A., Bruck, C., Chantrenne, H., Cleuter, Y., Dekegel, D., Ghysdael, J., Kettmann, R., Leclercq, M., Leunen, J., Mammerickx, M. and Portetelle, D., 1980. Bovine Leukemia Virus: molecular biology and epidemiology. In: Viral Oncology. Klein, G. (ed.) Raven Press, New York, pp. 231-289.

Mammerickx, M., Portetelle, D., Burny, A. and Leunen, J., 1980. Detection by radioimmunodiffusion- and radioimmunoassay-tests of antibodies to bovine leukemia virus antigens in sera of experimentally infected sheep and cattle. Zentralbl. Veterinaermed. Reihe B, 27: 291-303.

Portetelle, D., Bruck, C., Burny, A., Dekegel, D., Mammerickx, M. and Urbain, J., 1978. Detection of complement-dependent lytic antibodies in sera from Bovine Leukemia Virus-infected animals. Ann. Rech. Vet., 9: 667-674.

Portetelle, D., Bruck, C., Mammerickx, M, and Burny, A., 1980. In animals infected by Bovine Leukemia Virus (BLV), antibodies to envelope glycoprotein gp51 are directed against the carbohydrate moiety. Virology, 105: 223-233.

Schmerr, M.J., Miller, J.M. and Van der Maaten, M.J., 1980. Antigenic reactivity of a soluble glycoprotein associated with Bovine Leukemia Virus. Virology, in press.

DISCUSSION

M. Mussgay *(FRG)*

Did you treat your lymphocytes with tunicamycin to observe cytotoxic activity.

A. Burny *(Belgium)*

If you take the lymphocytes fresh from the blood and check, there is no cytotoxic activity. If you put them in culture, you get it right away.

M. Mussgay

But if you use tunicamycin?

A. Burny

We haven't done this on lymphocytes.

M. Mussgay

Could it be that removing the carbohydrates means only that you are changing the conformation of the proteins?

A. Burny

And that the antigenic site would still be a protein part? That cannot be excluded at present.

D. Portetelle *(Belgium)*

We have some competition radioimmunoassay with sugar.

A. Burny

Mannose is the best competitor in the assay but it does not compete everything.

D.H. Roberts *(UK)*

Can you relate cytotoxicity in serum to, say, complement fixation? With complement fixation, the IgG_1 fixes complement whereas the IgG_2 does not fix complement - or the other way around. So, is there any relationship between cytotoxicity and complement fixation?

D. Portetelle

IgG_1 is cytotoxic.

D.H. Roberts

I know that one is cytotoxic and the other is not. What about your rabbit sera? Does that fix complement?

D. Portetelle

We had a control with rabbit antilymphocyte, antimembrane and it lysed the cells.

R. Schön *(DDR)*

Did you try to raise antisera in rabbits against the gp51 within the viral membrane? If your explanation is right then you should only get antisera directed against the carbohydrate part of the molecule.

A. Burny

It is probably the same result.

R. Schön

You could do the reverse experiment, trying to immunise a goat or a sheep against the isolated glycoprotein.

A. Burny

The indication is that if you don't treat the virus you get an antibody that is directed against the sugar part; if you treat it with a detergent then you get an antibody directed against the protein part of the molecule.

R. Schön

You have tried this then; you have got rabbit antisera against the glycoprotein part by immunising with a virus membrane?

A. Burny

Yes, that is what you get.

HUMORAL AND CELLULAR IMMUNE RESPONSES TO BOVINE LEUKAEMIA VIRUS INFECTION IN SHEEP

M. Suneya, M. Onuma, T. Mikami and H. Izawa
Department of Epizootiology, Faculty of Veterinary Medicine, Hokkaido University, Sapporo, 060, Japan

ABSTRACT

Sheep were experimentally infected with either bovine leukaemia virus (BLV) from 3178 cells or together with BLV from adult lymphosarcoma cells. None of the infected sheep developed leukaemia or lymphosarcoma during the experimental period of 22 months. However, all of them developed both humoral and cellular immune responses against BLV related antigens. The antibody against glycoprotein (gp) of BLV appeared earlier than the antibody against p24. The antibody titres of gp were higher than those of p24. The complement-dependent antibody cytotoxicity (CDAC) test was performed for the detection of antibody against BLV-related cell membrane antigen by using two different types of target cells; FLK cells which were persistently infected with BLV and SF-28 cells which were sheep fibroblasts transformed by BLV. Comparing the development patterns of antibody titres, the titres against SF-28 cells were different from those against FLK cells which express gp of BLV on their surface. The lymphocyte-mediated immunity assay showed that peripheral blood lymphocytes of BLV infected sheep had the effect of colony reduction against SF-28 cells. The nature of this effective lymphoid cell was nylon non-adherent cells, presumably T cells. The possible role of the immune response of the host against tumour cells is discussed below.

O.C. Straub (ed.), Fourth International Symposium on Bovine Leukosis

INTRODUCTION

The development of lymphoid neoplasms in sheep inoculated with bovine leukaemia virus (BLV) material has been reported from several laboratories (Olson et al., 1972; Ressang et al., 1976; Van der Maaten and Miller, 1976). Attempts to transfer BLV to goats and calves have been successful, however the efficacy of BLV to induce tumours in them seems rather weak (Ressang et al., 1976).

Animals infected with BLV developed humoral antibodies against the structural proteins of BLV (glycoprotein; gp and p24 antigens). The development of antibody titres in BLV-infected sheep showed that antibody titres of gp and p24 increase continuously up to the animal's death due to tumours (Bex et al., 1979). This evidence suggested clearly that strong humoral response to p24 and gp antigens of BLV does not hinder the progress of the disease. Seroepidemiological studies in Japanese cattle showed that about 30% to 50% of clinically normal cattle in an enzootic area became infected with BLV, while the incidence of lymphosarcoma or leukaemia in such an area was less than 0.1% of the cattle (Onuma et al., 1979). This observation suggested that an immunosurveillance mechanism may be operated to prevent the advance of the disease in BLV infected cattle.

The purpose of the present study is to examine the humoral and cellular immune responses in sheep infected with BLV and to understand the roles of both types of immunity in their resistance to lymphoma formation.

MATERIALS AND METHODS

Experimented animals and inoculum

Five 3 month old lambs (Nos. 19, 21, 23, 28 and 31) were inoculated intraperitoneally with BLV materials i.e. 50 ml of supernatant fluids from cultured 3178 cells (Onuma et al., 1978).

Six weeks later, two of them (21 and 23) were further inoculated by the same method with 50 ml of whole blood from cattle with adult lymphosarcoma. Two other 3 month old lambs (26 and 30) were inoculated with culture fluids from normal sheep fibroblasts to act as a control.

Haematological examinations

Following infection, blood counts were performed and serum samples were collected at one month intervals for a period of 22 months.

Complement fixation (CF) test

The CF test was performed with purified gp and p24 antigens.

Complement-dependent antibody cytotoxicity (CDAC) test

The CDAC test was performed by the trypan-blue dye exclusion method as described previously (Honma et al., 1980) with minor modifications. Briefly, two µl of target cells (6×10^5 cells/ml), 2 µl of test serum and 2 µl of rabbit complement were mixed together in a Terasaki plate and incubated at $37^{\circ}C$ for 45 min. After incubation, 1 µl of 0.5% trypan-blue solution was added and the viability of cells was compared with the control cells. As a control of the complement and test serum, they were replaced by Eagle's minimal essential medium for each test. Sera negative for BLV antibodies collected from 48 normal sheep were used to examine the non-specific reaction in this test system. When compared with the control cells, none of these sera reduced the viability of the target cells by less than 75%. Therefore, in this test system, a cell-viability of less than 50% was considered to be positive for cytotoxicity.

For the CDAC test, 2 different kinds of cells were used as target cells; FLK cells and SF-28 cells which were sheep fibroblasts transformed by BLV (Onuma et al., 1981).

Since sera from sheep 21 and 23 had cytotoxicity against normal bovine cells, these sera were absorbed with normal bovine lymphoid cells (1×10^8 cells/1 ml of serum) before use. All sera tested had no cytotoxicity against normal sheep or bovine cells.

Detection of BLV

Syncytia assays were performed to detect BLV in peripheral blood lymphocytes from sheep as described previously (Onuma et al., 1980).

Lymphocyte-mediated immunity (LMI) assay

Sensitised lymphocytes were obtained from sheep which were infected with BLV 10 to 12 months previously. Lymphocytes were isolated from peripheral blood by flotation in Ficoll-Conray and were washed three times in PBS before use. Transformed sheep fibroblasts (SF-28 cells) formed a colony in semi-solid agar culture and colony efficiency was 56.4%.

Sensitised lymphocytes (5×10^5 to 50×10^5 per 0.1 ml) and SF-28 cells (target cells, 5×10^4 per 0.1 ml) were mixed together in a suspension and incubated at 37°C for 24 hours. After incubation, the mixtures were plated in 35 mm Petri dishes with soft agar medium (0.35% Bact Agar). The plates were incubated in a CO_2 incubator at 37°C. Colonies were counted 12 days after incubation.

Separation of adherent and non-adherent cells

Lymphocytes were separated on a nylon-wool column, using a method previously described (Paul et al., 1977).

RESULTS

Haematology and detection of BLV

According to Paulsen's haematological criteria for sheep lymphocytes, the lymphocyte level of all the 5 BLV-infected sheep, as well as that of the 2 control sheep, was normal during the experimental period. Furthermore, all 7 sheep were clinically and haematologically normal.

BLV was first detected 2 - 3 months after inoculation and has persisted to date (22 months). BLV could not be detected in sheep No. 26 and No. 30 which were inoculated with culture fluids from normal sheep fibroblasts.

Humoral antibody response

CDAC and CF antibodies were found in all 5 sheep 4 weeks after infection. The typical development pattern of antibody titres are given in Figure 1. Sera collected at one month intervals from all 5 BLV-infected sheep showed by the CF test that antibody against gp appeared earlier than that against p24. Antibody titre of gp was higher than that of p24 during the course of the experiment. CF and CDAC antibodies generally appeared simultaneously one month after inoculation. Gp antibody in sheep 19 gradually decreased 2 months after inoculation and finally disappeared 8 months after inoculation (Figure 1a). Antibody against p24 in the same sheep could not be detected throughout the experimental period. The other sheep, No. 21, maintained its gp and p24 titres during the course of the experiment (Figure 1b). The development of antibody titres of No. 23 and No. 28 were similar to that of No. 21 while that of No. 31 was similar to No. 19.

The evolution of CDAC antibody titres against FLK cells were similar to those of gp antibody in the sera which were collected from each of the inoculated sheep at one month intervals for 2 years. On the other hand, the evolution of CDAC antibody titres against SF-28 cells was different from that against FLK cells (Figure 1).

Two lambs, inoculated with culture fluids from normal bovine embryonic cells remained serologically negative.

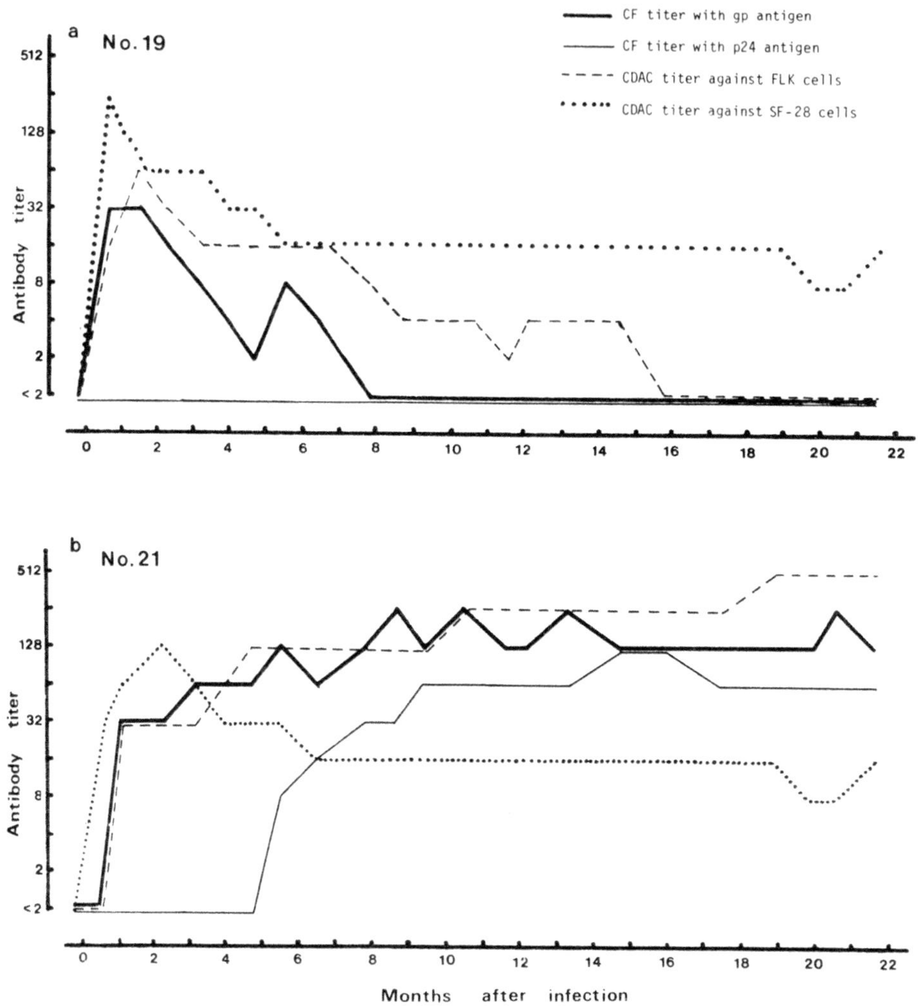

Figure 1ab. Results of CF and CDAC tests on serum from sheep inoculated with BLV materials.

a : No. 19 b : No. 21

TABLE 1

REDUCTION OF COLONY FORMATION BY LYMPHOCYTES FROM SHEEP

Sheep No.	% reduction in colony formation[1] at conc (lymphocytes/plate) of 5×10^5	25×10^5	50×10^5
BLV infected			
19	67.3[2]	73.9	86.9
21	44.0	76.0	ND
28	52.0	80.0	100
Control			
26	11.5	12.6	20.6
30	7.5	18.3	23.7

1) Percentage reduction in colony formation was calculated by the following formula:

$$\frac{\text{average number of colony per media control well} - \text{average number of colony per lymphocyte-treated well}}{\text{average number of colony per media control well}} \times 100$$

2) Average of 2 experiments in which triplicate petri plates were assayed

ND = Not determined

Cellular immune response against transformed cells

The effects of lymphocytes from 3 BLV-infected and two BLV-free control sheep against transformed SF-28 cells were tested with the reduction of colony formation of the target cells (Table 1). A dose response effect was observed in that an increase in the number of lymphocytes from 5 x 10^5 to 50 x 10^5 cells per plate resulted in a decrease in the number of colony per well. Lymphocytes from another 2 BLV-infected sheep also significantly reduced the number of colony formations of SF-28 cells when compared to the lymphocytes from sheep 26 and 30.

Sensitised lymphocytes were separated into nylon-adherent and nylon non-adherent cells by nylon-wool column. In this method, nylon-adherent cells were enriched (56.3% surface immunoglobulin positive cells) in B cells, whereas the non-adherent cells were markedly enriched for non-B lymphocytes, presumably T cells (1.9% surface immunoglobulin positive cells). Non-adherent cells from sensitised lymphocytes significantly reduced the colony formation of SF-28 cells when compared to that of the adherent cells (95% vs 58%).

DISCUSSION

Although all of the sheep inoculated with BLV materials were clinically and haematologically normal during the course of the experiment, they showed humoral and cellular immune responses. The appearance of gp antibody was earlier than that of p24 antibody and the CF antibody titres of the former were systematically higher than that of the latter.

Two different kinds of target cells were used for the detection of CDAC antibodies. From the results of serological comparison of cell surface antigens of FLK and transformed sheep cells (SF-28), it appeared that the major antigen of FLK cells was gp antigen of BLV while that of SF-28 cells was a new antigen that might be associated with transformations, for instance the tumour-associated cell surface antigen (Onuma et al., 1981). Previous papers showed that the CDAC test using FLK cells detected mainly the antibody against gp antigen of BLV (Honma et al., 1980). In the present experiments, the same results were obtained in the sera collected monthly from each sheep infected with BLV. However, the evolution of CDAC antibody titres against FLK cells was different from that of the titres against SF-28 cells. These results suggest that the CDAC test with SF-28 cells may be able to detect antibody different from that against BLV structural proteins.

The results of a lymphocyte-mediated immunity assay revealed that the peripheral blood lymphocytes from BLV-infected sheep had the effect of colony reduction against transformed SF-28 cells. Similar effects were observed in lymphocytes from cattle naturally infected with BLV (our unpublished data). The lymphoid cells which were effective for colony reduction were nylon non-adherent cells, presumably T cells in nature. Despite the fact that more than 64% of the total SF-28 cell population expresses the new antigen, the expression of BLV antigen was low (about 8%) (Onuma et al., 1981). Therefore, sensitised lymphocytes from BLV-infected sheep seem to react specifically to cells expressing this new antigen. There is a possibility that this immune response may also be directed against other antigens including gp antigen of BLV, histocompatibility antigens, and possibly others expressed on the surface of the transformed sheep cells.

The evidence that genetic and immunologic deficient diseases result in an increased risk of developing lymphoid leukaemia led Burnet to propose the immunosurveillance mechanism (Burnet, 1970). Many studies in rodents and felines support the hypothesis that the immunosurveillance mechanism may be operated under natural conditions to eliminate malignant cells (Essex et al., 1975; Hirsch and Murphy, 1968). Previous observations by Bex et al. (1979) suggested that antibodies against p24 and gp did not hinder the progress of the disease. As explained in our previous paper, the CDAC antibody against the new antigens expressed on SF-28 cells was found in half of the sera from BLV-infected healthy cattle, whereas the same antibody was found in only one of the 23 sera from cattle with lymphosarcoma (Onuma et al., 1981). These observations suggest that a humoral response directed against transformed SF-28 cells may play a similar role in immunosurveillance for tumours to that suggested in the feline oncornavirus system (Essex et al., 1975). In the present experiment, all of the BLV-infected sheep showed a humoral immune response against SF-28 cells but they developed no tumour. There are at least two possibilities to fight against tumorous lymphocytes:

1. A humoral response directed against the new antigen expressed on transformed sheep cells.
2. A cellular immune response against the transformed cells.

Much attention should be devoted to the identification of this new antigen.

REFERENCES

Bex, F., Bruck, C., Mammerickx, M., Portetelle, D., Ghysdael, J., Cleuter, Y., Leclercq, M., Dekegel, D. and Burny, A., 1979. Humoral antibody response to bovine leukemia virus infection in cattle and sheep. Cancer Res., 39: 1118-1123.

Burnet, F.M., 1970. The concept of immunological surveillance. Prog. Exp. Tumor Res., 13: 1-27.

Essex, M., Sliski, A., Cotter, S.M., Jakowski, R.M. and Hardy, W.D. Jr., 1975. Immunosurveillance of naturally occurring feline leukemia. Science, 190: 790-792.

Hirsch, M.S. and Murphy, F.A., 1968. Effects of anti-thymocyte serum on Rausher virus infection of mice. Nature (Lond.), 218: 478-479.

Honma, T., Onuma, M., Suneya, M., Mikami, T. and Izawa, H., 1980. Cytotoxic antibody in cattle and sheep exposed to bovine leukemia virus. Archiv. Virol., In press.

Olson, C., Miller, L.D., Miller, J.M. and Hoss, H.E., 1972. Transmission of lymphosarcoma from cattle to sheep. J. Natl. Cancer Inst., 49: 1463-1467.

Onuma, M., Ishihara, K., Ohtani, T., Honma, T., Mikami, T. and Izawa, H., 1979. Seroepizootiological survey on antibodies against bovine leukemia virus in Japanese Black cattle. Jpn. J. Vet. Sci., 41: 601-605.

Onuma, M., Okada, K., Yamazaki, Y., Fujinaga, K., Fujimoto, Y. and Mikami, T., 1978. Induction of C-type virus in cell lines derived from bovine lymphosarcoma. Microbiol. Immunol., 22 683-691.

Onuma, M., Watarai, S., Mikami, T. and Isawa, H., 1981. Cell surface antigens on transformed sheep fibroblasts by bovine leukaemia virus. IV International Symposium on Bovine Leukosis, Bologna, Nov. 5-7, 1980 (this publication).

Onuma, M., Watarai, S., Sonoda, M., Mikami, T. and Izawa, H., 1980. Detection of bovine leukemia virus by syncytium assay. Can. J. Comp. Med., 44: 289-293.

Paul, P.S., Pomeroy, K.A., Johnson, D.W., Muşcoplat, C.C., Handwerger, B.S., Soper, F.F. and Sorensen, D.K., 1977. Evidence for the replication of bovine leukemia virus in the B lymphocytes. Am. J. Vet. Res., 38: 873-876.

Ressang, A.A., Baars, J.C., Calafat, J., Mastenbroek, N. and Quak, J., 1976. Studies on bovine leukaemia. III. The hematological and serological response of sheep and goats to infection with whole blood from leukaemic cattle. Zent. Vet. Med. (B)., 23: 662-668.

Van der Maaten, M.J. and Miller, J.M., 1976. Induction of lymphoid tumors in sheep with cell-free preparations of bovine leukemia virus. Bibl. Haemat., 43: 377-379.

DISCUSSION

J.F. Ferrer *(USA)*

The paper that you presented this morning, and the paper you have presented now, show that two sheep cell cultures infected with BLV express different membrane antigens when they are transformed. How does this fit in with your hypothesis that at least one of these antigens is an equivalent to the FOCMA antigen in the feline system?

M. Onuma *(Japan)*

The major antigens expressed on FLK cells are BLV antigens like gp. Other antigens are antigenically different from BLV antigens. So my speculation is that this new antigen expressed on transformed sheep cells and 3178 cells might be a transformation associated antigen. You can say BOCMA but it looks like a non-structural protein.

J.F. Ferrer

But the FLK cells are transformed and yet do not express this antigen. So apparently it is not a transformation antigen.

M. Onuma

With FLK cells the major antigen is a glycoprotein and p24 but the minor antigens, we don't know; they may be expressed like a FOCMA antigen.

J.F. Ferrer

Therefore, it does not seem to be a transformation antigen.

DETECTION OF ANTIBODIES AGAINST SKIN LYMPHOSARCOMA CELLS IN SHEEP

M. Onuma, M. Suneya, K. Matsumoto, T. Mikami and H. Izawa
Department of Epizootiology, Faculty of Veterinary Medicine, Hokkaido University, Sapporo, 060, Japan

ABSTRACT

Three sheep inoculated with tumour cells from the skin form of lymphosarcoma showed no haematological and clinical changes during the 2 year observation period. Neither bovine leukaemia virus (BLV) nor antibodies against BLV could be detected in these sheep. When athymic nude mice were used for heterotransplantation of skin lymphosarcoma cells, transplantable tumour cells were established in these mice. All three sheep inoculated with skin lymphosarcoma cells developed specific cytotoxic antibodies against these transplantable cells from nude mice.

O.C. Straub (ed.), Fourth International Symposium on Bovine Leukosis

INTRODUCTION

The four forms of bovine lymphosarcoma; the adult (ALS), calf (CLS), thymic (TLS) and skin (SLS) forms, are clinically distinct from each other. Sporadic bovine leukosis (SBL) consisting of CLS, TLS and SLS is rare and its aetiology is unknown. Experimental transmission of SBL to sheep and calves has never been successful, whereas that of enzootic bovine leukosis (EBL) or ALS have been reported (Olson et al., 1972; Miller et al., 1972). Therefore it was desirable to transplant SBL cells in laboratory animals.

In our previous paper, we reported the first successful heterotransplantation of the 4 forms of natural bovine lymphosarcoma cells to athymic nude mice (Onuma et al., 1980a). The transplantable SLS cells were maintained for 18 passages in nude mice.

Sheep inoculated with SLS cells showed no clinical sign during the 2 years. However, sera from these sheep showed a specific reaction against the transplantable SLS cells in nude mice. In the present paper, we will describe the specific immune response to SLS inoculation in sheep and the usefulness of nude mice in the study of SBL.

MATERIALS AND METHODS

Heterotransplantation in athymic nude mice

BALB/c nude mice were used in the transplantation of SLS cells according to the method described previously (Onuma et al., 1980a). Tumours were passed from mouse to mouse by surgically removing tumour tissues after anaesthesia by ether. About 0.1 ml of cell suspensions were injected into the subcutaneous layer of the back.

Experimentally inoculated sheep

Three 3 month old lambs (22, 24 and 27) were inoculated with tumour cells from a SLS case. They were inoculated intraperitoneally with 50 ml of whole blood from cattle with SLS. Two months later, they were inoculated intraperitoneally with 5 ml of packed tumour cells (at 1 000 rpm, 5 min) from the same cattle. Two other 3 month old lambs were inoculated with culture fluids from normal sheep fibroblasts to act as a control. Blood samples were then collected on a monthly basis and the total leukocyte counts were made. Sera were tested for bovine leukaemia virus (BLV) antibodies by the complement fixation test and the complement-dependent antibody cytotoxicity (CDAC) test. Sera were also tested for antibodies against SLS cells by the CDAC test. Blood lymphocytes were examined for BLV by syncytium assay (Onuma et al., 1980c).

Complement-dependent antibody cytotoxicity (CDAC) test

A microcytotoxicity test was performed by the trypan-blue dye exclusion method as described previously (Honma et al., 1980). FLK and SF-28 cells were used as target cells in the detection of antibodies against BLV related cell membrane antigens. Transplantable tumour cells from nude mice were used. in the detection of antibodies against SLS cells. Fresh tumours in nude mice were teased out with scissors and forceps. The suspension was filtered with gauze and the single suspended tumour cells were used as target cells for the CDAC test.

RESULTS

As shown in Figure 1, the growth curves of SLS cells in nude mice were similar to each other at different passage levels. Tumour growth was rapid, resulting in the eventual death of the mice.

Histological examinations of these transplanted tumours in nude mice revealed lymphoblastic lymphosarcoma. Karyological analysis showed that the tumours induced in the nude mice were of bovine origin and not of mouse origin.

Three sheep inoculated with SLS cells were clinically and haematologically normal during the 2 years after inoculation.

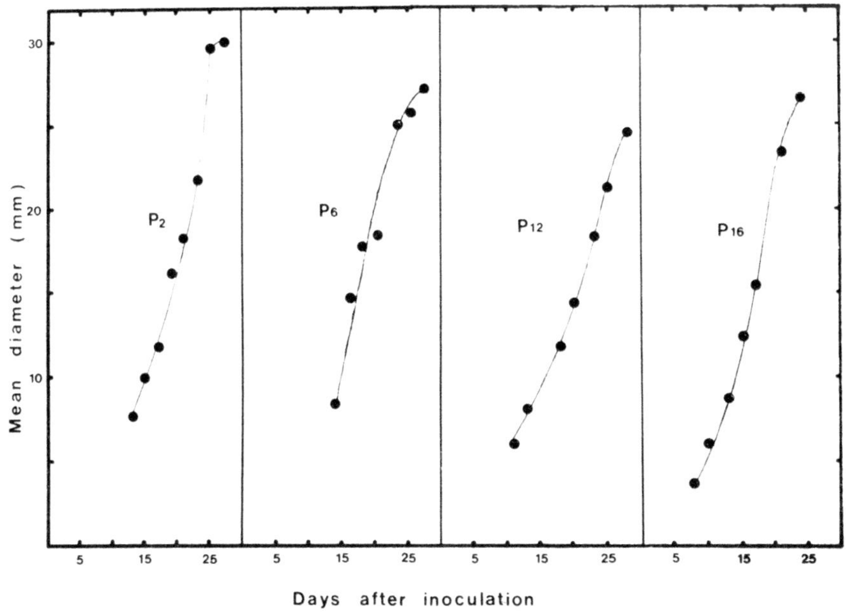

Fig. 1. Growth curves of bovine skin lymphosarcoma implanted in nude mice. P2, 6, 12, 16 : Passage number in nude mice.

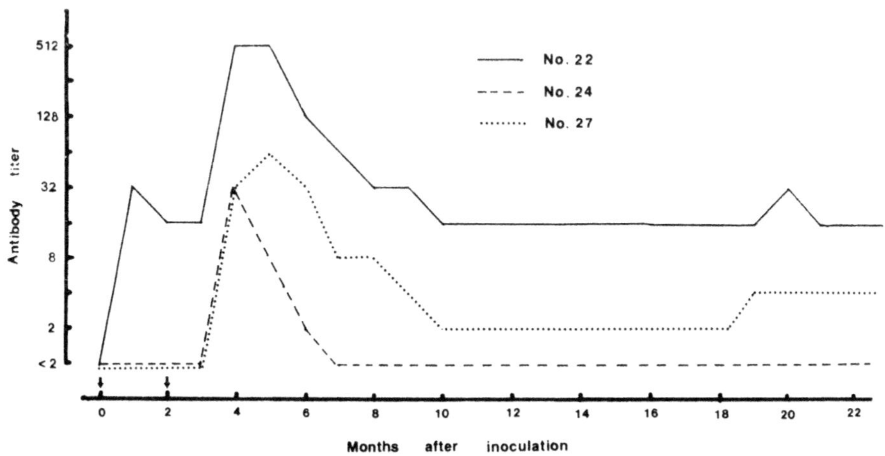

Fig. 2. Results of CDAC tests on sera from sheep inoculated with SLS cells against transplantable SLS cells in nude mice.
Arrow indicates the times of inoculation of SLS cells.

Neither BLV nor antibodies against BLV could be detected. The results of CDAC test using transplantable SLS cells and FLK cells are shown in Table 1. Sera from these 3 sheep had cytotoxic activity against transplantable SLS cells in nude mice but not against BLV producing foetal lamb kidney (FLK) nor SF-28 cells.

TABLE 1

DETECTION OF ANTIBODIES AGAINST THE TRANSPLANTABLE SKIN LYMPHOSARCOMA AND FLK CELLS IN VARIOUS SERA

Sera from		Cytotoxicity against SLS cells	Cytotoxicity against FLK cells
Cattle with natural bovine lymphosarcoma	ALS [1]	0/4 [2]	4/4
	CLS	0/6	0/6
	TLS	0/8	0/8
	SLS	0/3	0/3
Sheep experimentally inoculated with	BLV	0/6	6/6
	SLS	3/3	0/3
Nude mice with transplanted SLS cells		3/8	0/8

1) ALS : adult lymphosarcoma, CLS : calf lymphosarcoma, TLS : thymic lymphosarcoma, SLS : skin lymphosarcoma

2) No. positive / No. tested

3) All sera were absorbed with normal bovine lymphoid cells before test to eliminate the non-specific reaction

No cytotoxicity against transplanted SLS cells was observed in sera from cattle with lymphosarcoma and in sera from sheep experimentally infected with BLV. Three of the 8 sera from nude mice bearing SLS tumours had cytotoxic activity against SLS cells. Cytotoxic activity against FLK cells could be detected in all sera from cattle with ALS, and also in sera from sheep experimentally infected with BLV. Sera from the 2 control sheep had no antibody against BLV and SLS cells.

Figure 2 shows the evolution patterns of CDAC antibody titres against transplanted SLS cells in sera collected monthly from 3 sheep inoculated with SLS cells. The sheep inoculated with SLS cells developed specific serological responses in 1 to 4 months after inoculation, and these responses have persisted in 2 of the 3 sheep (Nos. 22 and 27). In sera from sheep No. 27, cytotoxic antibody could not be detected 7 months after the first inoculation. Serum from sheep No. 21 which was inoculated with culture fluids from 3178 cells and ALS cells (Suneya et al., 1981) was cytotoxic both against normal bovine cells and SLS cells. However absorption of the serum (sheep No. 21) with normal bovine lymph node cells (2 x 10^6/ml serum) completely removed the above mentioned cytotoxic activity. Absorption of sera from sheep 22, 24 and 27 with the same number or more of normal bovine lymph node cells resulted in no decrease in the antibody titres against the SLS cells.

DISCUSSION

SBL is very rare and the aetiology of the disease is still unknown. EBL could be transmitted in sheep and cattle under experimental and natural conditions, respectively. In sporadic leukosis, however, neither experimental nor natural transmissions have been observed in sheep and cattle. The usefulness of heterotransplantation of SBL to athymic nude mice has been reported by Onuma et al. (1980a). The establishment of transplantable skin lymphosarcoma cells in nude mice is an excellent tool for studying sporadic leukosis.

Comparison of cell surface antigen of EBL and SBL cells revealed the following evidence:

1. The origin of neoplastic cells of EBL is the B cells but that of SBL may be the lymphoid stem cell (Onuma et al., 1979).
2. Specific tumour associated antigen was found on tumour cells from EBL but not on tumour cells from SBL (Onuma and Olson, 1977).

3. The presence of different cell surface antigens on EBL and SBL cells was suggested by the sera from nude mice bearing transplanted tumours (Onuma et al., 1980b).

Inoculation of SBL cells into sheep gave neither clinical, haematological nor serological changes. In the present experiment, 3 sheep inoculated with SLS cells showed cytotoxic activity against transplantable SLS cells which were transplanted into nude mice. The immune response of 2 sheep (Nos. 22 and 27) have persisted for about 2 years after inoculation. The following evidence proves that the reaction should be specific to SLS cells:

1. The sera from 3 sheep had no antibodies against BLV and BLV-related cells membrane antigens.
2. Absorption of the sera with normal bovine lymphoid cells could not remove the reaction.
3. Transplantable SLS cells in nude mice showed bovine karyotype and no reaction against anti-murine leukaemia virus serum.

Although the exact reason for the persistency of the immune response in sheep inoculated with SLS cells is not known, SLS cells or an infectious agent which should be an aetiological agent of SLS may replicate in sheep. Present studies show that the establishment of transplantable SLS cells in nude mice is extremely important for further investigation of sporadic leukosis.

REFERENCES

Honma, T., Onuma, M., Suneya, M., Mikami, T. and Izawa H., 1980. Cytotoxic antibody in cattle and sheep exposed to bovine leukemia virus. Archiv, Virol., In press.

Miller, L.D., Miller, J.M. and Olson, C., 1972. Inoculation of calves with particles resembling C-type virus from culture of bovine lymphosarcoma. J. Natl. Cancer Inst., 48: 423-428.

Olson, C., Miller, L.D., Miller, J.M. and Hoss, H.E., 1972. Transmission of lymphosarcoma from cattle to sheep. J. Natl. Cancer Inst., 49: 1463-1467.

Onuma, M., Honma, T., Mikam, T., Ichijo, S. and Konishi, T., 1979. Studies on the sporadic and enzootic forms of bovine leukosis. J. Comp. Path., 89: 159-167.

Onuma, M., Matsumoto, K., Kodama, H., Fujimoto, Y., Moriguchi, R., Mikami, T. and Izawa, H., 1980a. Heterotransplantation of natural bovine lymphosarcoma to nude mice. Europ. J. Cancer, In press.

Onuma, M., Matsumoto, K., Mikami, T. and Izawa, H., 1980b. Heterotransplantation of natural bovine lymphosarcoma and established cell lines to nude mice. In: Yohn, Lapin, Blakeslee (Editors), Adv. Comp. Leuk. Res., 1979, Elsevier North Holland, Inc., New York, pp 43-44.

Onuma, M. and Olson, C., 1977. Tumor-associated antigen in bovine and ovine lymphosarcoma. Cancer Res., 37: 3249-3256.

Onuma, M., Watarai, S., Sonoda, M., Mikami, T. and Izawa, H., 1980c. Detection of bovine leukemia virus by syncytium assay. Can. J. Comp. Med., 44: 289-293.

Suneya, M., Onuma, M., Mikami, T. and Izawa, H., 1981. Humoral and cellular immune responses to bovine leukaemia virus infection in sheep. IV International Symposium on Bovine Leukosis, Bologna, Nov. 5-7, 1980 (this publication).

DISCUSSION

G.H. Theilen *(USA)*

You showed a photograph of the cytogenetics of a transplantable tumour in mice and it had a normal chromosome composition. Most of the tumours that I have analysed in bovine leukosis, whether they are of the adult, thymic, or cutaneous form, were hypo- or hyperdiploid and I do not recall finding more than one or two that had normal chromosome sets. Did all the transplantable tumours you had have normal sets, or did that just represent one?

M. Onuma

I did not check very many different natural skin and other lymphosarcoma cases, but some were normal karyotypes and some were very different from the natural bovine. These skin lymphosarcoma cases were natural ones.

O.-R. Kaaden *(FRG)*

How many cells did you implant or transplant into the sheep? This question relates to the fact that the onset of the cytotoxic antibody production was relatively late, beginning about two months after the implantation. Did you see any tumours, or how do you explain this late onset of cytotoxicity?

M. Onuma

We inoculated 50 ml of whole blood per sheep first and then 3 ml of packed cells. So it was a huge number of cells.

O.R. Kaaden

This was from a case of sporadic skin leukosis, wasn't it?

M. Onuma

Yes.

A.A. Ressang *(Netherlands)*

I have a comment on the last opinion you expressed, that in the study of juvenile leukosis use should be made of athymic mice. In the last five years we have investigated some 16 to 20 juvenile cases of bovine leukosis using all kinds of experimental animals, including athymic mice, with no results whatsoever. I think that your case of skin lymphosarcoma, judging from the histological picture, might be related to the lymphosarcoma in the dog.

M. Onuma

At first we used very young nude mice, next time irradiated ones. After several transplants we did not need irradiation and we used young nude mice.

A.A. Ressang

Yes, but have you done inoculation experiments with nude mice with material obtained from juvenile cases? If so, have you achieved any results so far?

M. Onuma

Juvenile cases are very hard to transplant. We implanted four or five nude mice and only one had a tumour.

B.S. Samagh *(Canada)*

Did you check any sera from sporadic cases to see whether they have cytotoxic activity to these transplantable cells?

M. Onuma

There was no cytotoxic activity against skin lymphosarcoma cells. Serum from cattle with natural lymphosarcoma shows no cytotoxicity activity against skin lymphosarcoma cells.

<u>A. Burny</u> *(Belgium)*

How does the antigen you find now relate to the one you find in SF-28 cells? Are they related at all?

<u>M. Onuma</u>

No. I checked against SF-28 cells but serum from the inoculated sheep and nude mice showed no cytotoxic activity against the SF-28 cells. So it is a completely different antigen.

INFLUENCE OF COLOSTRAL ANTIBODY ON SUSCEPTIBILITY OF SHEEP TO BOVINE LEUKOSIS VIRUS

C. Olson and R.W. Kaja
Department of Veterinary Science, University of Wisconsin, Madison, Wisconsin, USA

ABSTRACT

Calves born to nursing cows infected with bovine leukosis virus (BLV) seldom show evidence of infection after colostral antibodies have disappeared. Such calves have potential exposure to BLV from contact with their infected dam and from BLV infected lymphocytes in the milk. This suggested a possible protective influence of colostrum. Four groups of sheep which had received colostrum from their BLV infected ewes were inoculated with BLV in sheep lymphocytes at 2 weeks, 4 months, 17 months and up to 4.5 years of age. Evidence of BLV infection has been measured by BLV antibodies in agar gel immunodiffusion tests. In the first group, 5 of 7 sheep have remained serologically negative after disappearance of colostral antibodies. The other two sheep have been persistently positive and BLV infected. The sheep exposed when older in the other 3 groups have persistent BLV antibodies with one exception. It appears that BLV colostral antibodies, if present at time of exposure to BLV, will usually prevent infection.

O.C. Straub (ed.), Fourth International Symposium on Bovine Leukosis

INTRODUCTION

Transmission of bovine leukosis virus infection appears to occur from some form of contact exposure between those cattle infected with the virus and those susceptible to the virus. Such contact transmission of bovine leukosis virus (BLV) has not been demonstrated in sheep. In herds of cattle, where BLV infection is present, most cattle do not show evidence of the infection until they are 2 or more years of age (Olson et al., 1978). It is quite probable that some lymphocytes of cows infected with BLV are shed in the milk. This is a potential source of infection to calves born from these cows when they nurse. The colostrum has a high concentration of antibody to BLV which could neutralise the virus. This would suggest some protection by colostral antibody during the early months of life.

An opportunity arose to investigate the influence of colostral antibody on susceptibility of sheep to bovine leukosis virus.

MATERIALS AND METHODS

Ewes experimentally infected with BLV provided 27 lambs used in this study. The lambs were allowed to nurse their dams until weaned. All lambs were inoculated with 2 to 10 x 10^6 peripheral blood leukocytes from BLV infected sheep either intraperitoneally, intravenously or intradermally. Colostral antibodies were still present when 7 of the lambs were inoculated at 1 - 2 weeks of age. In 19 other lambs, colostral antibody had disappeared when they received BLV infected leukocytes at 4 to 55 months of age. One sheep had colostral antibodies when it was inoculated at 5 months of age. Nineteen susceptible lambs born to BLV negative ewes received inocula similar to those given to the test sheep. These sheep served as controls.

Seroconversion to a positive test for BLV antibodies by agar gel immunodiffusion (AGID) served as evidence for BLV infection following the inoculations already described. Agar gel immunodiffusion (AGID) tests were performed using glycoprotein antigen either prepared as described previously (Onuma et al., 1975) or as furnished by Pitman-Moore Inc., Washington Crossing, N.J. The BLV glycoprotein antigen was placed in a central well surrounded by 6 peripheral wells. Test sera were adjacent to a well with BLV positive control serum. Control sera were obtained from BLV infected sheep negative for other common bovine and ovine viruses.

RESULTS

Five of 7 lambs receiving BLV infective leukocytes during the first 2 weeks of life remained negative after the colostral antibody disappeared (Table 1). The colostral antibody titre of these 5 lambs ranged from 4 to 32 and disappeared at 12 to 14 weeks of life. These lambs have remained negative up to 1.5 years of age. Two lambs, K-02 and L-104, receiving BLV infective lymphocytes at one and two weeks of age respectively, were persistently positive for 2.5 and 1.5 years, respectively. In one lamb (K-02, Figure 1) the titre was 8 at 4 months of age, 2 weeks later it was 1, and no colostral antibody could be detected by AGID at the age of 5 months but reappeared with a titre of 8 at the age of 8 months. In the other lamb (L-104, Figure 1) there was a reduction in titre but no break between colostral antibody and antibody which apparently was derived from active BLV infection.

Seven lambs were challenged at the age of about 4 months with peripheral blood leukocytes from BLV infected sheep (Table 1). In 6 of these lambs colostral antibodies had disappeared at the time they received the infective BLV. All 6 lambs seroconverted one month after exposure. One of the 7 lambs inoculated at 19 weeks of age had a low titre of BLV antibody by AGID test and never did become completely negative. After infection, its titre increased from 1 to 32.

TABLE 1

CHALLENGE OF COLOSTRAL PROTECTION OF 27 SHEEP EXPOSED TO BLV AT VARIOUS AGES. ALL TEST SHEEP WERE BORN FROM EWES INFECTED WITH BLV AND CHALLENGED WITH BLV INFECTED LEUKOCYTES.

	Seroconversion			
Age	Negative		Positive	
at challenge	No.	At months	No.	At months
2 weeks	5	17	2	3,8
4 months	0		7	1
17 months	1	11	3	1,2.5
48 months	0		9	1,2
Controls			19	1,2

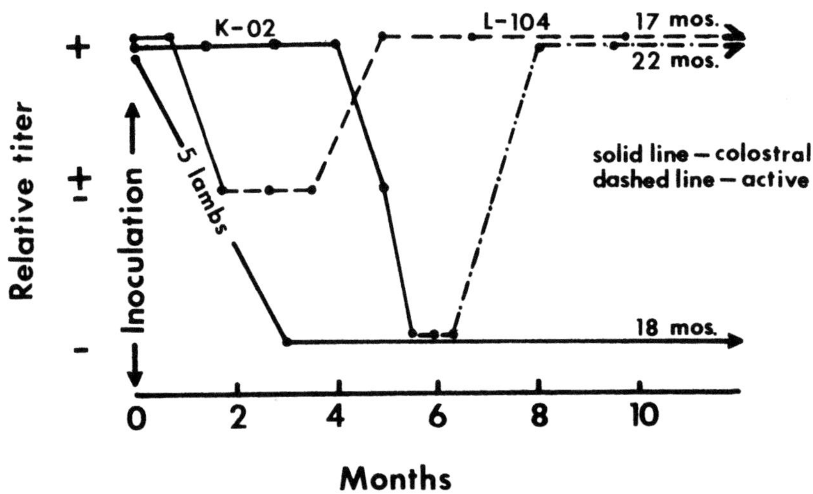

Fig 1. BLV antibody in sheep inoculated when 1 to 2 weeks old. Note the complete disappearance of antibody in 5 sheep and the development of persistent antibody in sheep K-02 and L-104.

Four lambs were 17 months of age when they were challenged with infective BLV in sheep leukocytes (Table 1). None of these 4 lambs had colostral antibody persisting at the time they received the challenge. Three of these seroconverted at 1 to 2.5 months after challenge. One lamb, K-12, remained negative at 11 months following challenge.

Nine lambs were challenged at the age of 48 months and these lambs were all serologically negative at the time of challenge having lost their colostral antibody. All 9 lambs developed antibody as measured by AGID test 1 to 2 months after exposure (Table 1).

Nineteen susceptible sheep born to BLV negative ewes, ranging in age from young lambs to about 5 years old, received inocula similar to and at the same time as the test sheep. These sheep serving as controls all seroconverted 1 to 2 months after inoculation.

DISCUSSION

In January 1978 one week old lambs were inoculated with BLV. One of these (K-02, Figure 1) had received colostral antibodies and the other (K-01) had not. K-01 developed active BLV infection as evidenced by development of persisting strong antibody 6 weeks later. Colostral antibodies persisted in K-02 to 4 months, were not found at 5 to 6 months, then antibodies reappeared and persisted at 8 months. Active BLV infection was demonstrated twice at 13.5 and 14 months when peripheral blood lymphocytes from K-02 produced BLV infection in two susceptible sheep. What appeared to be a latent infection in K-02 may have been due to suppression by colostral antibodies. This led to the further investigation as presented in this report.

It would seem colostral antibodies had prevented BLV infection in 5 of 6 additional lambs when inoculated with BLV at two weeks of age. Evidence of infection as measured by seroconversion in the lamb K-02 and increase of relative titre in the lamb L-104 was delayed for 8 and 5 months respectively. This is in contrast to seroconversion in the susceptible control lambs or sheep at 1 to 2 months.

There was no influence of previous colostral antibodies in sheep inoculated at 4 months or 48 months of age.

A peculiar observation was made in one of four sheep inoculated at 17 months of age. It has remained negative for antibodies for 11 months. Three other sheep inoculated at the same age seroconverted at 1 to 2.5 months.

Colostral antibodies seemed to neutralise BLV and prevent infection in 5 of 7 lambs. The mechanism of suppression is of interest since it could neutralise and destroy infectivity of the virus in 5 of 7 lambs while in 2 lambs the virus was only temporarily neutralised during a prolonged latent period.

In these experiments a relatively large number of cells was used as the infective inoculum. The protective effect of colostrum probably exists for longer than 2 weeks and may extend to 3 months against a smaller infective dose. The route of exposure could also be a factor, although the routes used in this study seemed to have no influence. Oral exposure was not tested. Mammerickx et al. (1980) had found colostral antibodies to protect lambs from oral exposure.

ACKNOWLEDGEMENT

This work was supported in part by the College of Agriculture and Life Sciences, University of Wisconsin, Madison, Wis.

The diligent technical assistance of Ms. Jody Baumgartner is much appreciated.

REFERENCES

Mammerickx, M., Portetelle, D., Burny, A. and Leunen, J. 1980. Detection by immunodiffusion - and radioimmunoassay - tests of antibodies bovine leukemia virus antigens in sera of experimentally infected sheep and cattle. Zbl. Vet. Med. B., 27: 291-303.

Olson, C., Kaja, R., Stauffacher, R. and Zehner, E., 1978. Development of bovine leukosis virus infection in cattle. A preliminary study. Ann. Rech. Vét., 9(4): 845-849.

Onuma, M., Olson, C., Baumgartener, L.E. and Pearson, L.D., 1975. An ether-sensitive antigen associated with bovine leukemia virus infection. J. Natl. Cancer Inst., 55: 1155-1158.

DISCUSSION

F. Bürki *(Austria)*

What exactly do you mean by seroconversion? Which test did you use?

C. Olson *(USA)*

This was the agar gel immunodiffusion test only.

F. Bürki

Did you try at least to quantitate this one? I am interested in the quantity of maternal antibodies that might be protective.

C. Olson

No, and neither do we know what type this is, whether it is an Igl or Ig2. The antibody in the colostrum is certainly very high and these lambs nursed immediately, or soon after, they were born, in the normal fashion. The colostral antibody titres must have been quite high.

F. Bürki

And when would the titres have been lost, if you had not challenged these animals?

C. Olson

The sheep were losing antibodies at about the age of three to four months.

J.F. Ferrer *(USA)*

Do you think the sheep might have had antibodies before colostrum?

C. Olson

No. They received colostral antibodies only from their own dams.

<u>J.F. Ferrer</u>

How did you exclude the possibility of prenatal infection of these sheep?

<u>C. Olson</u>

I am not sure that Mother Nature allows this, but there may have been.

<u>J.F. Ferrer</u>

So you cannot rule out the possibility that these lambs were infected before birth?

<u>C. Olson</u>

The sera from these lambs were not tested prior to their receiving colostrum but had they been infected prior to birth I would have anticipated a persisting antibody level.

<u>J.F. Ferrer</u>

I asked the question because you had two sheep that were not protected. I was wondering whether these two had been infected prenatally.

<u>C. Olson</u>

I do believe that those two evidenced a partial protection because their seroconversion was delayed so long.

<u>J.F. Ferrer</u>

But they may still have been infected prenatally?

<u>C. Olson</u>

It is possible of course, yes.

<u>A.A. Ressang</u> *(Netherlands)*

Did you check the colostrum for the presence of BLV?

C. Olson

No.

A.A. Ressang

Why not? I think this is a crucial question.

C. Olson

I am not sure how one could do this.

A.A. Ressang

It is very simple. You isolate the lymphocytes after digestion of proteins in the colostrum and then you get a nice layer of lymphocytes.

C. Olson

What difference would that make? Certainly, in these young lambs we gave them plenty of lymphocytes.

A.A. Ressang

I am interested in the fact of whether, besides your antibodies, you also administer virus.

C. Olson

There probably is virus, or at least pro-virus, in the lymphocytes that we give.

A.A. Ressang

All right. But now a practical point. What do you advise in the case of enzootic bovine leukosis in a herd? If you slaughter all the positive reactors, what is your advice concerning the calves from such a herd?

C. Olson

This is a very practical point and perhaps we do not have the definitive answer. From what we have observed in infected herds calves can nurse the colostrum from their infected dams and they will remain negative until one or two years later. Is this a suppression of virus or is it a new infection, and they are seroconverting at a later date from exposure to BLV from other sources? I don't know that answer. All I know is that, in practice, these calves can apparently be raised in many herds and remain negative.

IMMUNOGLOBULIN AMOUNTS AND LEUKOSIS-SPECIFIC ANTIBODIES IN COLOSTRUM, MILK AND SERUM IN THE PERIPARTURIENT PERIOD AND THEIR LEVELS IN THE NEWBORN

W. Matthaeus and O.C. Straub
Federal Research Institute for Animal Virus Diseases,
D-7400 Tübingen, Federal Republic of Germany.

ABSTRACT

The absolute amounts of immunoglobulins of the dams and their offspring were determined by the radial immunodiffusion test and the rocket immunoelectrophoresis.

The immunoglobulins in colostrum and milk of the individual quarters in general show a decrease from shortly before parturition until the second week when they level off. The most remarkable reduction occurs in most animals between days 1 and 3 pp. A comparison of the amounts of immunoglobulins in the individual quarters of some animals show a similar composition and decrease; in others marked differences could be observed. Shortly before and after parturition the immunoglobulin amounts were extremely high.

There was no distinct variation in the serum immunoglobulins of dams during the periparturient period. In the calves variation could be related to the intake of colostrum of different quality.

Antibody titres in the sera of some dams were found to be higher before rather than after parturition. At parturition, extremely high antibody titres were observed in colostrum samples, and only then were there no differences between individual quarters. During the following days they decreased with differing rapidity. In most cases, antibodies against gp70 antigen predominated.

O.C. Straub (ed.), Fourth International Symposium on Bovine Leukosis

INTRODUCTION

The correlation between the level of passively acquired immunoglobulins in the newborn and disease resistance, including information on this correlation in bovines, is documented in numerous publications (Gay et al., 1965; Graves, 1963; Matthaeus and Bögel, 1964; McEwen, 1950; McEwen et al., 1970; Penhale et al., 1973; Straub, 1969; Straub and Matthaeus, 1978). It has been established that the serum titre of specific antibodies in the calf is dependent on the volume of colostrum, its composition and the time of administration *post partum*. It was found, for example, that 1 000 ml colostrum given within the first twelve hours were sufficient to produce the same antibody titre in the newborn as in the dam (Straub and Matthaeus, 1978).

This study deals with the transmission of immunological protection against bovine leukosis. Thus, the following parameters were determined: composition of the colostral and milk immunoglobulins of the cow's individual quarters, antibody titres against bovine leukosis virus (BLV) in milk and blood serum from dam and offspring for the periods indicated in the Tables.

MATERIALS AND METHODS

Experimental animals

Six cows in the periparturient period which were haematologically and serologically positive for bovine leukaemia, as well as one normal animal without clinical symptoms, were used, the latter as a control. Following parturition the newborn calves were included in the experiments.

Serum, colostrum and milk

Both blood for serum and colostrum/milk (taken separately from each quarter of the mammary gland) were collected before and at various times after parturition as shown in Tables 1 - 3.

TABLE 1 ABSOLUTE AMOUNTS OF IMMUNOGLOBULINS IN COLOSTRUM AND MILK OF THE INDIVIDUAL QUARTERS FROM SIX COWS INFECTED WITH BLV AND A NON-INFECTED CONTROL, DETERMINED ACCORDING TO THE RADIAL IMMUNODIFFUSION TEST (FOR IgG AND IgA) AND THE ROCKET IMMUNOELECTROPHORESIS (FOR IgM). Cows Nos.2 and 4 suffered from tumours and persistent lymphocytosis

Quarter	Time of sampling	B L V - i n f e c t e d c a t t l e																			Non-infected control			
		No 1			No 2			No 3			No 4			No 5			No 6							
		IgG	IgA	IgM	IgG	IgA	IgM	IgG	IgA	IgM	IgG	IgA	IgM	IgG	IgA	IgM	IgG	IgA	IgM		IgG	IgA	IgM	hours p.p.
RF	d.a.p. 1-4				10550	320	710													RF				
RR					11300	340	638													RR				
LF					11300	340	496													LF				
LR					10550	310	568													LR				
RF	h.p.p. 1-2	1)												8100	320	528	11850	1085	430	RF				
RR		12400	270	1123										9100	340	566				RR				
LF		11850	235	1110										9100	365	655	13400	1200	546	LF				
LR		12400	223	1085										9600	420	568	12900	1140	486	LR				
RF	h.p.p. 1-2				12400	420	647				5720	700	730	6000	255	533	8600	840	441	RF	10400	425	566	6
RR		11300	235	996	13400	446	643				2470	790	776	7400	284	521				RR	10200	500	572	
LF		10300	184	941	13400	446	620				2740	745	800	7050	270	532	9600	950	567	LF	10300	500	476	
LR		10550	165	977	12900	380	657				2900	600	842	7400	320	427	8100	895	522	LR	10100	560	474	
RF	1				9100	223	436	9600	270	317	2000	210	256	1730	53	157	5400	600	354	RF	4200	228	252	12
RR		7050	165	672	10550	255	468	10300	310	529	750	270	514	1930	63	170				RR	4000	158	219	
LF		6000	137	628	10550	270	493	9100	255	350	980	184	210	1930	67	176	7050	745	468	LF	3550	98	176	
LR		6300	155	656	10300	235	540	10550	284	365	1140	137	640	1825	59	177	6300	700	426	LR	3800	126	200	
RF	2				4400	76	215	7400	71	157				265	20	56	3000	255	96	RF	1140	48	114	24
RR		740	20	212	5100	91	381	7780	97	221				280	21	45				RR	1840	64	115	
LF		470	17	152	4880	76	162	6690	76	213				280	21	48	4000	380	397	LF	1840	87	116	
LR		525	19	168	4630	91	230	7780	91	312				280	20	67	2600	284	116	LR	1350	43	111	
RF	3				3540	51	200	4000	29	176	1640	20	108	158	17	68	225	91	77	RF	660	26	83	36
RR		470	18	139	4200	56	285	4200	42	184	495	37	180	143	18	60				RR	895	28	105	
LF		380	18	104	4000	51	80	3780	33	149	680	20	96	185	19	51	470	175	282	LF	598	28	96	
LR		380	19	127	3200	42	67	4630	37	250	740	21	96	165	19	51	225	114	94	LR	545	29	100	
RF					710	27	50				470	20	133	143	18	50				RF	380	22	74	48
RR	d.p.p. 4	328	18	123	870	37	68				174	29	117	150	18	52				RR	370	22	74	
LF		214	17	94	1030	33	57				158	19	96	150	18	53				LF	230	24	63	
LR		279	18	109	990	29	44				122	18	91	136	17	51				LR	248	28	70	
RF	5							1075	24	33	206	14	99							RF				
RR		252	16	88				1190	26	57	165	21	112							RR				
LF		158	16	78				990	23	38	136	18	101							LF				
LR		186	16	83				1140	27	47	136	17	127							LR				
RF	6										136	17	0							RF				
RR				76							110	19	0							RR				
LF				62							186	17	0							LF				
LR				71							186	18	0							LR				
RF	7							265	21	19	165	16	0				165	76	97	RF				
RR								363	26	27	158	18	0							RR				
LF								252	27	20	165	16	0				193	209	114	LF				
LR								310	21	23	174	15	0				150	109	93	LR				
RF	14																122	51	43	RF				
RR																				RR				
LF																	174	109	51	LF				
LR																	122	44	55	LR				
RF	21																104	39	43	RF				
RR																				RR				
LF																	116	63	55	LF				
LR																	122	34	47	LR				
RF	m.p.p 3.5							165	18	0										RF				
RR								214	19	0										RR				
LF								186	16	0										LF				
LR								195	21	0										LR				

Explanation: 1) Amounts in mg/100 ml. d.a.p. - days ante partum; h.a.p. - hours ante partum; h.p.p. - hours post partum; d.p.p. - days post partum; m.p.p. - months post partum

RF - right front quarter; RR - right rear quarter; LF - left front quarter; LR - left rear quarter.

TABLE 2 ABSOLUTE AMOUNTS OF SERUM IMMUNOGLOBULINS DETERMINED BY THE ROCKET IMMUNOELECTROPHORESIS OF 6 BLV INFECTED CATTLE AND A NON-INFECTED CONTROL AND THEIR CALVES. THE FIRST SAMPLES FROM THE CALVES WERE TAKEN BEFORE THE INTAKE OF COLOSTRUM. Cows Nos.2 and 4 suffered from tumours and persistent lymphocytosis.

Time of sampling		No 1			Calf from No 1			No 2			Calf from No 2			No 3			Calf from No 3		
		IgG	IgA	IgM	IgG	IgA	IgM	IgG	IgA	IgM	IgG	IgA	IgM	IgG	IgA	IgM	IgG	IgA	IgM
d.a.p.	1-4							2055	47										
h.a.p.	1-2	3000	44																
h.p.p.	1-2	2710	48		105	0		2050	53		0	0							
	1	2800	50		2630	184		2140	58		3150	138		3650	26		2360	83	
	2	2750	53		2735	122		2550	57		2990	96		4150	28		2820	74	
	3	2730	56		2810	77		2555	54		2745	80		4300	29		1350	70	
	4	2640	56		2250	53		2545	55		2535	59							
d.p.p.	5	2350	53		2240	51								4450	25		1900	59	
	6																		
	7													5250	23		2500	51	
	14																		
	21																		
m.p.p.	3.5													3200	23		1740	19	

Time of sampling		No 4			Calf from No 4			No 5			Calf from No 5			No 6			Calf from No 6		
		IgG	IgA	IgM	IgG	IgA	IgM	IgG	IgA	IgM	IgG	IgA	IgM	IgG	IgA	IgM	IgG	IgA	IgM
d.a.p.	1-4																		
h.a.p.	1-2							1820	63										
h.p.p.	1-2	2400	40		300	35		2330	62		150	0		3400	158		0	0	
	1	3310	43		4150	143		2340	65		1200	187		3450	154		2260	175	
	2							2330	60		1300	184		3400	155		2400	165	
	3	2990	38		5700	86		2320	61		1240	96		3300	157		2300	147	
	4	2650	39		5800	77		2350	62		1250	58							
	5	2415	38		5650	71		2310	59		1190	33							
	6	1950	40		5730	62													
	7	1600	37		5600	26								3420	153		2080	134	
	14													3440	156		1750	71	
	21													3650	156		1650	44	

Control			Calf from Control			
IgG	IgA	IgM	IgG	IgA	IgM	h.p.p.
1660	57	213	51	0	48	6
1980	57	214	1335	87	150	12
2175	57	215	1335	77	150	24
2280	55	214	1200	40	142	36
2225	53	220	1140	35	135	48

For explanation see Table 1

TABLE 3 ANTIBODY TITRES IN COLOSTRUM AND MILK OF THE INDIVIDUAL QUARTERS OF 3 BLV INFECTED COWS (NUMBERS REFER TO THESE LISTED IN TABLES 1 AND 2). Cows Nos. 2 and 4 suffered from tumours and persistent lymphocytosis.

Quarter	Time of sampling	No 1 gp	No 1 p_{24}	No 2 gp	No 2 p_{24}	No 4 gp	No 4 p_{24}
RF	d.a.p. 1-4			1:32	1:64		
RR				1:16	1:64		
LF				1:32	1:64		
LR				1:32	1:64		
RF	h.a.p. 1-2						
RR		1:32	-				
LF		1:32	-				
LR		1:32	-				
RF	h.p.p. 1-2			1:32	1:64	1:128	1:16
RR		1:32		1:32	1:32	1:128	1:8
LF		1:32	-	1:64	1:64	1:128	1:16
LR		1:32	-	1:32	1:64	1:128	1:16
RF	d.p.p. 1			1:16	1:16	1:16	1:2
RR		1:8	-	1:32	1:16	1:32	1:4
LF		1:8	-	1:16	1:16	1:8	1:1
LR		1:8	-	1:32	1:64	1:32	1:1
RF	2			1:4	1:8	1:4	1:1
RR		(1:1)	-	1:8	1:32	1:8	1:1
LF		1:2		1:4	1:4	1:4	1:1
LR		(1:1)	-	1:4	1:8	1:1	1:2
RF	3			1:4	1:8	-	-
RR		-	-	1:4	1:8	1:4	-
LF		-	-	1:2	1:4	-	-
LR		-	-	(1:1)	1:4	1:1	-
RF	4			-	1:1	-	-
RR		-	-	1:1	1:4	1:1	-
LF		-	-	1:1	1:2	-	-
LR		-	-	-	1:4	-	-
RF	5					-	-
RR		-	-			1:1	-
LF		-	-			-	-
LR		-	-			-	-
RF	6					-	-
RR		-	-			-	-
LF		-	-			-	-
LR		-	-			-	-
RF	7					-	-
RR		-	-			-	-
LF		-	-			-	-
LR		-	-			-	-
RF	14					-	-
RR		-	-			-	-
LF		-	-			-	-
LR		-	-			-	-

Explanation:
gp - antibody titre against the glycoprotein antigen
p_{24} - antibody titre against the internal p_{24} antigen
d.a.p. - days ante partum; d.p.p. - days post partum
h.a.p. - hours ante partum; h.p.p. - hours post partum

Antisera and immunoglobulins

Rabbit antisera to bovine serum IgG, IgA and IgM as well as control and reference samples of the corresponding bovine serum immunoglobulins were purchased from Miles Laboratories GmbH (Frankfurt). Another preparation of anti-IgM rabbit serum was a kind gift from Dr. Z. Trainin, Bet Dagan, Israel.

Determination of the absolute amounts of the different immunoglobulin classes

The radial immunodiffusion test (RIDT) according to Mancini et al. (1965) and the electroimmunoassay (EIA, rocket immunoelectrophoresis) described by Laurell (1966) were employed for the determination of the absolute amounts of immunoglobulins in serum, colostrum and milk samples respectively. The RIDT was performed in pre-formed kits (Miles Laboratories) without any dilution of the samples. For the EIA (employed only for the determination of IgM levels) the samples tested were diluted with PBS (1 : 10). Further technical details were given in a previous paper (Matthaeus and Straub, 1968).

Estimation of the antibody titre by immunodiffusion

This was performed as previously described (Straub, 1978a; Straub, 1978b).

Immunoelectrophoresis

Details of the conditions used have been described previously (Matthaeus and Straub, 1976).

RESULTS

Extremely high values for the three classes of immunoglobulins were reached shortly before parturition (average mg/100 ml: IgG - 12 000, IgA - 400, IgM - 600). A marked drop occurred between the first and second day *post partum* (pp) (generally about 70 - 80%). 'Normal' values seemed to be reached at the end of the first week pp. There were some distinct differences noted among the values of the individual quarters, but they were synchronous as far as their composition of immunoglobulins was concerned. No significant difference was found between the absolute amounts of the three classes of immunoglobulins of the BLV infected cows and the control (Table 1).

There were no noticeable changes during the periods of examination as far as the absolute amounts of serum IgG and IgM were concerned, but the readings from the calves varied according to the intake of colostrum, as has been shown previously (Straub and Matthaeus, 1978). Details may be taken from Table 2.

In immunoelectrophoretic studies comparing the intensity of the precipitation reactions from colostrum/milk and blood serum samples a correlation was found between the intensity and the absolute contents of the individual immunoglobulins. Precipitations could no longer be observed below a certain level.

Determination of the specific antibodies in the blood sera revealed that some animals had slightly higher titres (average 1 : 8) before rather than after parturition (average 1 : 2). Colostral antibodies at calving time were extremely high (maximum 1 : 128) and there was no difference among the individual quarters. The decrease in antibody titres varied from one animal to the other. Three days pp was the earliest day pp, 6 the latest date after which no antibodies could be detected. Three examples are summarised in Table 3. There was, however, a difference in the concentration of antibodies against the major antigens. The antibodies against gp antigen were in general 4 - 8 times higher than those against p24. Details to be published later.

DISCUSSION

The extremely high immunoglobulin contents present at calving time confirm earlier results (Matthaeus and Bögel, 1964) and are in good agreement with the results of other studies; the immunoglobulin levels of the adult animals were within the range shown in the literature (summarised in Table 4). The dependence of the levels in the newborn on the colostral parameters has also been mentioned already (Graves, 1963; Lamotte, 1977; Straub and Matthaeus, 1978).

TABLE 4

ABSOLUTE AMOUNTS OF THE DIFFERENT BOVINE SERUM IMMUNOGLOBULIN CLASSES DESCRIBED (mg/100 ml) (Taken from Matthaeus and Straub, 1978).

Authors	IgM	IgG	IgA
Mach, Pahud	250 (112-308)	1850 (1540-2160)	60 (7-110)
Roesti, Fey	250 (130-370	1700 (990-2410)	30 (10-50)
Williams, Maxwell, Spooner	271 (149-393)	2070 (1380-2760)	32 (16-48)
Porter, Noakes			78 (51-115)
Trainin et al. normal cattle	260 (230-290)	2590 (2370-2810) immunized	
leukotic cattle	135 (60-210)	1760 (1100-2400)	
Matthaeus, Straub +) normal cattle			
before inoculation with IBR-IPV virus	284 (231-368)	2161 (1685-2600)	47 (37-53)
after inoculation with IBR-IPV virus	299 (180-465)	2336 (1683-1710)	56 (40-75)
leukotic cattle			
before inoculation with IBR-IPV virus	222 (124-386)	1869 (950-3070)	44 (23-65)
after inoculation with IBR-IPV virus	279 (135-437)	2180(975-4025)	52 (29-95)

+) Matthaeus and Straub, 1978.

Immunoelectrophoresis demonstrated the presence of all bovine immunoglobulin classes in the colostrum, milk and blood serum samples. There was no difference between the 2 animals with tumour involvement and persistent lymphocytosis and the others which were only sero-positive. Most of the calves lacked serum IgA and IgG before the uptake of colostrum. Those animals which had come into contact with BLV prenatally had therefore most probably done so earlier rather than during the period immediately prior to parturition. There may be a special period during gestation when it is easier for BLV to pass through that barrier than at other periods.

It is remarkable, however, that there is such variation from quarter to quarter during the first days pp but not in the colostrum. It had also been anticipated, from earlier data (Straub et al., 1978), that the antibodies would persist for much longer periods. It could therefore be quite acceptable to conclude that viruses could easily be shed and transmitted by milk after the first week pp.

ACKNOWLEDGEMENT

The authors gratefully acknowledge the technical assistance provided by Miss G. Kuebart and Mr. E. Schlotterer.

REFERENCES

Gay, C.C., Anderson, N., Fisher, E.W. and McEwen, E.W., 1965. Gammaglob ulin levels and neonatal mortality in market calves. Vet. Rec., 77: 148-149.

Graves, J.H., 1963. Transfer of neutralizing antibody by colostrum to calves born of foot-and-mouth disease vaccinated dams. Immunology, 90: 251-256.

Lamotte, G.B., 1977. Total serum protein, serum protein fractions and serum immunoglobulins in colostrum-fed and colostrum-deprived calves. Am. J. Vet. Res., 38: 263-268.

Laurell, C.B., 1966. Quantitative estimation of proteins by electrophoresis in agarose gel containing antibodies. Anal. Biochem., 15: 45-52.

Mancini, G., Carbonara, A.O. and Heremans, J.F., 1965. Immunochemical quantitation of antigens by single radial immunodiffusion. Immunochem., 2: 235-254.

Matthaeus, W. and Bögel, K., 1964. Vergleichende elektrophoretische Untersuchungen der Serumproteine und immunologische Betrachtungen nach experimenteller Virusinfektion beim kolostrumfrei aufgezogenen Kalb. Zbl. Vet. Med. B 11: 273-288.

Matthaeus, W. and Straub, O.C., 1976. Studies on the distribution of γ-globulins and on abnormal globulins from serums of leukotic cattle and sheep. Vet. Microbiol., 1, 363-373, Straub, O.C. (ed.) Elsevier Publishing Company, Amsterdam and CEC, Luxembourg.

Matthaeus, W. and Straub, O.C., 1978. Die neutralisierenden Serumantikörper normaler und leukotischer Rinder nach der Infektion mit IBR-IPV-Virus. (The immune response of normal and leukotic cattle to IBR-IPV-virus). Zbl. Bakt. Hyg. I, Abt. Orig. A 240: 152-164.

McEwen, A.D., 1950. The resistance of the young calf to disease. Vet. Rec. 62: 83-93.

McEwen, A.D., Fischer, E.W. and Selman, I.E., 1970. Observations on the immunoglobulin levels of neonatal calves and their relationship to disease. J. Comp. Path., 80: 259-265.

Penhale, W.J., Logan, E.F., Fisher, I.E. and McEwen, A.D., 1973. Observations on the absorption of colostral immunoglobulins by the neonatal calf and their significance in colibacillosis. Ann. Rech. Vét., 4: 223-233.

Straub, O.C., 1969. Die Übertragung viraler Antikörper durch das Kolostrum. Tierärztl. Umschau, 24: 571-573.

Straub, O.C., 1978a. Diagnosis of enzootic bovine leukosis: a comparison of haematological and immunodiffusion tests. Res. Vet. Sci., 25: 13-15.

Straub, O.C., 1978b. Horizontal transmission studies on enzootic bovine leukosis. Ann Rech. Vét., 9: 808-813.

Straub, O.C. and Matthaeus, W., 1978. The immunoglobulin composition of colostrum and the persistence of acquired immunoglobulins and specific antibodies in the calf. Ann. Rech. Vét., 9: 269-275.

Straub, O.C., Fischer, W. and Frerking, H., 1978. Über die Zunahme leukose-seropositiver Reagenten in einem hämatologisch negativen Rinderbestand. Tierärztl. Umschau, 33: 657-661.

DEMONSTRATION OF BOVINE LEUKAEMIA VIRUS SPECIFIC PRECIPITATING IgM ANTIBODIES IN IMMUNE COMPLEXES

W. Matthaeus, O.C. Straub and E. Schlotterer
Federal Research Institute for Animal Virus Diseases
D-7400 Tübingen, Federal Republic of Germany.

ABSTRACT

Immune complexes produced between BLV antigen and bovine leukaemic sera as well as colostra, were analysed by SDS-PAGE. The tests applied have demonstrated the presence of IgG and IgM antibodies. Corresponding immunoprecipitates with ovine leukaemic sera showed only immunoglobulins of the IgM class. The principal detectable reacting viral structural protein was gp 60.

O.C. Straub (ed.), Fourth International Symposium on Bovine Leukosis

INTRODUCTION

The precipitating antibody classes against bovine leukaemia virus (BLV) isolated from bovine leukaemic sera revealed precipitating activities with the IgG1 subclass and the IgA class (Matthaeus, 1978; Matthaeus and Weiland, 1976; Matthaeus et al., 1978). Neither IgG2 nor IgM entered into precipitation reactions following isolation.

The present study deals with the analysis of immune complexes produced in immunodiffusion tests (IDT) between leukaemia virus antigens and bovine leukaemic sera and colostra as well as ovine leukaemic sera.

MATERIAL AND METHODS

Serum and colostrum

Precipitating antibody-containing sera and colostra were isolated in the periparturient period from several cows haematologically and serologically positive for bovine leukaemia (Matthaeus and Straub, 1981). Sera and colostra were mixed separately. Blood for ovine serum was collected after experimental infection with BLV-containing milk. Serum from bull no. 78 (Matthaeus, 1978; Matthaeus and Weiland, 1976; Matthaeus and Straub, 1981; Matthaeus et al., 1978) was used as control for specific precipitation reactions in the IDT (Straub, 1978).

BLV antigen

An antigen preparation containing principally gp60 (Matthaeus and Straub, 1980) was kindly provided by Behringwerke A.G. (Marburg, FRG).

Isolation and analysis of immune complexes

For the analytical identification of precipitating immunoglobulins and viral structural proteins involved in the IDT precipitation reactions, the immunoprecipitates were prepared for the gel-containing plates and subjected to SDS-polyacryl-

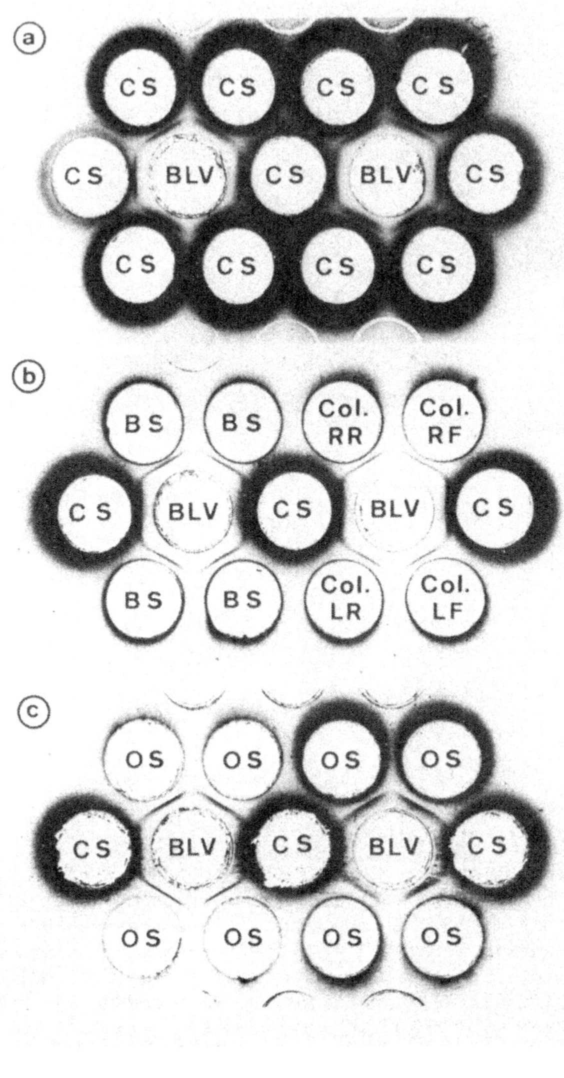

Fig. 1. Immunodiffusion tests showing immunoprecipitates between BLV antigen preparations and sera from leukaemic cattle and sheep as well as colostra from corresponding cows

(BLV = bovine leukaemia virus preparation; CS = control serum from bull no.78; BS = mixture of bovine leukaemic sera; col. RR, RF, LF, LR = bovine colostrum from the individual quarters - right rear, right front, left front, left rear; OS = sero-positive ovine serum).

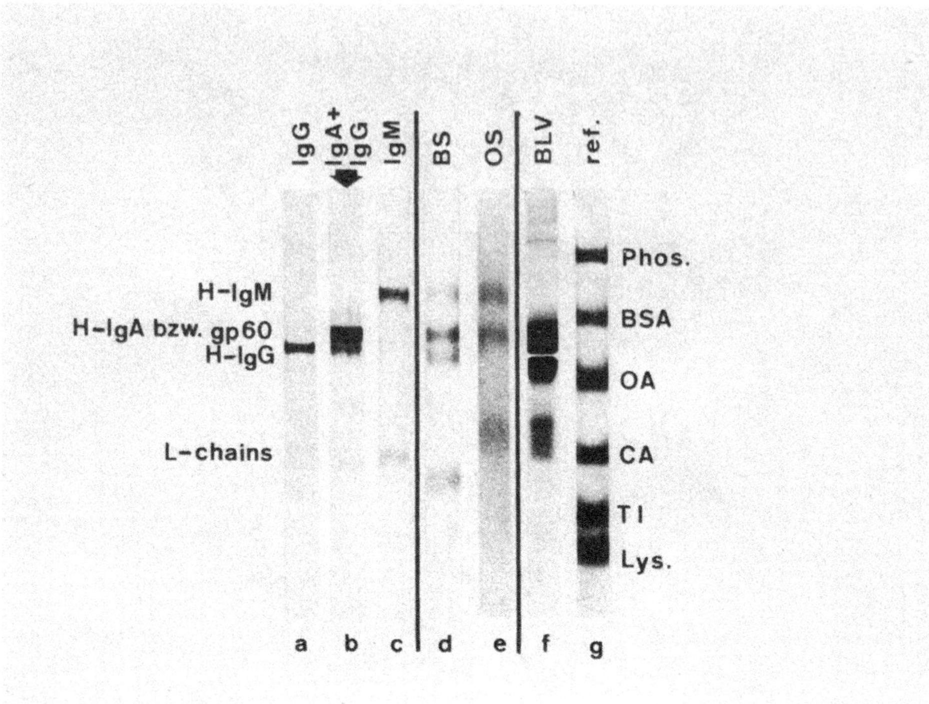

Fig. 2. SDS-PAGE of chemically degraded immune complexes isolated from immunodiffusion tests

(a-c = immunoglobulin controls; d = components of an immune complex formed by bovine leukaemic sera or colostra with BLV; e = analysis of immune complexes produced between BLV and ovine leukaemic sera; BLV = bovine leukaemic virus preparation; H-IgM, H-IgG, H-IgA = heavy chains of the corresponding immunoglobulins; L-chains = light chains; BS = bovine leukaemic sera or colostra; OS = seropositive ovine serum; ref. = mixture of the reference proteins phosphorylase B 92 kd -Phos-, bovine serum albumin 67 kd -BSA-, ovalbumin 45 kd -OA-, carbonic anhydrase 30 kd -CA-, trypsin inhibitor 21 kd -TI-, lysozome 14.7 kd -Lys-; the conditions for SDS-PAGE have been described previously (Matthaeus, 1980, 1981)) amide gel electrophoresis (SDS-PAGE) as previously described (Matthaeus, 1980, 1981).

RESULTS

Figure 1 shows precipitation lines with the BLV antigen preparation which coalesce between the control serum, bovine leukaemic sera and colostrum on the one hand (Figure 1b) and control serum and ovine leukaemic sera on the other (Figure 1c).

Following separation and degradation of the immune complexes the identification of their constituents by SDS-PAGE demonstrated from the reacting bovine body fluids the heavy chains of both the immunoglobulins IgG and IgM and their light chain band beside the viral structural glycopolypeptide gp60 (Figure 2d). In the case of ovine leukaemic sera, only IgM antibodies represented by their heavy and light chains (Figure 2e) could be shown to precipitate with viral gp60 and another viral structural polypeptide ranging with a molecular weight of about 30 kd (probably gp30).

DISCUSSION

Precipitating activities obtained in the IDT with 19 S fractions from bovine leukaemic sera after gel filtration (Straub and Matthaeus, 1979) suggested that in horizontal transmission studies the production of precipitating IgM antibodies might be the first step, or one of the first steps, in the reaction of the host against infection with bovine leukaemic virus. The present analytic studies of degraded immune complexes confirm not only the participation of IgM in precipitation reactions with bovine and ovine leukaemic sera, but also with colostra from leukaemic cows. The question as to why isolated leukaemia-specific bovine IgM antibodies did not precipitate BLV antigen preparations immunoelectrophoretically or in the IDT cannot be answered clearly at present. From the results of previous experiments it can be suggested that either the formation of insoluble IgM-containing immune complexes is restricted to a very narrow and limited region of equivalence (Matthaeus, 1978;

Matthaeus and Weiland, 1976; Straub and Matthaeus, 1979; Matthaeus and Straub, 1980; Matthaeus et al, 1978) or that for precipitation reactions this antibody class requires the immunoglobulin classes IgG and IgA or one of them, respectively, or any auxiliary proteins. The IgM antibody of the ovine serum is most likely due to the short interval between inoculation and collection of serum. IgA antibody shown to precipitate BLV (Matthaeus, 1978; Matthaeus et al., 1978) could not be demonstrated satisfactorily in the present studies as its heavy chain (58 kd) was superimposed in the SDS-PAGE by the viral glycoprotein gp 60.

From these results it can be concluded that all known bovine immunoglobulin classes show precipitating activities with BLV.

REFERENCES

Matthaeus, W. and Weiland, F., 1976. Studies on leukotic bovine and ovine precipitating serum antibodies and the electrophoretic behaviour of the antigen specific for leukotic cattle. Vet. Microbiol. 1, 263-274, O.C. Straub, (Ed.) Elsevier Scientific Publishing Company, Amsterdam and CEC, Luxembourg.

Matthaeus, W., 1978. Heterogeneous properties of BLV-precipitating immunoglobulins in bovine leukemic sera. Ann. Rec. Vét. 9, 635-641.

Matthaeus, W., Kaaden, O.R., Frenzel, B. and Schlotterer, E., 1978. Identification and behaviour of the precipitating BLV antibodies in sera of leukotic cattle. Int. J. Cancer 22, 166-173.

Matthaeus, W., 1980. Analysis of soluble bovine viral diarrhoea virus antigens and serological relationship to virus structural glycoproteins. Zbl. Vet. Med. B 27, 734-741.

Matthaeus, W. and Straub, O.C., 1980. Detection of precipitating antibodies and identification of bovine leukemia virus antigens by micro countercurrent immunoelectrophoresis. Zbl. Vet. Med. B 27, 61-69.

Matthaeus, W. and Straub, O.C., 1981. Immunoglobulin amounts and leukosis specific antibodies in colostrum, milk and serum in the periparturient period and their levels in the newborn. Fourth International Symposium on Bovine Leukosis, Bologna, November 1980 (this publication).

Matthaeus, W., 1981. Differences in reaction behaviour of bovine viral diarrhoea virus (BVDV) structural polypeptides with antisera against BVDV and hog cholera virus (HCV). Zbl. Vet. Med. B (in press).

Straub, O.C., 1978. Diagnosis of enzootic bovine leukosis: a comparison of haematological and immunodiffusion tests. Res. Vet. Sci. 25, 13-15.

Straub, O.C. and Matthaeus, W., 1979. Observations during a serologically controlled horizontal transmission study of bovine leukosis. Paper presented at the Workshop on Bovine Leukosis, November 1979, Weybridge.

DISCUSSION

F.W. Schmidt *(FRG)*

I have just a small comment on the question of serum antibody titre and parturition. A member of our group, Ingrid Bause, just published some results on her work which is along the same lines as the work described by Straub. Concerning the serum antibody titres of pregnant cows, she found a distinct, and statistically verified, influence of parturition. About 6 to 4 weeks before calving, all the 28 cows in the study showed a slow decrease in antibody titre against BLV, as detected by AGID. In timing and quantity this is paralleled by a decrease in IgGl in the serum of these cows. The decrease is lowest at the actual day of parturition, or one or two days later. Then the titres increase slowly again. We found that the decrease during parturition might result in negative AGID tests in a cow with a low antibody titre. Cows with a high antibody titre just show a decrease but may still stay AGID positive.

BOVINE LYMPHOSARCOMA: ELECTROPHORETIC STUDY OF BOVINE SERUM PROTEINS FROM A FARM IN THE SABANNA OF BOGOTA

L.R. Neira, F. Lozano A. and O. Mariño
Laboratorio de Investigaciones Médicas Veterinarias
Instituto Colombiano Agropecuario ICA.
Apartado Aéreo 29743, Bogotá, Colombia.

ABSTRACT

Electrophoretic variations in the bovine serum proteins of 3 groups of Holstein Friesian cattle from a farm in the Sabanna of Bogota, known to have had bovine lymphosarcoma are described. In group 1 which was made up of 26 cattle serologically negative to bovine lymphosarcoma the mean values of the total serum proteins, albumin, alphaglobulins, betaglobulins and gammaglobulins were found to be within the normal levels. Group 2 integrated by 61 cattle serologically positive to bovine lymphosarcoma showed a slight decrease in the mean albumin concentration and a moderate increase in the alphaglobulin mean values. Group 3 which consisted of 8 cattle showing antibodies against bovine lymphosarcoma and which had developed clinical and histological lymphosarcoma, presented moderate decreases in the mean total serum proteins and gammaglobulins. A relevant increase in the mean alphaglobulin concentration was observed. The experimental data showed an increase in the level of serum alphaglobulins during infection with bovine lymphosarcoma virus and clinical posterior development of the disease. Serological diagnosis of bovine lymphosarcoma was determined using the immunodiffusion test.

O.C. Straub (ed.), Fourth International Symposium on Bovine Leukosis

INTRODUCTION

In human as well as in veterinary medicine electrophoretic patterns in serum proteins from subjects with pathological conditions have been established for some time. Human lymphoid leukaemia (Kelsey, 1971) and bovine lymphosarcoma are two diseases where changes occur (Matthaeus et al., 1976a) Matthaeus et al., 1976b). The electrophoretic changes in bovine serum proteins from cows with lymphosarcomas were analysed in the present study.

MATERIALS AND METHODS

Serum samples from 87, 3 to 6 year old Holstein cows were studied. These samples came from clinically normal cattle from a dairy farm where bovine lymphosarcoma had been present. Serum samples from 7 bovines with clinical lymphosarcomas were also analysed. In the latter bovines the adult form of the disease was diagnosed histologically. Specific serum antibodies against bovine leukaemia virus (BLV) were detected using the immunodiffusion test (Miller et al., 1971); control positive and negative sera were used with each sample. According to the presence or absence of specific antibodies, the cattle were distributed in three groups: group 1 without serum antibodies, group 2 with serum antibodies; both these groups were clinically normal. Group 3 consisted of 7 cattle with lymphosarcoma and also with serum antibodies. Total serum proteins were determined using the Goldberg's refractometer. Serum protein electrophoresis was undertaken using cellulose acetate. The quantification of protein fractions was carried out using the densitometric technique and the electrophoretic profiles were done using the Digiscreen Scanner-R Gelman Instrument Co. Duplicate serum samples were used and the protein concentrations were given in mg/100 ml. Mean values were recorded.

RESULTS

From the 87 cattle, 26 did not present specific serum

antibodies and they formed group 1. Group 2 was composed of 61 bovines with specific serum antibodies. Group 3 consisted of 7 cattle with specific serum antibodies and clinical lymphosarcoma. Albumin concentrations in group 2 decreased whereas, in groups 1 and 3, the concentrations were within the normal range (Table 1). Alphaglobulin concentrations in group 1 were observed to be within the normal range whereas the concentrations in group 2 were abnormally high; this increase was more marked in group 3 (Table 1). Betaglobulin concentrations were found to be normal in all groups. Gammaglobulin concentrations were lower in Group 3 than in groups 1 and 2.

TABLE 1

BLV ELECTROPHORETIC FRACTIONS OF SERUM PROTEINS FROM 94 HOLSTEIN CATTLE

Groups	No. bovines	Albumin	Globulins			Total serum proteins
			Alpha	Beta	Gamma	
		mg/100	mg/100 ml	mg/100 ml	mg/100 ml	mg/100 ml
1	26	3 059.50	904.09	814.36	2 779.74	7 557.69
2	61	2 786.56	1 156.41	835.41	2 867.52	7 645.90
3	7	2 874.23	1 410.63	781.98	2 033.16	7 100.00

CONCLUSIONS

The presence of specific antibodies indicates viral infection which may or may not produce the disease. Recent studies show that abnormal serum proteins (paraproteins) type gamma G can be demonstrated by immunoelectrophoresis in cases of bovine lymphosarcoma. The decrease in albumin concentration in group 2 is associated with an increase in the globulin fraction. This increase is made at the expense of albumin in the alphaglobulin concentration observed in groups 2 and 3 and agrees with the work of Kelsey et al., 1971 in cases of human lymphoid leukaemia. In cattle, this increase is progressive according to the development of the disease. The increase in the gammaglobulin fractions in group 2 was due to the presence of abnormal gamma proteins (paraproteins) which are produced and increase in this fraction. Conversely a marked decrease of gammaglobulins was observed in group 3 and indicates a humoral immunosuppression phenomenon, which is evident in severe cases of this disease. Decrease in gammaglobulins has been described in human lymphoid leukaemia patients.

REFERENCES

Butler, J.E., 1971. Review of the bovine immunoglobulins. Journal of Dairy Science. 54, 1315-1316.

Ganong, W.F., 1973. Review of Medical Physiology. 6th ed. Lange Medical Publications. San Francisco. pp. 830-832.

Kelsey, R.L., 1971. Interpretation of routine electrophoresis patterns of serum proteins in health and disease. Clinical Electrophoresis. Masonic Medical Center. Illinois. pp. 5-34.

Lowenstein, J., Bjerum, O.J., Weeke, E. and Weeke, B., 1975. Characterization of bovine whey proteins by crossed immunoelectrophoresis. Scandinavian Journal of Immunology. 4, 155-161.

Matthaeus, W. and Weiland, F., 1976. Studies on leukotic bovine and ovine precipitating serum antibodies and the electrophoretic behaviour of the antigen specific for leukotic cattle. Veterinary Microbiology. 1, 263-274, O.C. Straub (Ed.), Elsevier Scientific Publishing Company, Amsterdam and CEC Luxembourg.

Matthaeus, W. and Straub, O.C., 1976. Studies on the distribution of gamma globulins and on abnormal globulins from serums of leukotic cattle and sheep. Veterinary Microbiology. 1, 363-373, O.C. Straub (Ed.), Elsevier Publishing Company, Amsterdam and CEC Luxembourg.

Miller, J.M. and Olson, C., 1972. Precipitating antibody to an internal antigen of the C-Type virus associated with bovine lymphosarcoma. Journal of the National Cancer Institute. 49, 1459-1461.

Millipore Biomedica, 1974. Immunoglobulin abnormality detection by immunoelectrophoresis. Millipore Corporation. Massachusetts.AR 710, 1-3.

Olson, C. and Baumgartener, L.E., 1975. Lymphosarcoma (Leukemia) of cattle. Bovine Practitioner. 10, 15-22.

Pfeiffer, N.E., McGuire, T.C., Bendel, R.E. and Weikel, J.M., 1977. Quantitation of bovine immunoglobulins: comparison of single radial immunodiffusion, zinc sulfate turbidity, serum electrophoresis and refractometer methods. American Journal of Veterinary Research. 38, 693-698.

Schalm, O.W., Jain, N.C. and Carrol, E.J., 1975. Veterinary Hematology 3rd ed. Lea and Febiger Philadelphia. pp. 602-616.

Tyler, L., 1978. Enzootic Bovine Leucosis. The Veterinary Record, 103, 194-198.

DEVELOPMENT OF BOVINE LEUKOSIS VIRUS INFECTION IN CATTLE OF AN EXPERIMENTAL STATION

M. Severini[1], D. Rutili[2], F. Titoli[2], L. Rampichini[1] and A. Vizzani[1]

([1]) Istituto di Ispezione degli Alimenti di Origine Animale - Facoltà di Medicina Veterinaria - Perugia, Italy.

([2]) Istituto Zooprofilattico Sperimentale dell'Umbria e delle Marche - Perugia, Italy.

ABSTRACT

Cattle from infected breeds were put under observation for 5 years in an experimental station. The results of haematological, serological and virological examinations conducted on the above mentioned animals and their progeny are reported.

O.C. Straub (ed.), Fourth International Symposium on Bovine Leukosis

INTRODUCTION

This investigation started in 1974 immediately after the first report of the existence of enzootic bovine leukosis (EBL) in Italy (Rampichini et al., 1975). It has been carried on for six years simultaneously with the development of epidemiologic studies in our region (Rutili et al., 1977; Rutili et al., 1978). The purpose of this research was to study some aspects of the spontaneous development of BLV infection through prolonged and continuous observation of a group of naturally infected animals and their progeny, calved and nursed in high risk conditions.

MATERIALS AND METHODS

Animals

A group of 14 Holstein-Friesian dairy cattle was kept under observation in the experimental station of our Institute. The age, sex, origin and the length of the observation period of each animal are reported in Tables 1 and 2. All the animals studied were kept in adjacent tied stalls. The calves born in this herd were nursed by their dams for three months and then housed in stalls several metres from the stalls of the other animals. Calf number 3 was constantly near its mother.

Examinations

Blood was collected monthly (occasionally every two or three months for the adult cattle) from the jugular vein of each animal for the following tests:

a) White blood cell count and differential leukocyte count;

b) Electron microscope observation of short-term lymphocyte cultures for the presence of BLV.

Beginning in 1976, the sera were collected and stored at -30°C until used in the agar gel immunodiffusion (AGID) test which was conducted according to the method described elsewhere

TABLE 1

CHARACTERISTICS OF THE CATTLE UNDER OBSERVATION

Animal no.	Sex	Age at start of observation	Present age	Length of observation period	Notes
2	F	5 years	died at 9 years	4 years	
9	F	4 years	6 years	26 months	coming from a herd with a
10	F	4 years	6 years	26 months	case of lymphosarcoma
3	F	birth	died at 5 years	5 years	born from cow number 2
4	F	birth	40 months	40 months	born from cow number 2
30	F	8 years	11 years	3 years	
273	F	5 years	8 years	3 years	coming from a lymphosarco-
347	F	4 years	7 years	3 years	ma-free herd
361	F	4 years	7 years	3 years	
6	M	birth	removed at 15 months	15 months	born from cow number 30
7	F	birth	38 months	38 months	born from cow number 273
8	F	birth	29 months	29 months	born from cow number 361
11	F	birth	3 months	3 months	born from cow number 30
12	M	birth	2 months	2 months	born from cow number 347

TABLE 2

LENGTH OF TIME DURING WHICH ANIMALS WERE OBSERVED

Animal no.	1974	1975	1976	1977	1978	1979	1980
2	±	+	+	+	±		
9					±	+	±
10					±	+	±
3	±	+	+	+	+	±	
4				±	+	+	±
30				±	+	+	±
273				±	+	+	±
347				±	+	+	±
361				±	+	+	±
6				±	±		
7				±	+	+	±
8					±	+	±
11							±
12							±

+ = complete year

± = incomplete year

(Severini et al., 1981) utilising BLV glycoprotein antigen (Pitman Moore, USA) and p24 which we produced.

RESULTS

During the observation period one cow (number 2) died from lymphosarcoma (Rampichini et al., 1978). Another cow (number 3) died from a bacterial infection without any signs of lymphosarcoma. All the other animals were clinically normal The results of the various investigations are reported in Tables 3, 4 and 5. The data reported in Table 3 show that during the entire period of observation 3 cows had persistent lymphocytosis, constant presence of antibodies to BLV glycoprotein and p24, and the presence of BLV in short-term lymphocyte cultures. In three other cows the detection of

TABLE 3

RESULTS OF EXAMINATIONS CARRIED OUT IN THE ADULT CATTLE

Cow no	Lymphocytosis	Antibodies against gp	p24	BLV
2	persistent	+	3 months before death	+
9	persistent	+	-	+
10	transient	+	-	-
30	persistent	+	+	+
273	persistent	+	+	+
347	persistent	+	+	+
361	transient	+	±(*)	+

(*) Weak reaction only in few AGIDT during 1979.

antibodies to BLV glycoprotein and the presence of BLV in short-term lymphocyte cultures was constant, while lymphocytosis was persistent only in two animals. In these last three cows it was not possible to observe the constant presence of antibodies to p24 and, in fact, cow number 2 began to show these antibodies only when, three months before death, the first clinical signs of lymphosarcoma occurred. Cow number 361 presented a weak positive reaction only in some examinations during 1979. One cow (number 10) constantly had antibodies to BLV glycoprotein only.

From Table 4 it can be taken that the calves never developed persistent lymphocytosis. Six calves born in our herd (we do not have information on calf number 3) had BLV glycoprotein antibodies during the first months of life. In three animals these antibodies were present until four to seven months of age and they are still present in one, now 40 months old. In five calves p24 antibodies were observed until three months after birth (we do not have information on calf number 3), while in one calf these antibodies were never detected. BLV was not found in any of the calves during the first months of life and only observed occasionally in calf number 3 in the examinations carried out after four years of observation. This

TABLE 4

RESULTS OF EXAMINATIONS CARRIED OUT IN THE CALVES

Calf no	Lymphocytosis	Antibodies against gp	Antibodies against p24	BLV
3	-	+ (1)	- (1)	over 4 years old
4	-	from birth	-	over 8 months old
6	-	until 6 months old	until 3 months old	-
7	-	until 4 months old and over 27 months old	until 3 months old and over 30 months old	over 30 months old
8	-	until 7 months old	until 3 months old	-
11	-	+	+	-
12	-	+	+	-

(1) Tests started at the age of 32 months

calf presented BLV glycoprotein antibodies at the age of 32 months, when the first serological test was performed. Calf number 4, which had BLV glycoprotein antibodies from birth, showed BLV in short-term lymphocyte cultures at the age of 8 months. BLV was detected in calf number 7 at the age of 30 months. This calf had shown BLV glycoprotein antibodies at the age of 27 months and p24 antibodies at the age of 30 months.

Table 5 shows that 4 calves, born from dams with both BLV glycoprotein and p24 antibodies present just before and just after birth, presented the same antibodies just a few days after the beginning of nursing. One calf (number 4) only had glycoprotein antibodies as did the mother. Calf number 8 showed both types of antibodies, although p24 antibodies were absent in the mother's serum.

TABLE 5

DETECTION OF ANTIBODIES IN CALVES AND DAMS

Calves				
Animal no	Age in days	Antibodies against gp	Antibodies against p24	BLV
4	28	+	-	-
6	20	+	+	-
7	6	+	+	-
8	19	+	+	-
11	15	+	+	-
12	15	+	+	-

Dams				
Before calving				
Antibodies against gp	Antibodies against p24	BLV	Antibodies against gp	Antibodies against p24
+	-	+	+	-
+	+	+	+	+
+	+	+	+	+
+	-	+	+	-
+	+	+	+	+
+	+	+	+	+

CONCLUSIONS

Taking into consideration the results of examinations carried out on a total of 12 animals (introduced to, or born in, the experimental station) over the age of one year, one notes that two cattle were not BLV infected; one showed antibodies to glycoprotein only; five were BLV carriers and consistently showed antibodies to glycoprotein (two also showed persistent lymphocytosis); four were BLV carriers and consistently showed antibodies to both glycoprotein and p24 (three also showed persistent lymphocytosis).

Of the five animals which were BLV carriers and which had antibodies to glycoprotein only, one (number 2) died from lymphosarcoma at 9 years of age (after observation over 4 years) and showed antibodies to p24 as well during the last three months of life.

Another (number 361) occasionally showed a very weak positive reaction to p24 in 1 year out of the three years of observation.

From these initial observations it is not possible to draw any significant conclusion on the frequency of lymphosarcoma in BLV infected animals, given the small number of animals studied. One notes, however, that the infection may run a long course (3 - 4 years) without any clinical evidence of disease. It is also clear that the infection may frequently run its course without lymphocytosis and that in some animals there may be antibodies to glycoprotein present without BLV being apparent, at least by means of repeated EM examinations of short-term lymphocyte cultures.

In BLV carriers antibodies to glycoprotein were always present. While antibodies to p24 were consistently present in one group of the animals, in the other group they were either not present at all or the levels were too low to be detected by the AGID test. This variability in the finding of antibodies to p24 in BLV carriers has also been shown by other research workers (Baumgartener and Olson, 1978) and for the moment we are not able to explain this finding.

In the case of cow number 2, a BLV carrier which showed persistent lymphocytosis, during 4 years of observation it showed only antibodies to glycoprotein but three months before death it showed also antibodies to p24; we can only point out the coincidence between the beginning of the clinical symptoms and the appearance of antibodies to p24. At the actual stage of our knowledge we cannot say what relationship exists between the course of infection and the presence of antibodies to one or the other antigen.

BLV was never detected in lymphocyte cultures taken during the nursing period for those calves born in the experimental station. The animals born and nursed by mothers with antibodies to both glycoprotein and p24, had antibodies to both these antigens in the first months of life.

Calf number 8 was a peculiar case which showed antibodies to both antigens although the dam (number 361) had no demonstrable antibodies to p24 either before or after birth. It almost invariably showed negative reactions to tests for antibodies to p24 but on rare occasions gave a weak positive reaction. It is possible, therefore, that this animal had a very low quantity of antibodies in the serum which were probably concentrated in the colostrum and thus passed on to the daughter in a sufficient quantity to be detected in its serum. It has been found, in fact, that the colostrum of infected cows may present antibody titres to both glycoprotein and p24 which are much higher than those of the serum (Straub, 1980).

In three of the calves, more than 6 months old, it was noted that antibodies to p24 persisted until 3 months after birth, whereas antibodies to glycoprotein were present until 4 to 7 months after birth, as reported by other research workers (Seger et al., 1976). Due to the observation of the transitory presence of the antibodies and the lack of detection of BLV during the first year of life, we believe that these animals were born uninfected and that they assumed the antibodies from the dams' colostrum. It is known, in fact, that the progeny of BLV infected cows may be either uninfected or infected. In these infected calves the antigen is detectable from the first days of life, and the antibodies are persistent (Piper et al., 1979).

For two other calves that presented antibodies to both the antigens in the first months of life, we are not able to state with the same assurance that they were born uninfected. Given their present age of less than 4 months, we have not been able to ascertain the transitory presence of the antibodies, and the absence of BLV in the short-term lymphocyte cultures has been registered in too few samples for us to be sure of the validity of this test (Ferrer et al., 1977).

Of the three calves born uninfected, one (number 7) showed BLV and antibodies towards both the antigens at the age of 27 - 30 months. The infection probably occurred vertically via the dam's milk because the subject, after nursing, was no longer in close contact with infected animals. This type of transmission, though not frequent, is possible and has been demonstrated experimentally (Ferrer and Piper, 1978).

In contrast to the above subjects, calf number 4 showed only antibodies to glycoprotein from birth and for the whole observation period (40 months). In the first months of life the antibodies could be those received from the dam's colostrum, which contained only antibodies to glycoprotein. The same types of antibodies were subsequently produced by the calf which at the age of 8 months became virologically positive. It is not easy to identify accurately the way by which these animals were infected, but surely one must think of a vertical transmission. The calf persistently showed antibodies and, after the nursing period, was not in close contact with any infected animal. The sister (calf number 2) of this calf became virologically positive when she was more than 4 years old and was also positive to BLV glycoprotein starting from the first serological test performed at the age of 32 months. Antibodies to p24 were never found in this animal, which was nursed by the mother and lived for 34 months in contact only with her. We do not know if calf number 2 was infected horizontally or vertically, since we do not have information on the serological situation of the calf during the first two years of life. However, we can assume that BLV was transmitted by the mother which was a BLV carrier and which had antibodies only to glycoprotein.

The investigations performed over six years on the animals at the experimental station enable us to draw conclusions thought to be very useful for a correct and effective control of EBL in our country. From our data it appears that the AGID test is a reliable diagnostic method for the detection of BLV infected animals using the glycoprotein antigen.

Conversely, the sole use of p24 antigen may result in a relatively high rate of false negative tests. From our observations it can be seen that glycoprotein allowed us consistently to detect 9 animals out of 9 virologically positive, while p24 failed to detect 5 animals out of 9 with BLV. On the other hand, what seems to be important is the detection of BLV infected cattle showing antibodies to glycoprotein, because these animals are able to transmit BLV infection in the same way as those with antibodies to p24. We believe therefore, that it has been useful to begin, and that it is correct to continue, the epidemiological investigation in Italy using the AGID test with BLV glycoprotein antigen.

Our study also shows that calves born and nursed by infected dams show maternal antibodies for several months. It seems possible, therefore, to propose that serological examination for BLV antibodies be performed only on subjects older than one year. Furthermore, since calves can be infected vertically (*in utero* or via the milk), for effective control of BLV infection in a herd, it is necessary that animals born from infected dams are immediately isolated and nursed by negative cows.

However, in order to eliminate completely the risk of horizontal transmission of BLV from calf to calf, it would be useful, where possible, to detect and remove all BLV infected calves before contact with newborns may occur.

ACKNOWLEDGEMENTS

The authors thank S. Canalicchio, P. Proietti and L. Ferraguzzi for their technical assistance.

REFERENCES

Baumgartener, L.E. and Olsen, C. 1978. Immunodiffusion antibodies to p24 and gp antigens in Cattle. CEC Workshop Conference on the Serological Diagnosis of Enzootic Bovine Leukosis. Ed. A.A. Ressang, pp. 148-155 (Rotterdam, The Netherlands).

Ferrer, J.F., Piper, C.E., Abt, D.A. and Marshak, R.R. 1977. Diagnosis of Bovine Leukemia Virus Infection: Evaluation of serologic and hematologic tests by a direct infectivity detection assay. Am. J. Vet. Res. 38, 1977-1981.

Ferrer, J.F. and Piper, C.E. 1978. An evaluation of the role of milk in the natural transmission of the Bovine Leukemia Virus. Ann. Rech. Vét. 9, 803-807.

Piper, C.E., Ferrer, J.F., Abt, D.A. and Marshak, R.R. 1979. Postnatal and prenatal transmission of the Bovine Leukemia Virus under natural conditions. J. Natl. Cancer Inst. 62, 165-168.

Rampichini, L., De Castro Portugal, F.L., Severini, M. and Rutili, D. 1975. Leucosi Enzootica dei Bovini e Studio di Particelle di tipo C in una Bovina Adulta con Leucemia Linfatica Acuta e in Bovine dello stesso Allevamento con Linfocitosi Persistente. Tumori 61, 261-270.

Rampichini, L., Severini, M., Rutili, D., Titoli, F. and Cenci, G. 1978. Su di un Caso di Linfosarcoma in una Bovina Tenuta in Osservazione per quattro anni. Atti Soc. It. Buiatria 10, 303-311.

Rutili, D., Severini, M., Rampichini, L., Titoli, F. and Chicchini, U. 1977. Epidemiologic study on Enzootic Bovine Leukemia using serologic tests and hematologic examinations. Tumori 63, 407-413.

Rutili, D., Severini, M., Rampichini, L. and Titoli, F. 1978. Epidemiologic study on Enzootic Bovine Leukemia in Italy. Ann. Rech. Vét. 9, 761-764.

Seger, C.L., Hart, L. and Morgan, E. 1976. Incidence and persistence of Bovine Leukemia Virus antibody in calves fed pooled sour colostrum. Comparative Leukemia Research 1975, Bibl. Haemat. No. 43. Ed. J. Clemmensen and D.S. Yohn, pp. 375-376 (Karger, Basel).

Severini, M., Rutili, D., Fruganti, G., Rampichini, L. and Cenci, G. 1981. Experimental transmission of Enzootic Bovine Leukosis in calves. IV International Symposium on Bovine Leukosis, Bologna, Nov. 5-7, 1980 (this publication).

Straub, O.C. 1980. Bovine Leukosis: Etiology, Transmission and Epidemiology. Riv. Zootec. Vet. 1, 5-16.

SESSION IV

Diagnostic Procedures

Chairmen : R. Hoff-Jørgensen and A.A. Ressang

SENSITIVITY OF AN IMMUNODIFFUSION TEST FOR THE DETECTION AND QUANTITATION OF BOVINE LEUKAEMIA VIRUS INDUCED ANTIBODIES

T. Gauthier[1], B. Guillemain[2], T. Astier[2] and R. Mamoun[2]

[1] Institut Ronchèse - Laboratoire Cogla, Zone Industrielle de Libourne, F-33501 Libourne,

[2] Institut National de la Santé et de la Recherche Médicale, U-117, 229, cours de l'Argonne, F-33076 Bordeaux, France.

ABSTRACT

A dual antigen (p24 and gp51) was prepared and calibrated (in terms of BLV proteins content by competitive radioimmunoassays) for use in agar double immunodiffusion (AGID) tests. A quantification was obtained by using serial dilutions of BLV antibodies containing sera. The efficiency of the AGID test in detecting BLV infected cattle was compared to that of the early polykaryocytosis test (EPI), the anti p24 or the anti gp51 radioimmunological assays (RIAp24, RIAgp51). Highly significant correlations were observed when the antibody titres as obtained with the AGID test were plotted versus the titres obtained with highly sensitive techniques like RIAs and EPI tests. Furthermore, the threshold of sensitivity of the above mentioned AGID test was determined; it was observed that sera with relatively low EPI, RIAp24 or RIAgp51 titres were AGID reactors. Thus immunodiffusion may be used as a routine technique provided that the ultimate purpose is the detection of BLV infected herds but not that of individual cases. Of importance is the fact that some cattle were shown to react solely with p24 or gp51 antigens which thus favours the use of a dual antigen.

O.C. Straub (ed.), Fourth International Symposium on Bovine Leukosis

INTRODUCTION

Bovine leukaemia virus induced antibodies in the sera of BLV infected cattle may be detected by several serological techniques. The most commonly used have been immunodiffusion (ID) (Miller and Olson, 1972), immunofluorescence (Ferrer et al., 1972), complement fixation (Miller and Van der Maaten, 1974; Lévy et al., 1977a) radio-immunological assay (RIA) (Devare et al., 1976; McDonald and Ferrer, 1976; Lévy et al., 1977b) and to some extent, virus neutralisation tests (VNT) (Diglio and Ferrer, 1976) and early polykaryocytosis inhibition test (EPI) (Guillemain et al., 1978a). The use of these techniques by different laboratories showed that almost all animals with adult lymphosarcoma or persistent lymphocytosis are responders, but in addition a large number of apparently normal cattle which have been in contact with infected animals also carry BLV antibodies. Such animals are detected with a high probability by use of highly sensitive techniques like radioimmunoassays, VNT or EPI. The latter techniques were thought to be rather difficult to apply to field studies in laboratories which are not specifically equipped for their monitoring.

In view of its easiness and simplicity, immunodiffusion has been considered as the most practicable test and thus it is used in very large serological surveys in different countries. Using concentrated BLV p24 and/or BLV gp51 antigens, ID was found to be useful in practice although its sensitivity was found to be lower than that of other tests (Devare and Stephenson, 1978; Guillemain et al., 1978b).

It sounded logical, then, to appreciate quantitatively the sensitivity of the immunodiffusion test. In preliminary experiments we used a commercial antigen but because of a number of problems we decided to prepare a standard antigen containing both p24 and gp51 BLV proteins.

In order to make possible comparisons based on the sensitivity of different tests the antigen used in ID was calibrated for its content by radioimmunological procedures, namely radioimmunoprecipitations with iodinated p24 and gp51. In addition we conformed with the EC recommendations (Journal Officiel des Communautés Européennes, 1980).

The bovine serum content of BLV antibodies was measured in an immunodiffusion test by a dilution technique in which the serum titre was taken as the last (log_2) dilution giving a clear band with the antigen.

As most of our previous experiments had compared ID with EPI, we investigated the correlating factors binding RIAs, EPI and ID.

MATERIALS AND METHODS

Cell cultures

FLK-BLV cells, i.e. foetal lamb kidney cells, infected with and chronically producing the bovine leukaemia virus (BLV) were kindly supplied by Dr. M.J. Van der Maaten and Dr. J.M. Miller (Van der Maaten and Miller, 1976) (National Animal Disease Laboratory, U.S. Department of Agriculture, Ames, Iowa); there was evidence of mycoplasma as determined by the DNA stain technique (Barile, 1974) and of other viruses common in cattle upon electron microscopic examination. The murine infected cat cell line, CC81 (Fischinger et al., 1974) was the gift of Dr. Périès (Institut de Recherche sur les Leucémies et les Maladies du Sang, Laboratoire d'Hématologie Expérimentale, Hôpital St Louis, Paris, France).

The above cell lines were maintained as monolayers in RPMI 1629 culture medium supplemented with 5% (for FLK-BLV) or 10% (for CC81) heat inactivated (56°C, 30 min.) foetal calf serum, 100 units/ml penicillin, 100 µg/ml streptomycin and 100 µg/ml fungizone.

BLV antigen preparation for immunodiffusion (ID) test

The culture medium used to grow FLK-BLV cells was collected two days after the completion of the monolayer. After two centrifugations (3 000 g, 10 min; 10 000 g, 10 min) proteins were precipitated with ammonium sulphate, 30 g/100 ml; pH was then adjusted to 4.15 HCl 4N. After agitation at 4°C for 12 h, the solution was centrifuged (10 000 g, 30 min). The precipitate was then resuspended in distilled water (1 : 30 of the original volume) and extensively dialysed against phosphate buffered saline (PBS) at 4°C for 72 h. Finally the preparation was centrifuged (27 000 g, 10 min), the supernatant containing BLV p24 as well as BLV gp51 (dual antigenic preparation) was adjusted (see below) to 3 - 4 μg/ml gp51.

Agar gel immunodiffusion test

The agar used in this experiment was prepared according to the following formula: agarose, 1% in distilled water NaCl, 0.14 M; Tris-HCl, pH 8.3, 0.01 M; polyethylene glycol 6 000, 30 g/l; EDTA 0.37 g/l; sodium azoture, 0.2 g/l.

Six ml of dissolved gelose were distributed per 60 mm petri dish. The well pattern used was that recommended by the EEC. The central well was filled with 32 μl antigen and two opposite peripherical wells with 73 μl of a reference serum. The sera to be tested were placed in the other wells. After incubation for 24 - 72 h in a humid chamber at room temperature, the reactions were read.

The immunodiffusion test has been quantified by use of serial $\log_2$ dilutions of the antigen or of the sera to be tested. The titre of a serum was the value of the dilution factor at which a clear precipitation line was observed with an antigen containing 3 - 4 μg/ml gp51.

Early polykaryocytosis inhibition test

The procedure has already been described in detail (Guillemain et al., 1978b). In brief: serial $\log_2$ dilutions of the serum to be assayed (0.1 ml/well) were placed in Falcon Microtest II tissue culture plates; 5 x 10^3 FLK-BLV cells/well were added to 0.1 ml culture medium and the mixtures incubated at 37°C for one hour; finally, 2 x 10^4 CC81 cells/well were added to 0.1 ml culture medium; after 24 hours cocultivation at 37°C, the monolayers were fixed with methyl-alcohol and stained with Giemsa.

The titres of the sera were expressed as the reciprocal of the dilution which gave a 50% reduction of the number of syncytia as compared to non serum-treated control cultures (50% syncytia inhibitory dose or SID_{50}). The letter N in $SID_{50}N$ indicates that the titre is normalised for the number of syncytia, thus allowing a comparison between the relative potencies of different sera.

<u>Sera</u>

The sera used in this study were those of referred cases of bovine lymphosarcoma (enzootic or sporadic cases), those from field seroepidemiological studies and sera nos., 1, 3, 4 and 6 kindly supplied by Dr. Olson (University of Wisconsin, Madison, Wisconsin) used in a previous investigation (Guillemain et al., 1978b).

<u>Radioimmunological assay (RIAp24 and RIAgp51)</u>

Serial dilutions of bovine sera (200 µl) extending from 10^2 to 3 x 10^6 were prepared in Tris buffer, pH 7.9 0.01 M containing NaCl, 0.05 M; EDTA, 0.001 M; Triton-X 100, 0.1%; bovine serum albumin (BSA), 1%; normal bovine serum 2 µl (for all dilutions but the 10^2 dilution). After incubation (37°C for 3 h and 4°C for 12 h) with ^{125}I labelled purified p24 or gp51 (2 x 10^4 cpm), 150 µl goat anti-bovine Ig serum were added and the mixture further incubated (37°C, 1 h and 4°C, 2 h). The samples were then diluted with 500 µl Tris buffer, pH 7.9, 0.01 M containing NaCl, 0.01M; Triton-X 100, 0.1% and centrifuged (3 700 g, 15 mn). Radioactivity present in the pellet was determined. Serum titres were expressed as the reciprocal of the dilution of the bovine serum which bound 50% of the ^{125}I-labelled BLV antigen (p24 or gp51).

Competitive radioimmunoassay

Purified p24 antigen was iodinated (^{125}I) by the chloramine-T method (Greenwood et al., 1963) and purified gp51 was iodinated by the iodogen method (Devare and Stephenson, 1977).

The competitive radioimmunoassay was conducted as described (Mamoun et al., 1980) using the above p24 and gp51 as competitive antigens and a rabbit anti BLV serum. The precipitation was achieved with a 10% suspension of *Staphylococcus aureus* according to Kessler (1975).

Statistical analysis

This was carried out according to Finney (1952) and with the use of a computer.

RESULTS

Sensitivity of ID as compared to EPI

A number of 53 sera including leukotic animals, animals with persistent lymphocytosis and cattle from field surveys were tested by both techniques for their content in BLV induced antibodies. The log of the EPI titre ($SID_{50}N$) was plotted versus that obtained by ID.

Statistical analysis of the data presented in Figure 1 revealed that EPI titres and ID titres were linked by a linear regression according to an equation of the type:

(a) log (EPI titre) = a x log (ID titre) + b
in which a = 0.9672
and b = 2.1433

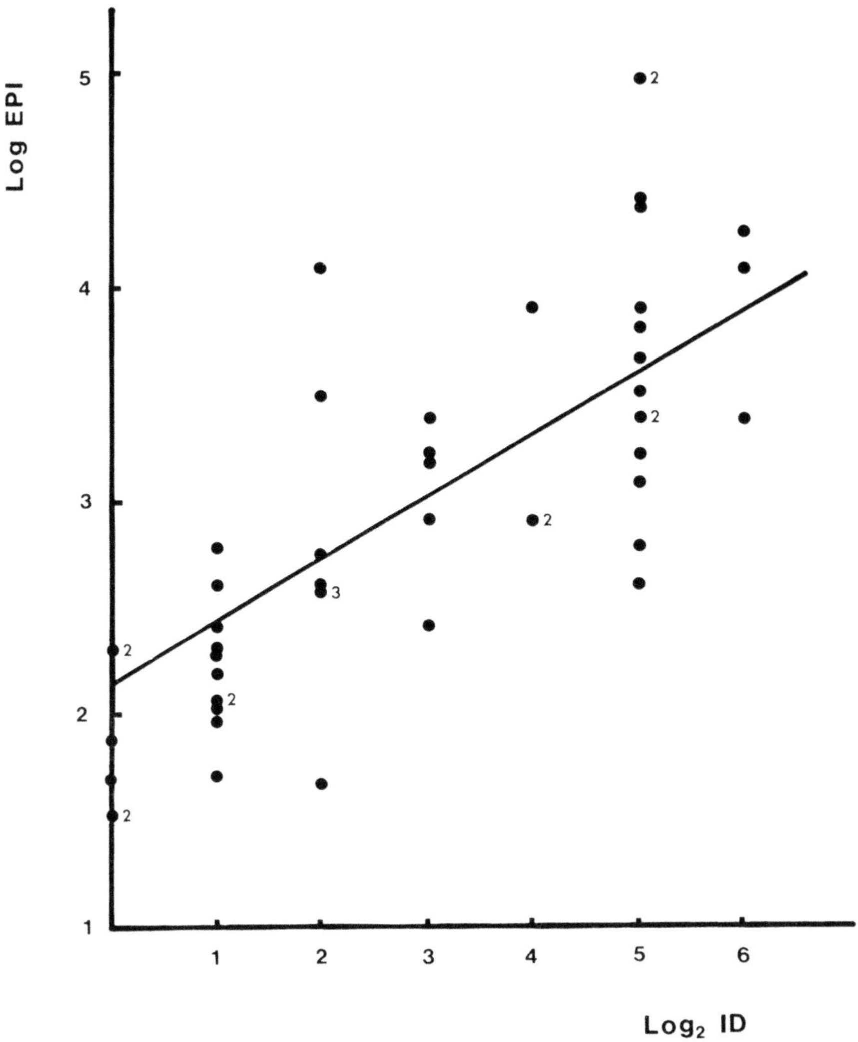

Fig. 1. Sensitivity of an immunodiffusion test for the detection and quantitation of bovine leukaemia virus induced antibodies.

The regression was found to be highly significant with a correlation coefficient $r = 0.6680$ ($P < 0.001$).

In these conditions one can consider that the ID test is less sensitive than the EPI test and that on the average a titre of 139 in the latter is the sensitivity threshold for ID.

Sensitivity of ID as compared to RIAp24

In the same conditions as above, 49 sera were assayed in RIAp24 and ID. A highly significant regression (Figure 2) was observed following the equation:

(b) $\log(\text{RIAp24 titre}) = 0.8085 \log(\text{ID titre}) + 2.8602$

the correlation coefficient (r) value was 0.5157 ($P < 0.001$).

As expected, this indicated that RIAp24 was a more sensitive test for the detection of BLV induced antibodies than ID.

On average, the ID test may be expected to be positive when RIAp24 titres exceed 583.

Sensitivity of ID as compared to RIAgp51

With 43 sera, a highly significant correlation (Figure 3) was observed between RIAgp51 titres and ID titres following the equation:

(c) $\log(\text{RIAgp51 titre}) = 0.7676 \log(\text{ID titre}) + 2.0640.$

with a correlation coefficient (r) value of 0.6820 ($P < 0.001$).

This indicates that, as expected, RIAgp51 is more sensitive than ID; on average, sera may be expected to be detected as positive in ID test when titrating at least 116 in the RIAgp51 test.

Conditions required for maximum sensitivity of the immunodiffusion test

According to the threshold of sensitivity for the detection of BLV infected antibodies of ID as compared to that of RIAp24 and RIAgp51, Figure 4 indicates that RIA positive sera may be classifi

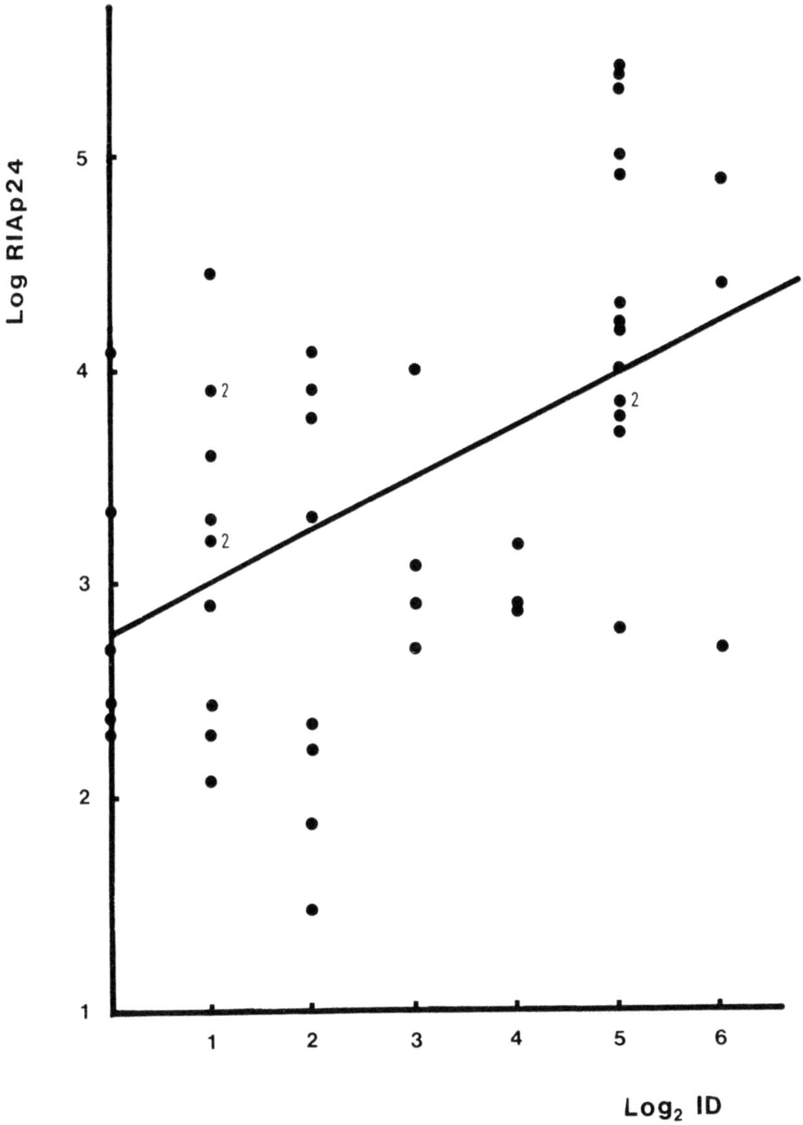

Fig. 2. Sensitivity of an immunodiffusion test for the detection and quantitation of bovine leukaemia virus induced antibodies.

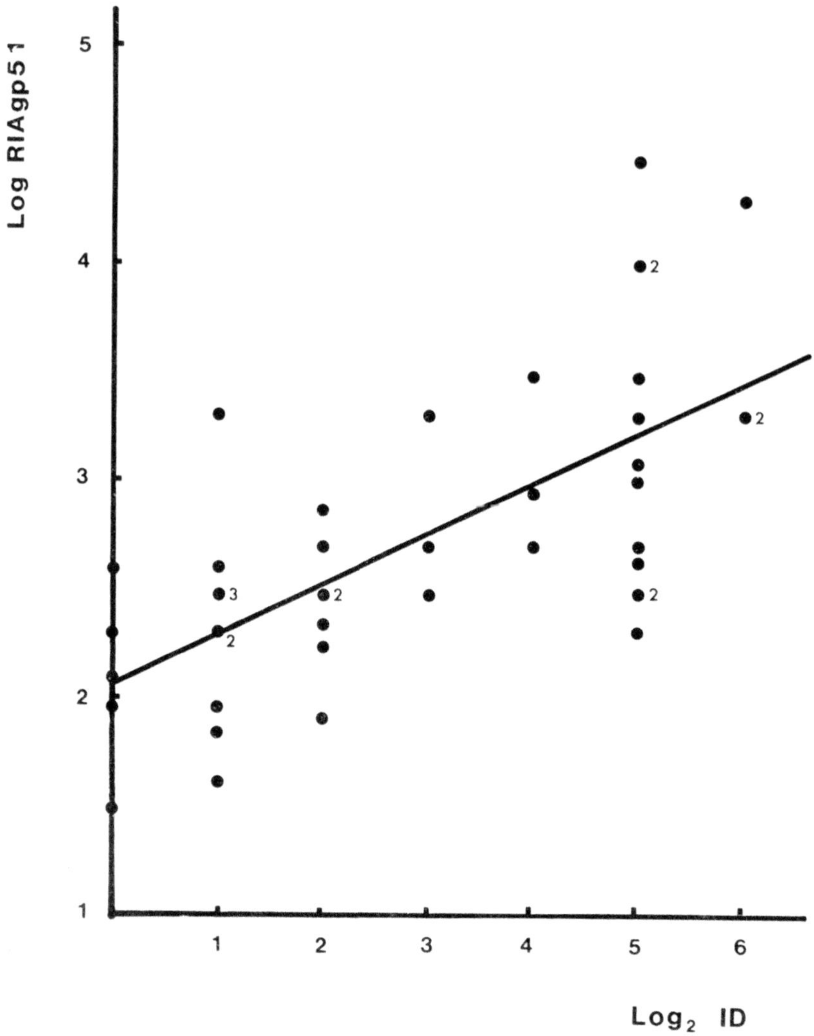

Fig. 3. Sensitivity of an immunodiffusion test for the detection and quantitation of bovine leukaemia virus induced antibodies.

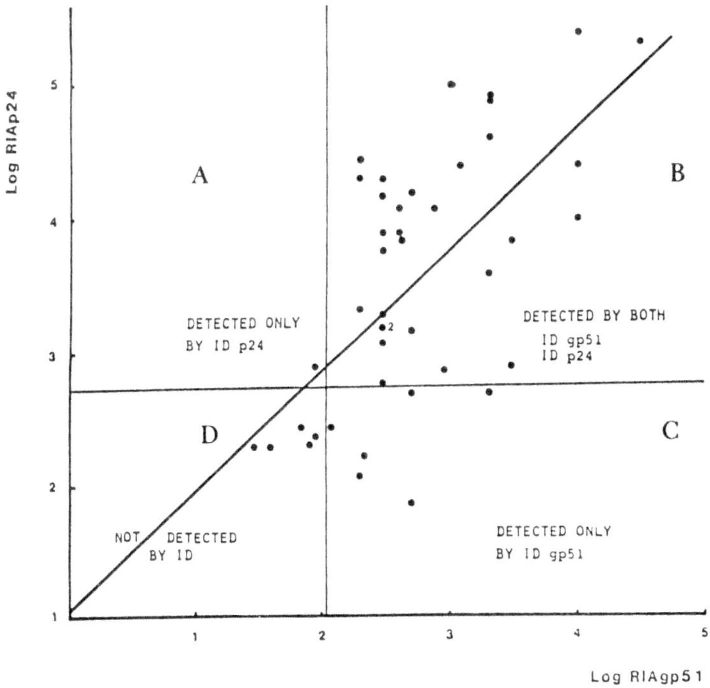

Fig. 4. Sensitivity of an immunodiffusion test for the detection and quantitation of bovine leukaemia virus induced antibodies.

in 4 categories. Compartment (A) corresponds to those sèra which contain enough anti p24 to be detected by ID but with only one precipitation line (p24), for such sera do not contain sufficient amounts of gp51 antibodies. Compartment (B) corresponds to the sera containing sufficient amounts of p24 and gp51 antibodies to be detected by ID; such sera should give rise to two precipitation lines (p24 and gp51). Compartment (C) corresponds to sera detectable by ID, but due to their low content of p24 antibodies they are detectable only by the precipitation line corresponding to gp51. Finally the sera of compartment (D), although positive by both RIAp24 and RIAgp51, do not contain sufficient p24 or gp51 antibodies to be detectable by ID. Although these results have only a statistical value and cannot be applied case by case they clearly indicate that in our serum sampling:

1.- 72% of the positive sera will be detected using IDp24 or IDgp51.

2-1.- 16% of the positive sera will be detected only by IDp24 or only by IDgp51.

2-2.- More importantly, if IDgp51 is far more sensitive than IDp24 for the detection of BLV infected cattle, few animals (2%) may be detected only by use of the p24 antigen.

3.- finally, due to the difference of sensitivity of RIAs as compared to immunodiffusion, 11% of RIA positive sera will not be detected by ID, whatever the antigen used.

DISCUSSION

Because the most sensitive techniques for the detection of BLV induced antibodies were thought to be rather difficult to apply in routine surveys, immunodiffusion has been selected by many countries in order to measure the incidence of viral infection, with the ultimate purpose of a complete eradication of the virus related disease. As many of our previous epidemiological studies were gathered with the EPI test and with radioimmunological assays, it seemed necessary to investigate the relative sensitivities of such techniques and of that of immunodiffusion. In preliminary investigations aimed at the comparison of the results obtained with radioimmunological procedures and with the immunodiffusion test, commercial antigen batches were used. Because such batches were found to be largely inconsistent in their antigen quantities and/or quality (e.g., detection of high percentages of false positive sera, almost complete absence of BLV antigens etc.) we decided to prepare our own antigen complying with several important criteria: 1.- in order to compare our results eventually with those obtained by other laboratories, the antigen preparation had to conform with the EC official recommendations (as is the case for the reference test sera); 2.- because it is generally agreed that immunodiffusion performed with BLV gp51 antigen is rather more sensitive than with BLV p24 antigen (Bex et al., 1979; Miller and Van der Maaten, 1976) and also because a number of positive sera were described as reacting only with the p24 antigen, we decided to include in the antigenic preparation both BLV gp51 and BLV 24 antigens; 3.- the antigenic preparation was standardised in terms of its antigenic content as determined by radioimmunological procedures; it was observed that the optimal value for the gp51 was between 3 and 4 μg/ml, and that with this value, the amount of p24 antigen was systematically adequate. As the comparisons of the results obtained with the different techniques required careful quantification of the titres, ID reacting sera were titrated by the limiting log_2 dilution which gave a clear precipitation line.

Our results clearly demonstrate that EPI - RIAp24 - RIAgp51 - ID are linked by highly significant correlating factors, thus indicating that all are specific of BLV induced antibodies. The differences observed in the b values of the different correlating equations mean that the different techniques mainly differ according to their threshold of sensitivity.

Whereas the EPI test was found to be as sensitive as RIAp24 and as RIAgp51 for the detection of BLV antibodies, it was observed that ID did not detect reactors with low titres in the other techniques. When analysing the correlation observed between the titres obtained by use of RIAp24 and of RIAgp51, it was found that all sera positive with one were also positive with the other technique; however a number of significant discrepancies were found for a number of sera in the two antibody specificities which they contained. This finding and the determination of the threshold of sensitivity of the ID test allowed us to classify positive sera in 4 categories. The majority, which contains large amounts of both BLV gp51 and BLV p24 antibodies, should be detected in ID by use of either one or the other corresponding antigen. A small percentage of sera should only be detected in ID tests by use of the gp51 antigen and an even smaller percentage would require the p24 antigen to react. Finally around 10% of BLV antibody containing sera would not be detected at all due to their low BLV p24 and BLV gp51 antibodies content. Thus it may be considered that, even when maximally sensitised, immunodiffusion may be used in a field survey for the detection of BLV infected herds but it cannot be expected to detect single cases.

These data agree with previously reported results which indicate that ID performed with the gp51 antigen is far more sensitive than ID performed with the p24 antigen. In addition the p24 antigen may be required for the detection of a limited number of positive sera. It is thus our conclusion that a calibrated (antigenic content determined with radioimmunological quantitative techniques) dual antigen has to be preferred to a single antigen for an optimal detection of reactors and should be used in large-scale surveys. It is our experimental inference that the antigens studied in this report fit best with the EC recommendations for large field sero-epidemiological surveys.

ACKNOWLEDGEMENTS

We gratefully acknowledge the excellent technical assistance of Ms D. Barrère, Mrs. C. Bourget and Mr. J.P. Portail. We also thank Mrs. N. Jaulin for her assistance in the preparation of the manuscript.

This work was supported in part by the Institut National de la Santé et de la Recherche Médicale (CRL n° 79-5-137-2) by the Institut National de la Recherche Agronomique (ATP 'Techniques Immunologiques') by the Institut Ronchèse (Zone Industrielle de Libourne) and by the Laboratoire Cogla (BP 45, 92360 Meudon-la-Fôret).

REFERENCES

Barille, M.F., 1974. General principles of isolation and detection of mycoplasmas. In: Les Mycoplasmes. INSERM., 33: pp. 135-142.

Bex, F., Bruck, C., Mammerickx, M., Portetelle, D., Ghysdael, J., Cleuter, Y., Leclercq, M., Dekegel, D. and Burny, A., 1979. Humoral antibody response to bovine leukemia virus infection in cattle and sheep. Cancer Res., 39: 1118-1123.

Devare, S.G., Stephenson, J.R., Sarma, P.S. and Aaronson, S.A., 1976. Bovine lymphosarcoma: Development of a radioimmunologic technique for detection of the etiologic agent. Science. 194: 1428-1430.

Devare, S.G. and Stephenson, J.R., 1977. Biochemical and immunological characterization of the major envelope glycoprotein of bovine leukemia virus. J. Virol., 23: 443-447.

Devare, S.G. and Stephenson, J.R., 1978. Radioimmunoassays for the major internal antigen (p24) and envelope glycoprotein (gp51) of bovine leukemia virus. In: The serological diagnosis of enzootic bovine leukosis, Ressang, A.A. (Ed.) ECSC-EEC-EAEC, Brussels, Luxembourg, pp. 43-55.

Diglio, C.A. and Ferrer, J.F., 1976. Induction of syncytia by the bovine C-type leukemia virus. Cancer Res., 36: 1056-1067.

Ferrer, J.F., Avila, L. and Stock, N.D., 1972. Serological detection of type C viruses found in bovine cultures. Cancer Res., 32: 1864-1870.

Finney, D.J., 1952. In: Statistical method in biological assay. Griffin, London.

Fischinger, P.J., Blevins, C.S. and Nomura, S., 1974. Simple quantitative assay for both xenotropic murine leukemia and ecotropic feline leukemia viruses. J. Virol., 14: 177-179.

Greenwood, F.C., Hunter, W.M. and Glover, J.S., 1963. The preparation of ^{131}I labelled human growth hormone of high specific radioactivity. Biochem. J., 89: 114-123.

Guillemain, B., Mamoun, R.Z., Astier, T., Duplan, J.F. and Parodi, A.L., 1978a. Early polykaryocytosis inhibition test: Evaluation of its performance in a seroepidemiological survey of bovine leukemia virus induced antibodies in cattle. Ann. Rech. Vét., 9: 709-720.

Guillemain, B., Mamoun, R.Z., Lévy, D., Astier, T., Irgens, K. and Parodi, A.L., 1978b. Early polykaryocytosis inhibition: A simple quantitative *in vitro* assay for the detection of bovine leukemia virus infection in cattle. Europ. J. Cancer. 14: 811-827.

Journal Officiel des Communautés Européenes. N° L51/30-33 (25-2-1980).

Kessler, S.W., 1975. Rapid isolation of antigens from cells with a staphylococcal protein A - antibody absorbent: Parameters of the interaction of antibody-antigen complexes with protein A. J. Immunology. 115: 1617-1624.

Lévy, D., Deshayes, L., Guillemain, B. and Parodi, A.L., 1977a. Bovine leukemia virus specific antibodies among French cattle. I. Comparison of complement fixation and hematological tests. Int. J. Cancer. 19: 822-827.

Lévy, D., Deshayes, L., Parodi, A.L., Lévy, J.P., Stephenson, J.R., Devare, S.G. and Gilden, R., 1977b. Bovine leukemia virus specific antibodies among French cattle. II. Radioimmunoassay with the major structural protein (BLV-p24). Int. J. Cancer. 20: 543-550.

MacDonald, H.C. and Ferrer, J.F., 1976. Detection quantitation and characterization of the major internal virion antigen of the bovine leukemia virus by radioimmunoassay. J. Nat. Cancer Inst., 57: 875-882.

Mamoun, R.Z., Astier, T. and Guillemain, B., 1980. In preparation.

Miller, J.M. and Olson, C., 1972. Precipitating antibody to an internal antigen of the C-type virus associated with bovine lymphosarcoma. J. Nat. Cancer Inst., 49: 1459-1462.

Miller, J.M. and Van der Maaten, M.J., 1974. A complement fixation test for bovine leukemia (C-type) virus. J. Nat. Cancer Inst., 53: 1699-1702.

Miller, J.M. and Van der Maaten, M.J., 1976. Serologic detection of bovine leukemia virus infection. Veterinary microbiology. 1: 195-202; Straub, O.C. (Ed.), Elsevier Scientific Publishing Company, Amsterdam amd CEC, Luxembourg.

Van der Maaten, M.J. and Miller, J.M., 1976. Replication of bovine leukemia virus in monolayer cell cultures. Bibliotheca Hematologica. 43: 360-362.

ELISA TEST FOR DETECTION OF ANTIBODIES TO ENZOOTIC BOVINE LEUKOSIS VIRUS

F. Biancifiori[1] and G. Cenci[2]

[1] Istituto Zooprofilattico Sperimentale dell'Umbria e delle Marche - Perugia, Italy.

[2] Istituto di Ispezione degli Alimenti di Origine Animale - Facoltà di Medicina Veterinaria - Perugia, Italy.

ABSTRACT

A total of 102 selected sera was examined by the ELISA. In order to study the sensitivity and specificity of the ELISA, the following groups of sera were examined:

1) Sera from leukosis-free herds,

2) AGID-positive sera,

3) AGID-negative sera from infected herds,

4) Sera from experimentally infected calves, collected at different intervals.

The results obtained seem to suggest that the ELISA is more suitable than the AGID test for large scale serological surveys.

O.C. Straub (ed.), Fourth International Symposium on Bovine Leukosis

INTRODUCTION

Enzyme-linked immunosorbent assay (ELISA) is one of the most sensitive serological methods developed for the detection and quantification of antibodies against a number of viruses (Bidwell, et al., 1977). Because of its sensitivity and reliability it is becoming a routine technique for use in diagnostic laboratories and for large scale screening.

In this brief report we describe an ELISA test for the serological diagnosis of enzootic bovine leukosis; we study its sensitivity and specificity and compare the results with those of the agar gel immunodiffusion (AGID) test, examining a total of 102 selected sera.

MATERIALS AND METHODS

A first commercial antigen (Enzygnost-Rinderleukose) was kindly supplied by Behringwerke (Marburg/GFR).

A second antigen was prepared in our institute from the supernatant of foetal lamb kidney (FLK) cell cultures chronically infected with BLV and grown in Hank's MeM supplemented with 10% foetal calf serum.

Culture fluids were clarified and the virus was pelleted by centrifugation at 60 000 g for 2 hours.

The pellet was resuspended in PBS containing 0.1% EDTA at a final (W/V) concentration of 1% of the original volume, layered on to a 10 - 40% gradient of sucrose in saline buffer and centrifuged at 100 000 g x 2 hours.

The opalescent virus band was collected, dyalised against PBS, and stored in small aliquots at -80°C until required.

Sera

The sera tested comprised the following groups:

1) Twenty pooled samples of 200 sera from leukosis-free herds.

2) Thirty-two AGID positive sera.

3) Thirty-eight AGID negative sera from infected herds.

4) Twelve sera from 3 experimentally infected calves, collected at various times.

5) Twenty AGID-negative sera found positive at the next test (six months later).

6) Positive and negative reference sera from commercial kits.

Enzyme-linked immunosorbent assay

The antigen was diluted x 400 (optimal work dilution previously determined) in 0.05 M carbonate buffer, pH 9.6 and dispensed in 100 µl volumes into each well of microtitreplates (Cook's-M 129 A). The plates were stored overnight at room temperature (about 20°C).

They were then washed four times with washing fluid (PBS containing 0.05% Tween 20) and used at once or stored at 4°C for a maximum of 48 hours.

Serum samples (100 µl) were diluted 1 : 8 with PBS containing 0.05% Tween 80 and distributed in duplicate to the plates. Sera of group 4 were diluted in twofold dilutions and titrated in the ELISA as well as in the AGID test.

After an incubation of 2 h at 37°C in a humid chamber, the plates were washed four times with washing fluid and 100 µl of conjugate (peroxidase-conjugated rabbit anti-bovine IgG; Nordic Immunological Laboratory) diluted 1 : 750 in PBS containing 0.05% Tween 80 and 4% lamb serum, dispensed into each well. After 1 h of incubation at 37°C the plates were washed thoroughly and the purified enzyme substrate, 5-amino-salicylic acid, adjusted to pH 6.0 and containing 0.05% H_2O_2, was added.

The reaction was stopped after 45 - 60 min by the addition of 2 N sodium azide (50 μl). Suitable controls were included in each plate.

The reactions were read by the naked eye.

Agar gel immunodiffusion test

This test was performed as previously described (Severini et al., 1980) using AGID kits obtained from Pitman-Moore Inc.

RESULTS AND DISCUSSION

Antigen

A 100% agreement between the two antigens used in our ELISA test was obtained.

Sera

Twenty pooled samples of 200 sera from leukosis free herds were negative by ELISA.

Thirty two sera positive by AGID were also positive by ELISA.

One sample from 38 AGID negative sera from infected herds, collected over a period of 5 years, always gave a positive reaction by ELISA.

One sample from the above group was scored doubtful by ELISA.

Five samples from 20 AGID negative sera which were positive 6 months later, were positive by ELISA.

In sera from 3 experimentally infected calves, collected at various times, antibodies were shown between 45 - 60 days after inoculation and the relative titres are shown in Table 1.

The ELISA appeared more sensitive and showed positive reactions up to three weeks earlier than the AGID test. These data show that it is at least as sensitive as the AGID test; moreover, it is technically simple, more easily read, the procedure is rapid, and the method is also adaptable to automation for processing of large numbers of sera.

TABLE 1

SEROLOGICAL REACTION IN EXPERIMENTALLY INFECTED CALVES

	ELISA (titre)	Difference in time (days) of appearance of antibodies	AGID (titre)
Calf 1	> 1 : 128	11	1 : 8
Calf 2	1 : 64	21	1 : 2
Calf 3	1 : 64	24	1 : 4

ACKNOWLEDGEMENTS

The authors would like to acknowledge the technical assistance of Mr. Francesco Vitelli.

REFERENCES

Bidwell, D.E., Bartlett, A. and Voller, A., 1977. Enzyme immunoassays for viral diseases. J. Infectious Diseases. 136: suppl. 274-278.

Severini, M., Rutili, D., Frùganti, G., Rampichini, L. and Cenci, G., 1981. Experimental transmission of enzootic bovine leukosis in calves. 4th International Symposium on Bovine Leukosis, Bologna, Italy, 1980 (this publication)

COMPARATIVE STUDIES ON THE ENZYME LINKED IMMUNO SORBENT ASSAY AND IMMUNODIFFUSION TEST IN THE DIAGNOSIS OF ENZOOTIC BOVINE LEUKOSIS

F. Behrens[1], R. Ziegelmaier[1], E. Forschner[2], D. Manz[3] and D. Wiegand[3]

[1] Research Laboratories of Behringwerke AG, D-3550 Marburg,

[2] Staatliches Veterinär-Untersuchungsamt, Eintrachtweg 17, D-3000 Hannover,

[3] Staatliches Veterinär-Untersuchungsamt, Marburger Strasse, D-6300 Giessen, Federal Republic of Germany.

ABSTRACT

The Enzyme Linked Immuno Sorbent Assay (ELISA) for the detection of antibodies against bovine leukosis virus in blood and milk serum is described. Comparison is made with the immunodiffusion test (ID test) in blood serum.

ELISA with blood serum is about 100-fold more sensitive than the ID test and positive earlier in approximately 50% of naturally infected animals, in specific cases up to 37 weeks prior to ID positive findings.

From 168 ELISA blood serum positive animals out of infected herds:

1) 128 ≙ 76% were positive in ID test on blood serum

2) 143 ≙ 85% were positive in ELISA on milk serum

3) 154 ≙ 91% were positive in combination of procedures 1) and 2)

ELISA titres in milk serum were usually lower than in blood serum.

O.C. Straub (ed.), Fourth International Symposium on Bovine Leukosis

INTRODUCTION

The routine diagnostic test for antibodies against the bovine leukosis virus (BLV) is the immunodiffusion test (ID) using gp-69-antigen of BLV (Forschner et al., 1978a; Forschner et al., 1978b; Forschner et al., 1979; Frank and Eberle, 1980).

More recent methods such as the anticomplement immunofluorescence (ACIF) (Frenzel et al., 1975), the radio immuno assay (RIA) (Chander et al., 1978) and the enzyme linked immuno sorbent assay (ELISA) (Behrens et al., 1979; Behrens et al., 1980; Todd et al., 1980) showed higher sensitivities than the ID test. Of these newer procedures which do not have the disadvantages of RIA, ELISA turned out to be the method of choice compared with ACIF and ID. It is more sensitive, easy to handle, and evaluation can be made visually as well as the more objective evaluation by photometric reading.

Furthermore, in the present study we analysed the potency of ELISA compared with ID in detecting BLV antibodies in blood serum; we also used ELISA to check for antibodies in milk serum (Manz et al., in press).

MATERIALS AND METHODS

The herds were selected for being negative or positive from routine diagnosis by haematology and later ID test. There were 22 herds with 328 animals negative by haematology and by the ID test, and 96 serologically positive herds with 2 669 animals. Thirty-two animals of one infected herd which seroconverted during their surveillance by the ID test were tested subsequently by ELISA. Milk samples were taken in 53 positive herds with 1 379 animals.

Preparation of Specimens

Blood serum was taken from clotted blood. Milk was frozen at -18° to $-20^{o}C$ and centrifuged (1 800 x g, 15 min) afterwards. The cream was skimmed and the milk serum decanted.

Performance of ID test

Bovine leukosis antigen from Behringwerke AG was used according to German Federal regulations in the ID test and was described in detail by Forschner et al. (1978a and 1978b). Semi-quantitative ID tests were performed as described by Behrens et al. (1979) using different serum dilutions and looking for the highest dilution which forms the specific precipitation line.

Performance of ELISA

ELISA was performed as described previously (Behrens et al., 1979) with the addition that milk serum was started undiluted. Briefly, BLV was propagated in foetal lamb kidney cell cultures and prepared according to Frenzel (1977). This antigen was absorbed to the wells of polystyrene microtitre plates according to Voller et al. (1975).

Anti bovine immunoglobulin from rabbit was purified by affinity chromatography and coupled with alkaline phosphatase according to Engvall and Perlman (1971). Paranitrophenylphosphate dissolved in 10% diethanoleamin buffer was used as substrate and stopped by a 2 molar solution of sodium hydroxide.

Four ELISA serum samples were diluted in phosphate buffered saline (PBS) pH 7.0 - 7.2 containing 4% Tween 20, titrated with a factor of 4 starting at a dilution of 1 : 8 for blood serum and undiluted for milk serum.

Serum incubation was performed for 2 h at +37°C. For the washing steps PBS plus 1% Tween 20 was used. Reading was done by naked eye or with a photometer at a wavelength of 405 nm. For visual reading every visible coloration was regarded as positive.

By photometry, using Titertek^{R}-Multiskan, an extinction of at least double the extinction of the negative controls in the same dilution, but not less than 0.2 E, was regarded as positive. Positive serum controls were always included and had to show their known titre.

RESULTS

From 22 negative herds with 328 animals, 327 reacted negative in both tests (Table 1). There was one animal with an ID doubtful and an ELISA positive reaction. It was bought from a flock not suspected of having leukosis (haematological testing). Repeated studies on this animal were impossible.

TABLE 1
22 NEGATIVE FLOCKS (HAEMATOLOGY), 328 ANIMALS

	Negative	Doubtful	Positive
ID test	327	1	-
ELISA	327	-	1

The results of the positive herds are summarised in Table 2. All ID doubtful reactors were ELISA positive. Additionally, there were 122 ID negative animals ELISA positive (4.6%).

TABLE 2
96 HERDS, 2 669 ANIMALS

	Negative	Doubtful	Positive
ID test	2 325	8	336
ELISA	2 211	-	458

Table 3 shows the results of a follow up study on 32 animals of one infected herd. Blood samples were taken at an interval of two weeks between nos. 1 - 11, 9 weeks between nos. 11 and 13, and 4 months between nos. 13 and 15. These 32 animals were first tested by the ID test and selected because of their seroconversion in this test during the survey. The results show that ELISA is approximately 100-fold more sensitive than the ID test and positive earlier in 17 of the 32 (53%) naturally infected animals; in case no. 314 for 37 weeks.

Table 4 demonstrates the results of 10 sera selected because of their low titres (1 : 8 - 1 : 64) by the ELISA technique. These sera were blind tested in the ID test and by Dr. Frenzel, Hannover, in the anticomplement immunofluorescence (ACIF) test described by Frenzel et al. (1975). The results show that the ACIF lies between the ID test and ELISA in its sensitivity.

The high sensitivity of the ELISA encouraged us to check milk serum for BLV antibodies. Table 5 shows the comparison of the ID test on blood serum and the ELISA on milk serum on 168 animals the blood serum of which had been ELISA positive. Milk samples were taken irrespective of the periods *post partum*.

One hundred and twenty eight animals could be detected by the ID test in the blood serum (76%); 143 animals were ELISA positive in the milk serum (85%); and 154 (92%) showed a positive reaction in the combination of blood serum ID test and milk serum ELISA. Neither method detected all blood serum ELISA positive animals. None of the negative animals classified by ELISA on blood serum gave a positive reaction in one of the other two tests.

The suitability of the ELISA technique using milk serum in the eradication programme for bovine leukosis has to be proven in further studies. The advantage of easier collection of samples is offset to some extent by the disadvantage that milk is not available from all animals.

TABLE 3

Animal No.	1	2	3	4	5	6	7	8	9	10	11	13	15
133	– –	– –	– 128	– 256	+/– >	1 >	1 >	4 >	4 >	4 >	4 >	6 >	6 >
178	– –	– –	– –	– –	– –	– –	– –	– –	– –	– –	– –	+/– 128	8 >
184	– –	– –	– –	– –	– –	+/– –	– –	+/– 512	4 >	4 >	4 x	4 >	6 >
185	– –	– –	– –	– –	– –	– –	– –	– –	– –	– 128	– –	4 >	6 >
187	– –	– –	– –	– –	– –	– –	– –	– –	– –	– 16	– 256	1 64	4 256
188	– –	– –	– –	– –	– –	– –	– –	– –	– 32	– 128	+/– x	1 >	1 >
212	– 128	– 128	– 128	– 128	+/– 128	1 >	2 >	1 >	1 >	4 >	1 >	4 >	2 >
213	– –	– –	– –	– –	– –	– –	– –	– –	– 128	1 >	10 >	4 >	2 >
219	– –	– –	– –	– –	– –	– –	– –	– –	– –	1 >	1 >	2 >	2 >
224	– –	– –	– –	– –	– –	– –	– –	– –	– –	– x	– x	6 >	x x
227	– –	– –	– –	– –	– –	– –	– –	– –	– –	1 128	2 >	4 >	4 >

TABLE 3 (CONTINUED)

Animal No.	1	2	3	4	5	6	7	8	9	10	11	13	15
228	- -	- -	- -	- -	- -	- -	- -	- -	- -	1 8	- 32	1 64	x x
229	- -	- -	- -	- -	- -	- -	- -	- -	- -	- -	- -	- -	12 >
230	- -	- -	- -	- -	- -	- -	- -	- -	- -	- -	- -	4 256	4 256
237	- -	- -	- -	- -	- -	- -	- -	- -	- x	1 64	2 256	6 256	4 >
242	- -	- -	- -	- -	- -	- 256	- 256	- 256	+/- 256	1 256	1 256	4 512	2 256
243	- 256	+/- 256	+/- >	1 >	+/- >	4 >	2 >	6 >	8 >	8 >	8 >	10 >	12 >
251	- -	- -	- -	- -	1 256	1 256	2 256	1 256	6 >	8 >	4 >	8 >	12 >
252	- -	- -	- -	- -	- -	- -	- -	- -	+/- 128	1 512	1 >	4 256	4 >
259	- -	- -	- -	- -	- -	- -	6 >	1 >	2 >	2 >	2 >	4 >	4 >
265	- 64	- 64	- 64	- 64	- 64	- 64	- 64	+/- >	+/- 256	1 >	1 >	1 >	1 256
270	- 128	+/- 256	+/- 256	+/- 256	- 64	1 256	1 256	1 256	2 256	2 256	1 256	2 256	1 256

TABLE 3 (CONTINUED)

Animal No.	1	2	3	4	5	6	7	8	9	10	11	13	15
272	- -	- -	- -	- -	- -	- -	- -	- -	- -	- -	- -	- -	1 >
275	- -	- x	+/- x	2 256	6 x	12 x	12 >	12 >	12 >	12 >	12 >	12 >	x x
282	- 64	- -	- -	- -	- -	- -	- x	- 256	- 256	x 256	x x	6 >	6 >
302	- -	- -	- -	- -	- -	- -	- -	- -	6 >	12 >	12 >	12 >	12 >
303	- 128	- 256	- 256	- 256	- 256	- 256	+/- 256	+/- 256	+/- 256	1 256	1 512	2 >	2 >
304	- -	- -	- -	- -	- -	- -	- -	- -	- -	- -	- -	4 >	1 256
306	- -	- -	- -	- -	- -	- -	- 64	- 64	+/- 256	- 256	1 256	4 256	12 >
307	- -	- -	- -	- -	- -	- -	- -	- 256	4 >	6 >	4 >	10 256	10 >
314	- -	- -	- -	- 16	- 16	- 16	- -	- -	- 64	- x	- -	- -	4 >
960	- -	- x	- x	- -	- x	- x	- -	- -	- 16	- 32	- 256	6 256	8 x

Upper line = ID values
Lower line = ELISA values
Figures = titre, dilution^{-1}
> = titre > 1 : 512

± = doubtful
- = negative (ID < 1 : 1)
(ELISA < 1 : 8)
x = not tested

TABLE 4

COMPARISON OF ID TEST, ELISA, AND ACIF

	Negative	Doubtful	Positive
ID test	7	3	-
ELISA	-	-	10(low titred)
ACIF	1	2	7

TABLE 5

COMPARISON OF ID TEST ON BLOOD SERUM AND ELISA ON MILK SERUM IN 168 ANIMALS POSITIVE IN ELISA ON BLOOD SERUM

		ELISA (milk serum)	
		Positive	Negative
ID test	positive	117	11
(Blood serum)	negative	26	14

CONCLUSIONS

1. All ID test positive sera are positive by ELISA.
2. All sera reacting doubtfully by ID test are positive by ELISA.
3. BLV antibodies can be detected in milk serum of infected animals by the ELISA technique at a higher rate than by ID test on blood serum. The applicability of this procedure for mass screening has to be evaluated in further studies.

REFERENCES

Bause, J., 1980. Die Persistenz präzipitierender Antikörper im Blutserum leukoseinfizierter Rinder mit besonderer Berücksichtigung des Kalbezeitpunktes. Inaugural-Dissertation. Göttingen.

Behrens, F., Knop, J., Weinmann, E., Maass, G., Baumeister, H.G., Majer, M. and Luthardt, T.H., 1977. Zur passiven oralen Immunisierung von Affen gegen den Erreger der infantilen Gastroenteritis des Menschen (Rotavirus). Vortrag: Deutsche Gesellschaft f. Hygiene u. Mikrobiologie, Sektion Virologie. 13. - 15.10.1977, Giessen.

Behrens, F., Ziegelmaier, R. and Forschner, E., 1980. Comparison of enzyme linked immuno sorbent assay and immunodiffusion-test in the diagnosis of enzootic bovine leucosis. Proceedings 2nd, International Symposium of Veterinary Laboratory Diagnosticians, Vol. 2, pp. 248-249, Lucerne.

Behrens, F., Ziegelmaier, R., Toth, T., v. Keyserlingk, M. and Forschner, E., 1979. Rinderleukose-Diagnostik: ELISA - ein neues Verfahren. Berl. Münch. Tierärztl. Wschr. 92, pp. 429-432.

Chander, S., Devare, S.G. and Stephenson, J.R., 1977. Comparison of radioimmunoassay and Bendixen's hematological evaluation in adult and calf forms of bovine lymphosarcoma. In Bovine Leucosis: Various Methods of Molecular Virology, A. Burny (Ed.), pp. 247-256, CEC, Kirchberg, Luxembourg.

Engvall, E. and Perlman, P., 1971. II. quantitative assay of protein antigen, immunoglobulin G, by means of enzyme labelled antigen and antibody coated tubes. Biochem. 259, pp. 427-434.

Forschner, E., Ewald, P., v. Keyserlingk, M., Röttgen, W. and Seidler, M.J., 1979. Nachweishäufigkeit von Leukose-Antikörpern in Abhängigkeit zum Alter der Rinder. Berl. Münch. Tierärztl. Wschr. 92, pp. 3-5.

Forschner, E., Seidler, M.J. and v. Keyserlingk-Eberius, M., 1978. Methodische Erfahrungen mit dem Agargelimmunodiffusionstest (ID-Test) bei der routinemässigen Massenuntersuchung von Blutproben zur Erkennung der enzootischen Rinderleukose. Berl. Münch. Tierärztl. Wschr. 91, pp. 447-450, 1978a, Berl. Münch. Tierärztl. Wschr. 91, pp. 453-456, 1978b.

Frank, W. and Buitkamp, J., 1979. Die serologische Leukose-Diagnostik in der Routineuntersuchung. Die Blauen Hefte für den Tierarzt 60, pp.526-531.

Frank, W. and Eberle, G., 1980. Fortschritte bei der Bekämpfung der Rinderleukose in Niedersachsen aus der Sicht der serologischen Überwachungsuntersuchungen. Dtsch. Tierärztl. Wschr. 87, pp. 176-178.

Frenzel, B., 1977. Reinigung eines präzipitierenden Glykoproteins des Rinderleukosevirus und vergleichende Untersuchungen über seine Verwendung bei der serologischen Diagnose der enzootischen Leukose des Rindes. Inaugural-Dissertation, Tübingen.

Frenzel, B., Mussgay, M., Schneider, L.G. and Straub, O.C., 1975. Immunofluorescence test for bovine leukosis-associated complement-fixing antibodies. Zbl. Vet. Med. B, 22, pp.519-523.

Kaaden, O.-R., 1980. Aktuelle Fragen der Rinderleukoseforschung und -bekämpfung. Dtsch. Tierärztl. Wschr. 87, pp. 41-43.

Levy, D., Deshayes, L., Parodi, A.-L., Levy, J.P., Stephenson, J.R., Devare, S.G. and Gilden, R.V., 1977. Bovine Leukemia virus specific antibodies among French cattle. II. Radioimmunoassay with the major structural protein (BLV p.24). Int. J. Cancer 20, pp. 543-550.

Manz, D., Wiegand, D., Behrens, F. and Ziegelmaier, R., (In press). Vergleichende serologische Untersuchungen an Blut und Milch zur Diagnostik der enzootischen Leukose des Rindes. Zbl. Vet. Med. B.

Miller, L.D. and Jones, N.K., 1980. Serological testing for enzootic bovine leukosis in the United States. Proceedings 2nd, International Symposium of Veterinary Laboratory Diagnosticians. Vol. 1, pp. 50-53. Lucerne.

Miller, J.M., Miller, L.D., Olson, C. and Gillette, K.G., 1969. Virus-like particles in phytohemagglutinin-stimulated lymphocyte cultures with reference to bovine lymphosarcoma. J. Natl. Cancer Inst. 43, pp. 1297-1305.

Miller, J.M. and Olson, C., 1972. Precipitating antibody to an internal antigen of the C-type virus associated with bovine lymphosarcoma. J. Natl. Cancer Inst. 49, pp. 1459-1462.

Paulsen, J., Best, E., Frese, K. and Rudolph, R., 1971. Enzootische lymphatische Leukose bei Schafen. Lymphozytose, pathologische Anatomie und Histologie. Zbl. Vet. Med. B. 18, pp. 33-43.

Paulsen, J. and Schliesser, Th., 1977. Zur Ätiologie und Diagnose der enzootischen Leukose bei Rind und Schaf. Tierärztl. Umschau 32, 343-347.

Piper, C.E., Ferrer, J.F., Abt, D.A. and Marshak, R.R., 1979. Postnatal and prenatal transmission of the bovine leukemia virus under natural conditions. J. Natl. Cancer Inst. 62, pp. 165-168.

Schmidt, F.-W., 1979. Erfahrungen nach der Umstellung der hämatologischen auf die serologische Leukoseuntersuchung beim Rind. Tierzüchter 11, pp. 452-453.

Seger, C.L. and Morgan, E., 1977. Differential incidence of bovine leukemia virus (BLV) antibody in yearling herdmates nursed on milk replacer or pooled sour colostrum. In Bovine leucosis: Various methods of molecular virology, A. Burny (Ed.), pp. 267-269, CEC, Kirchberg, Luxembourg.

Singh, V.K., 1975. Process of producing bovine milk products containing specific antibodies. US Patent No. 3.911.108.

Thoen, C.O., Hopkins, M.P. and Pietz, D.E., 1980. Detection of Brucella antibodies in cows milk using an automated enzyme linked immuno-sorbent assay. Proceedings 2nd, International Symposium of Veterinary Laboratory Diagnosticians. Vol. 2, pp. 228-231, Lucerne.

Todd, D., Adair, B.M. and Wibberley, G., 1980. An enzyme-linked immuno-sorbent assay for enzootic bovine leukosis virus antibodies. Vet. Rec. 107, pp. 124-126.

Voller, A. and Bidwell, D.E., 1975. A Simple method for detecting anti-bodies to Rubella. Br. J. exp. Path. 56, p. 338.

AUTOMATED METHODS FOR THE DETERMINATION OF BOVINE LEUKOSIS

D. Collet-Cassart*, C.G.M. Magnusson*,
R.F. Jay**, V. Reicher** and H.W. Holy**

*Unit of Experimental Medicine, International Institute of Cellular and Molecular Pathology, UCL 7430, Avenue Hippocrate 75, B-1200 Brussels, Belgium.

**Technicon International Division SA, 12 Chemin Rieu, CH-1208 Geneva, Switzerland.

ABSTRACT

Preliminary studies on positive and negative bovine leukosis control sera and test sera provided by the State Serum Laboratory, Copenhagen, Denmark, indicate that an automated system of complement fixation testing can be used in the diagnosis of bovine leukosis. The system described operates at 240 samples per hour and has been successfully employed for brucellosis eradication programmes.

The same samples were also run on a new fully automated non-isotopic immunoassay system (PACIA: Particle Counting Immunoassay) at 60 samples per hour. No sample pretreatment was required in this case and the sensitivity was up to 200 times greater.

The merits of the two methods are compared. Complement fixation testing is proposed for screening and the PACIA system for confirmatory testing of bovine leukosis.

O.C. Straub (ed.), Fourth International Symposium on Bovine Leukosis

INTRODUCTION

In the diagnosis of animal disease, automated analysis for diagnosis usually increases both the efficiency and scope of mass screening programmes. Automated determination of the brucellosis bacillus antibody has been an essential feature in the virtual eradication of this disease from the herds of many countries.

Recent legislation and proposed regulations restricting the movement of cattle not certified as free of bovine leukosis has led us to examine the feasibility of automating the determination for the presence of bovine leukosis virus.

We here report our preliminary results using two automated methods. The first is the automated complement fixation test (ACFT) used very successfully in the New Zealand brucellosis eradication programme and the second is a new non-isotopic immunoassay technique - PACIA, (Particle Counting Immunoassay), whose sensitivity and versatility equals radioimmunoassay.

1. AUTOMATED COMPLEMENT FIXATION TEST

MATERIAL

Sheep Red Blood Cells

Were purchased fresh from Tissue Culture Services Ltd., Slough, England, and prepared according to the Technicon method for ACFT.

Haemolysin

Purchased from bioMérieux, France, as a rabbit anti-sheep red cell serum.

Complement

Lyophilised guinea pig complement was purchased from

Tissue Culture Services Ltd., Slough, England, preserved in 20% Richardson's preservative.

Bovine Clq

Was prepared from calf sera according to the method of Eskildsen (1975).

Veronal Buffered Saline (VBS)

Was prepared according to the Technicon method for ACFT.

Serum Samples

One positive and one negative control serum, 4 positive test sera (Nos. 1 - 4) and 4 negative test sera (5 - 8) were the kind gift of Dr. R. Hoff-Jørgensen (State Serum Laboratory, Copenhagen, Denmark) and one control serum was provided by Behringwerke, Marburg, as used in their immunodiffusion kit for bovine leukosis.

Bovine Leukosis Antigen

Two antigens and a control antigen were also kindly given by Dr. Hoff-Jørgensen. One antigen (as used for the immunodiffusion test) consisted of concentrated supernatant from infected foetal lamb kidney cells; the control antigen was prepared similarly using non-infected cells.

The other antigen was purified by running the pelleted virus through a sucrose cushion and diluted 1/100 with phosphate buffered saline.

One further antigen was a gift of Behringwerke, Marburg, and again was that used in their bovine leukosis kit (Rinderleukose-Antigen OlPW14).

METHODS

Schematically, the analytical system is shown in Figure 1. The operational details are identical to those for the

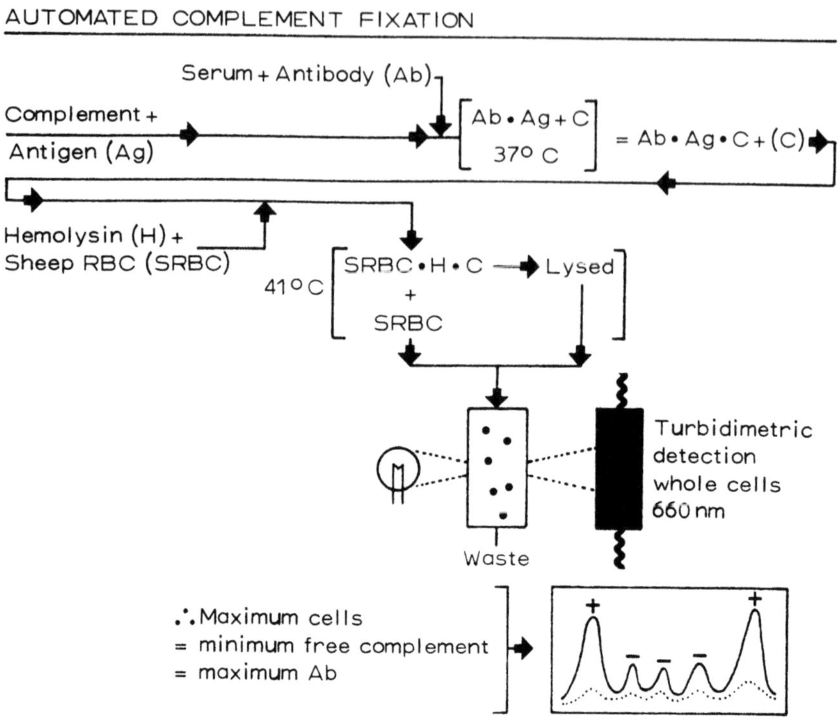

Fig. 1. Principle of automated complement fixation testing.

brucellosis screening system except that Clq, as above prepared, was added to the complement solution at a concentration of 1/240 to enhance the complement reaction according to the method of Hoff-Jørgensen (1977).

Optimum haemolysin concentration was determined automatically according to the Technicon Operation Manual as 1/12 000 dilution when measured against the 1% sheep red blood cells and 5% complement.

The haemolytic reagent was prepared from the sheep red blood cells and the optimum haemolysin concentration as described in the Technicon method.

Optimum complement concentration was also determined automatically as 2.5% by titration (Figure 2) according to the Technicon Operation Manual.

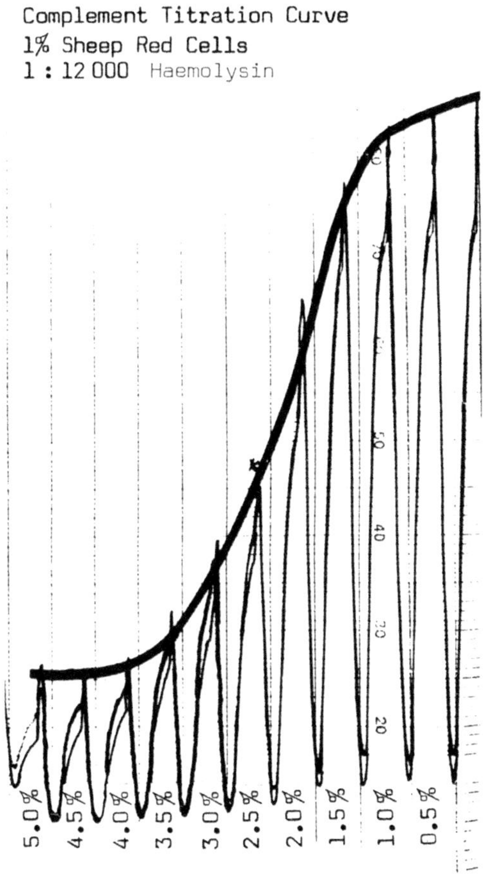

Fig. 2. Recorder traces for automated complement titration to determine the optimum concentration of complement for use in automated complement fixation testing of bovine leukosis virus antibodies.

SAMPLE PREPARATION

Series 1:

In the initial run, sera were diluted 1/10, 1/20 and 1/40 with VBS and inactivated at 56° for 30 minutes.

Series 2:

In the second run, all sera except the Behringwerke control were mixed with an equal volume of a 10% complement solution in VBS and incubated at 37°C for 30 minutes followed by heat inactivation at 56°C for 30 minutes as recommended by Hoff-Jørgensen (1977). The final dilutions of the sera were 1/20 and 1/5.

RESULTS

The first series run (Figure 3) showed that anti-complementary activity in most instances equalled or even exceeded the complement activity at all dilutions of the sera using the Copenhagen Antigen No. 1.

After serum pretreatment, Antigen No. 1 gave no significant response when used at a dilution of 1/160. The Behringwerke antigen, however, at a concentration of 1/20 correctly identified as positive the test sera 2 and 4 as well as the Behringwerke control serum (Figure 4).

Based on the peak height of the negative control (Figure 4) the ACFT failed to identify as positive sera 1 and 3. It correctly identified as negative sera 5, 6, 7 and 8 (Figure 5).

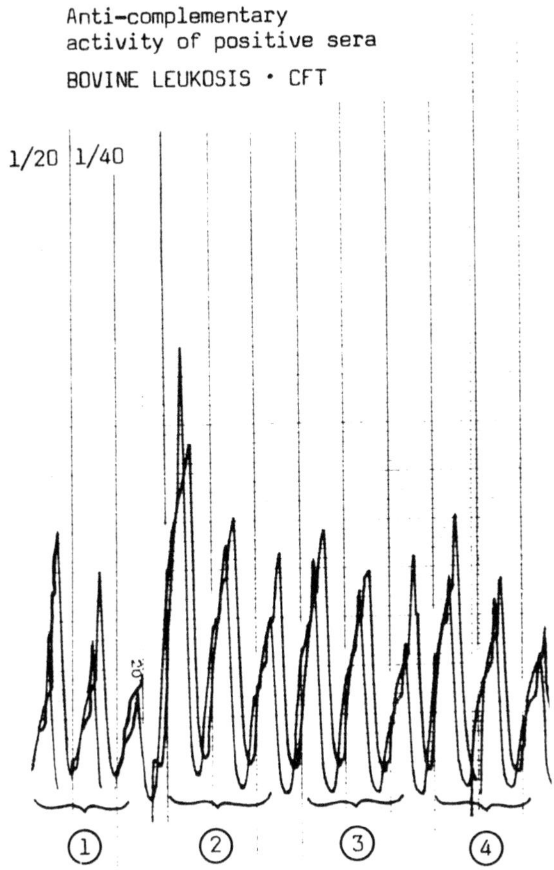

Fig. 3. Recorder trace showing anti-complementary activity in complement fixation test for bovine leukosis using Copenhagen antigen No. 1.

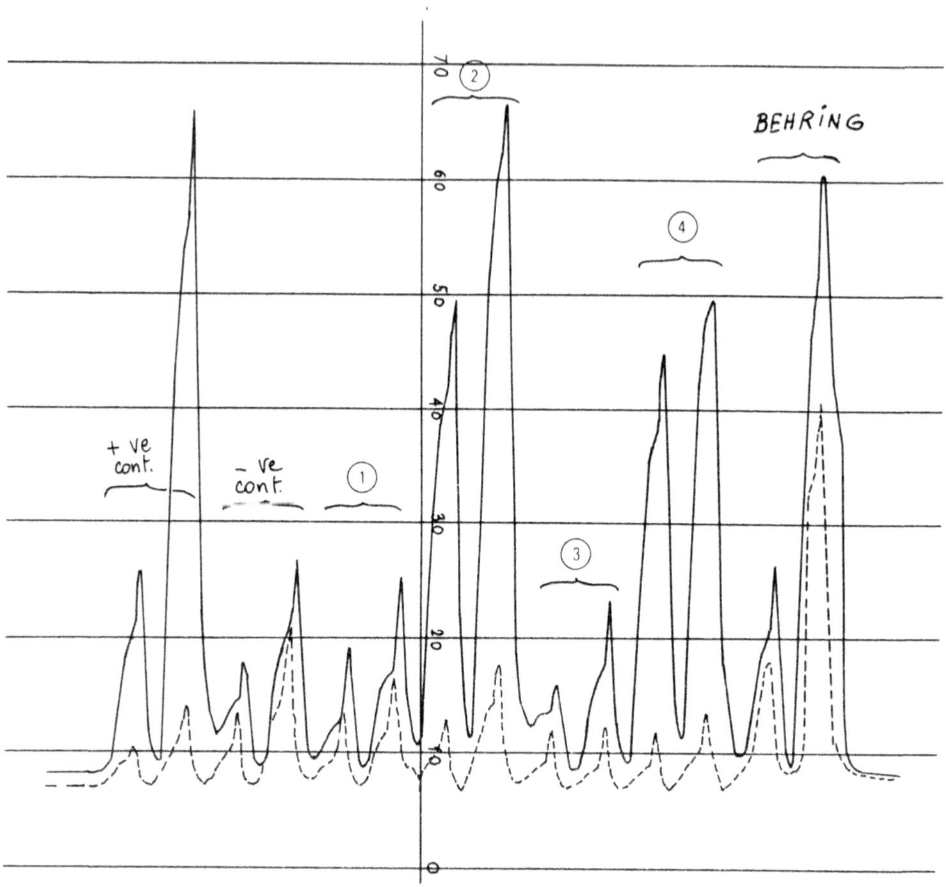

Fig. 4. Recorder trace showing results of the automated complement fixation test for bovine leukosis virus antibodies on positive and negative controls, positive test sera and Behringwerke control serum at 1/20 and 1/5 dilution using Behringwerke Rinderleukose antigen after sample pretreatment.

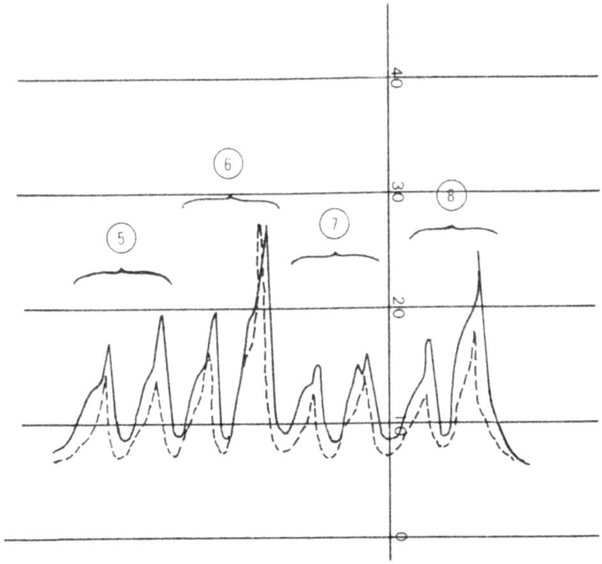

Fig. 5. Recorder trace showing results of the automated complement fixation tests for bovine leukosis virus antibodies on negative test sera at 1/20 and 1/5 dilution using Behringwerke Rinderleukose antigen after sample pretreatment.

2. PACIA

MATERIAL

Antigens

Were provided as for ACFT.

DTT (Dithiothreitol)

A 10 mg/ml solution of DTT was prepared in distilled water. 1 volume of this solution was mixed with 4 volumes of a 50 mM EDTA/GBS solution diluted 2 : 1 in distilled water.

Lx-Ag (1)

Adsorbed antigen latex was prepared according to the method of Limet et al. (1979) using the antigens provided.

Lx-Ag (2)

Antigen covalently coupled to latex was prepared according to the method of Sindic et al., (in press).

GBS-BSA (Glycine Buffered Saline)

0.1M glycine buffer pH 9.2 containing 0.17M NaCl and 0.1% bovine serum albumin.

Rheumatoid factor

The serum from a patient (Baker) with a high titre of rheumatoid factor was used at a 1/50 dilution.

SAMPLE PREPARATION

Samples were the same as those used for ACFT. They were diluted 1/10, 1/20, 1/40, 1/80 in GBS-BSA.

METHOD

The instrumental technique is detailed in Figure 6 and schematically represented (Figure 7). The method has been described in detail (Cambiaso et al., 1977; Collet-Cassart et al., in press; Technicon Monograph, 1979). Analysis rate was 60 samples/hour, incubation time about 36 minutes at 37°C.

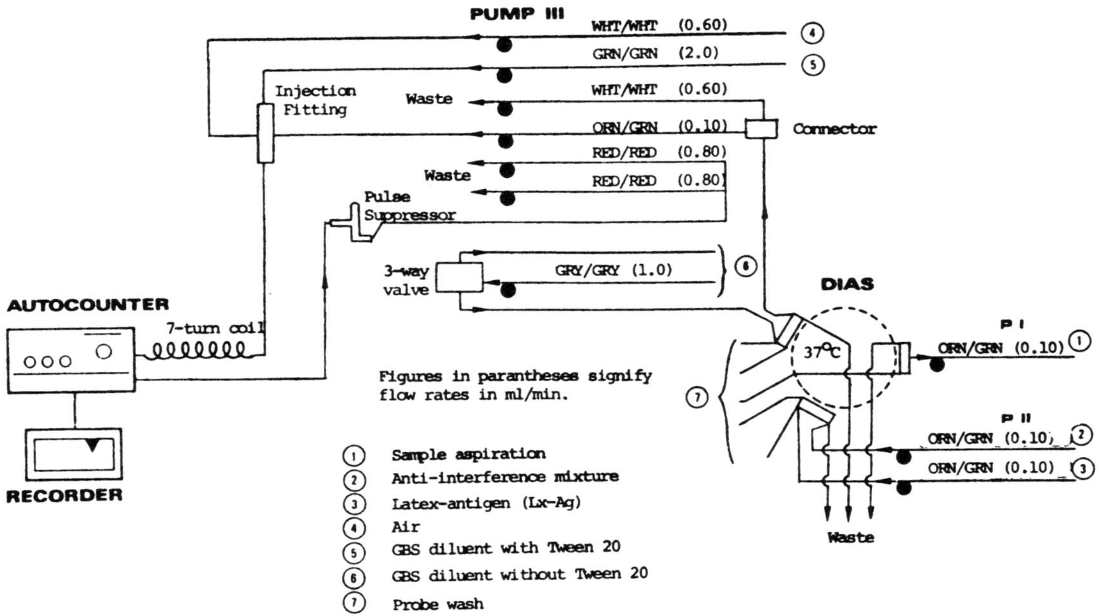

Fig. 6. Flow diagram for the automated particle counting immunoassay - PACIA - method for bovine leukosis virus antibodies.

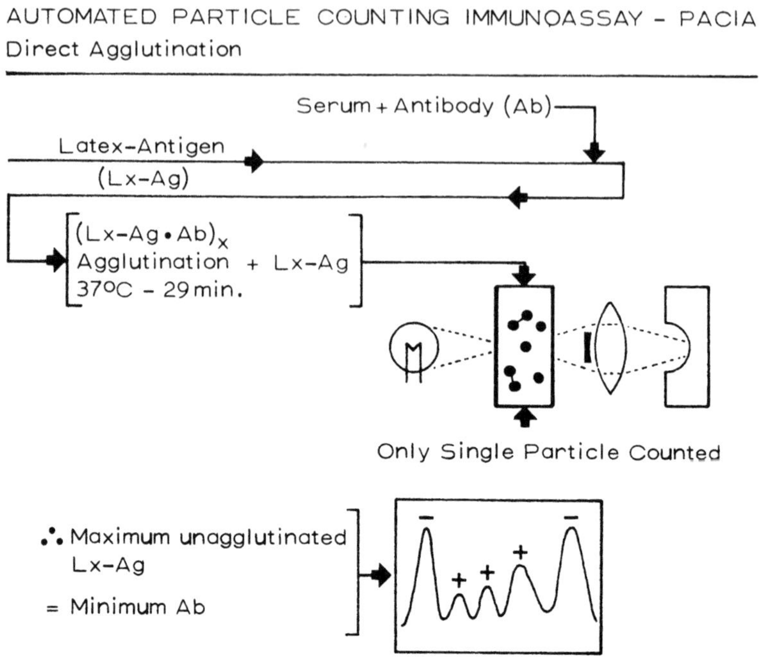

Fig. 7. Principle of Automated Particle Counting Immunoassay.

RESULTS

Figure 8 shows the results for the positive control serum and Figure 9 the results for the negative control serum using the Behringwerke antigen. Accepting the levels established as positive by this technique, the difference in reactivity between positive and negative controls correctly identifies test sera 1, 2, 3 and 4 as well as the Behringwerke control to be positive as labelled (Figure 10). Sera 5, 6, 7 and 8 were correctly shown to be negative (Figure 11). When covalently bound latex antigen was used (Figure 12), the response of the 1/60 diluted serum was approximately equivalent to the 1/15 diluted serum using the antigen adsorbed on to latex.

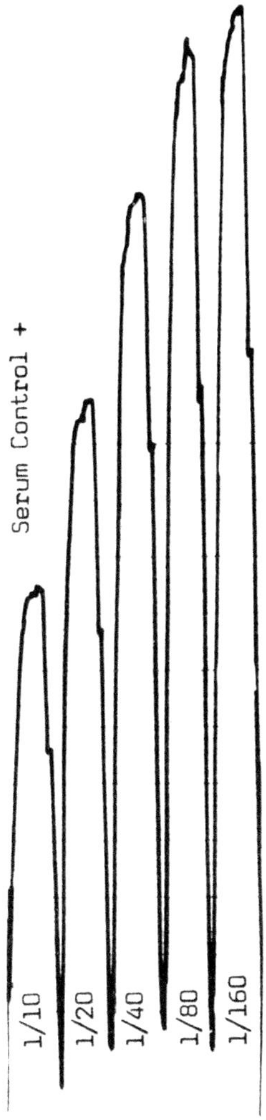

Fig. 8. Recorder traces for Automated Particle Counting Immunoassay of bovine leukosis virus antibodies. Positive control serum.

On the assumption that most antibodies to bovine leukosis are IgG (Portetelle et al., 1978) which is a poor agglutinator of latex particles, we sought to enhance the agglutination by the use of rheumatoid factor, which is mostly IgM. In principle, IgG antibodies attach to the latex-antigen and only in favourable circumstances (presumably sufficient molecules of IgG attached) will they cause agglutination. However, the IgM molecule by virtue of its large size (900 000 Daltons) and effectively 10 binding sites, is a powerful latex agglutinator when IgG-antigen complexes are on the latex surface (Figure 13).

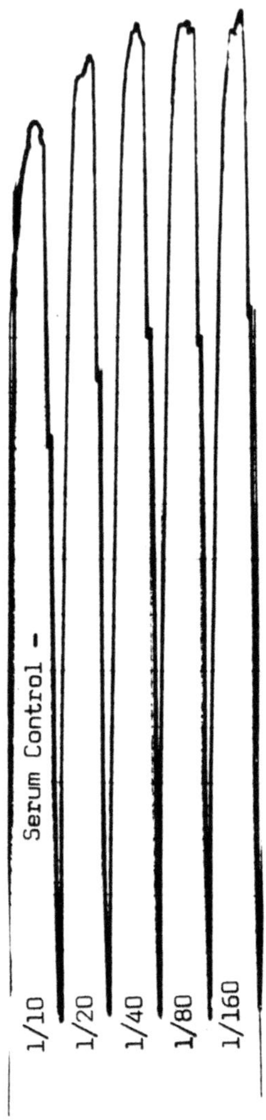

Fig. 9. Recorder trace for Automated Particle Counting Immunoassay of bovine leukosis virus antibodies. Negative control serum.

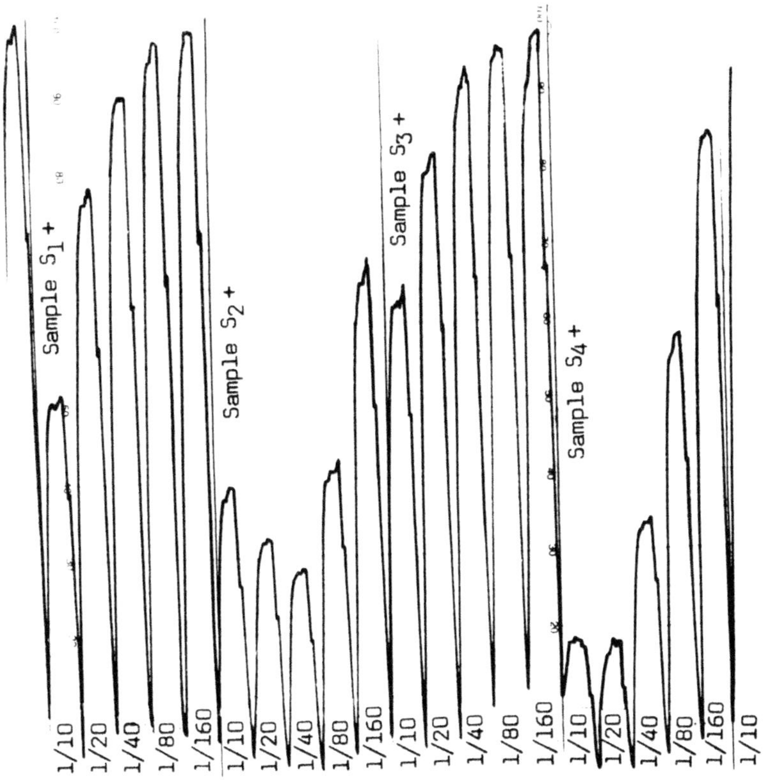

Fig. 10. Recorder traces for Automated Particle Counting Immunoassay of bovine leukosis virus antibodies. Positive test sera.

Accordingly, we repeated the assay on the 4 positive Copenhagen samples as well as the controls and the Behringwerke positive control using the following procedure:

30 µl sera were manually diluted in GBS-BSA 1/10, 1/20, 1/40, 1/80, 1/160 and inserted in sequence in the PACIA sampler. 30 µl of rheumatoid sera (Baker) followed by 30 µl Lx-Ag (2) were added to each dilution automatically.

We obtained a dramatic increase in sensitivity only in positive Copenhagen test sera No. 2 (Figure 14a) and No. 4 (Figure 15a). Serum No. 1 (Figure 16a), Copenhagen positive control (Figure 17a) and the Behringwerke positive control (Figure 18a) showed little if any significant enhancement.

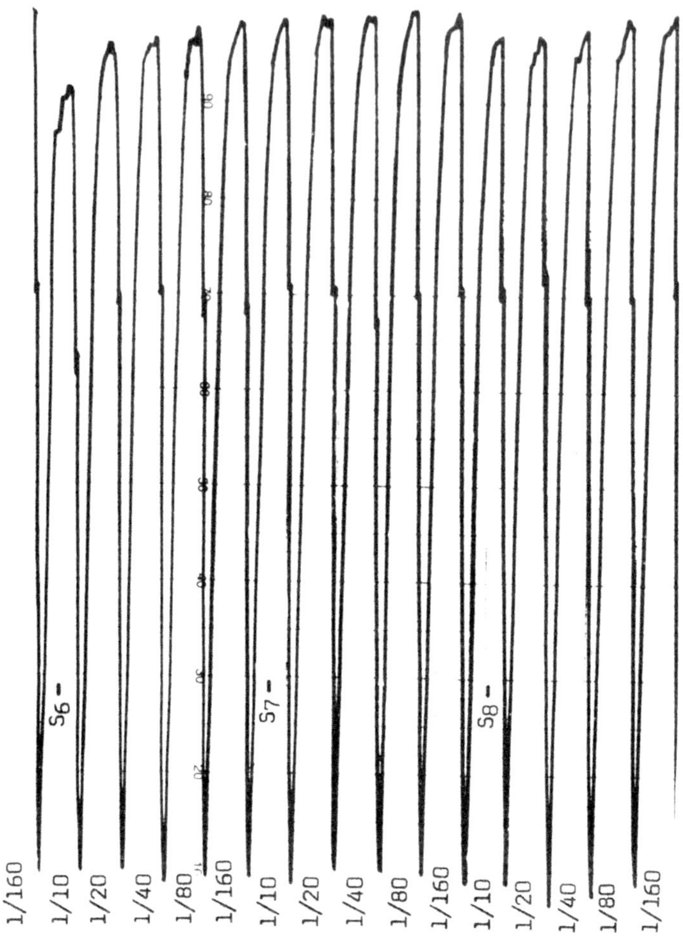

Fig. 11. Recorder trace for Automated Particle Counting Immunoassay of bovine leukosis virus antibodies. Negative test sera.

A possible (although admittedly unexpected) explanation would be that the antibodies were in fact IgM. Accordingly, following the procedure established for determination of immune complexes (Cambiaso et al., 1979) we decided to destroy IgM by pretreatment of the positive sera with dithiothreitol (DTT). We used the following procedure:

To 50 µl of serum diluted as above added 170 µl EDTA (50 mM) and 15 µl DTT (5 mg/ml in H_2O) and incubated for 30

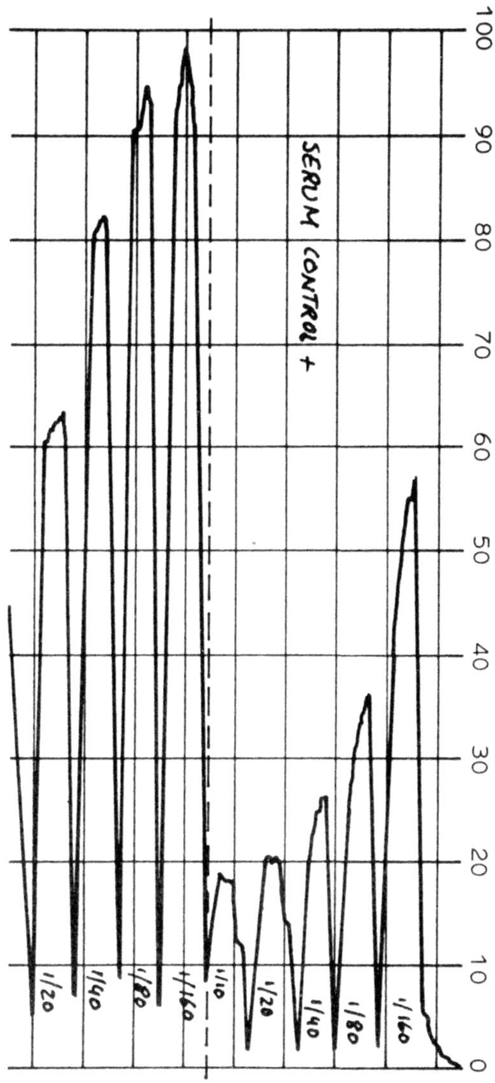

Fig. 12. Recorder traces for Automated Particle Counting Immunoassay of bovine leukosis virus antibodies. Comparison of results for the positive control sera using:

(a) antigen adsorbed on latex

(b) antigen covalently bound to latex

showing increased sensitivity of (b).

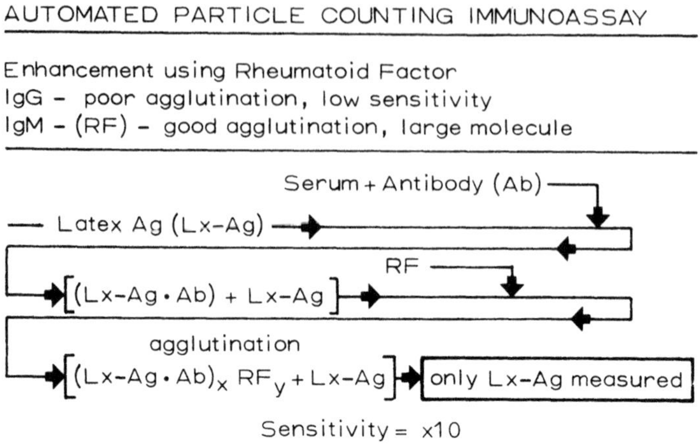

Fig. 13. Principle of using rheumatoid factor to enhance the agglutination of antigen coated latex by IgG antibodies.

minutes at 37°C. The reaction was stopped with 15 μl of hydrogen peroxide solution (1/180 dilution of a 30% solution). The samples were then analysed on the PACIA system as above.

We noted no significant difference in samples 2 (Figure 14b) and 4 (Figure 15b) nor in the Behringwerke control (Figure 18b). However, we lost all agglutinating activity in sample No. 1 (Figure 16b) and the Copenhagen positive control (Figure 17b).

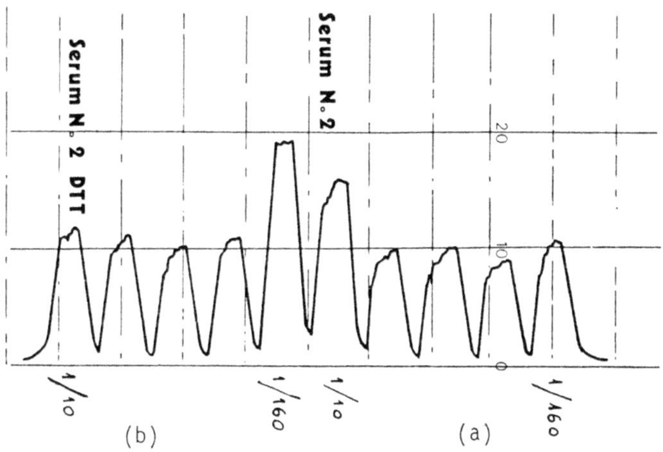

Fig. 14. Results of RF enhancement on test serum 2.
(a) Without DTT treatment of samples.
(b) With DTT treatment of samples.

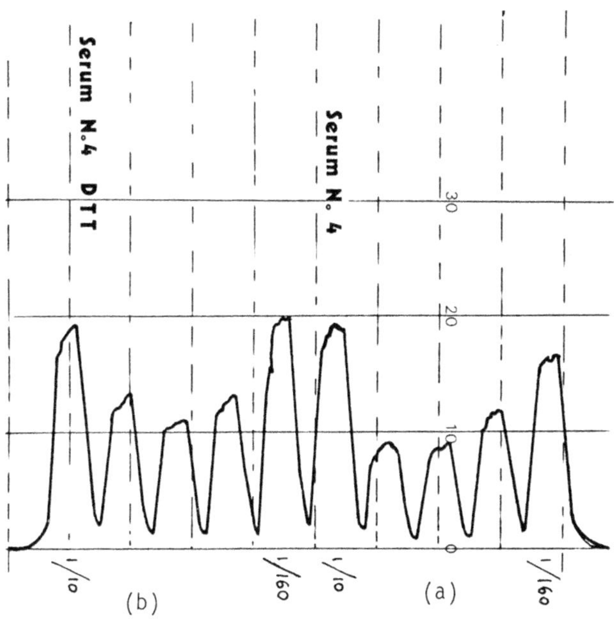

Fig. 15. Results of RF enhancement on test serum 4.
(a) Without DTT treatment of samples.
(b) With DTT treatment of samples.

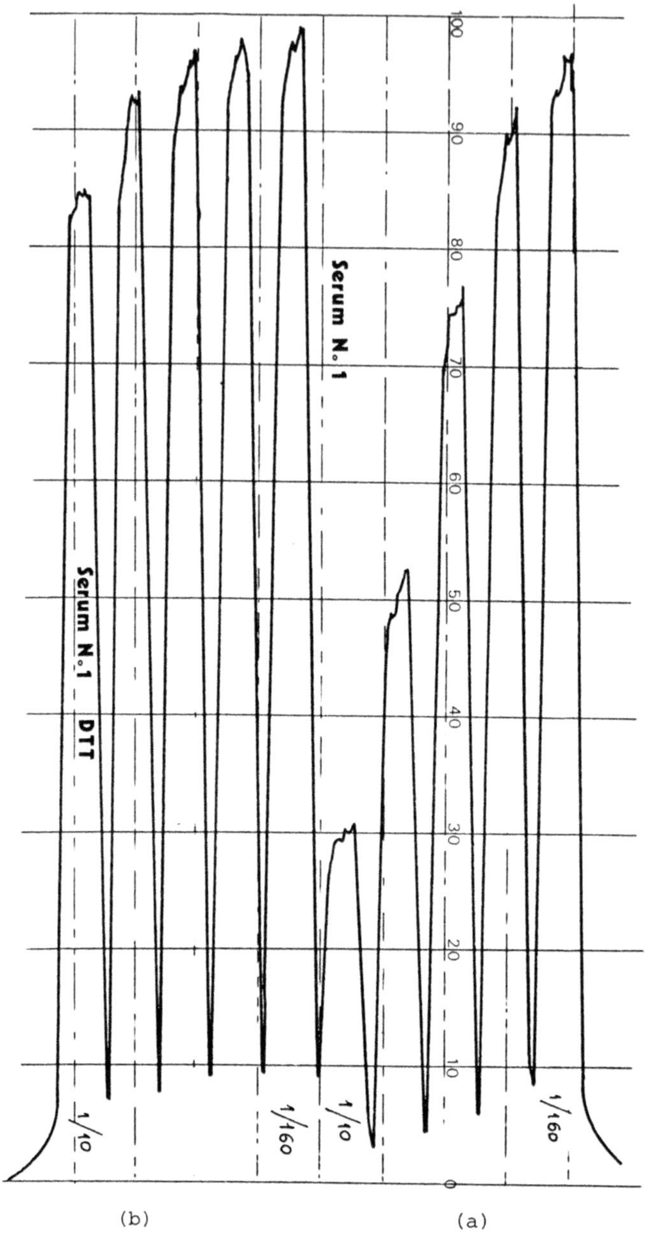

Fig. 16. Results of RF enhancement on test serum 1.
(a) Without DTT treatment of samples.
(b) With DTT treatment of samples.

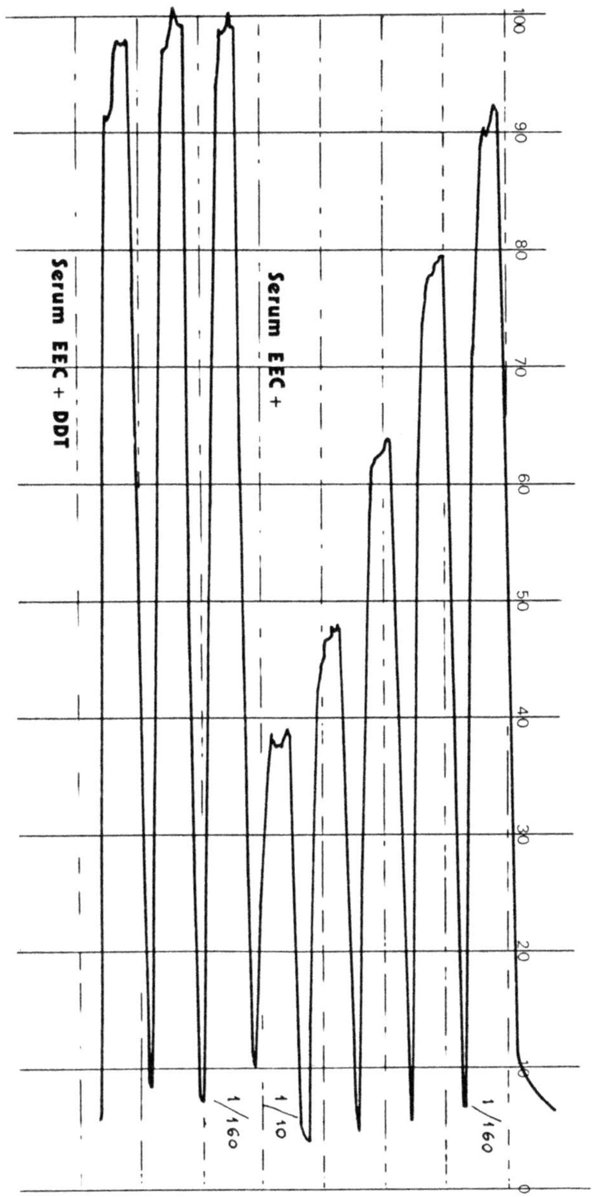

(b) (a)

Fig. 17. Results of RF enhancement on the positive control serum (Copenhagen)
(a) Without DTT treatment of samples.
(b) With DTT treatment of samples.

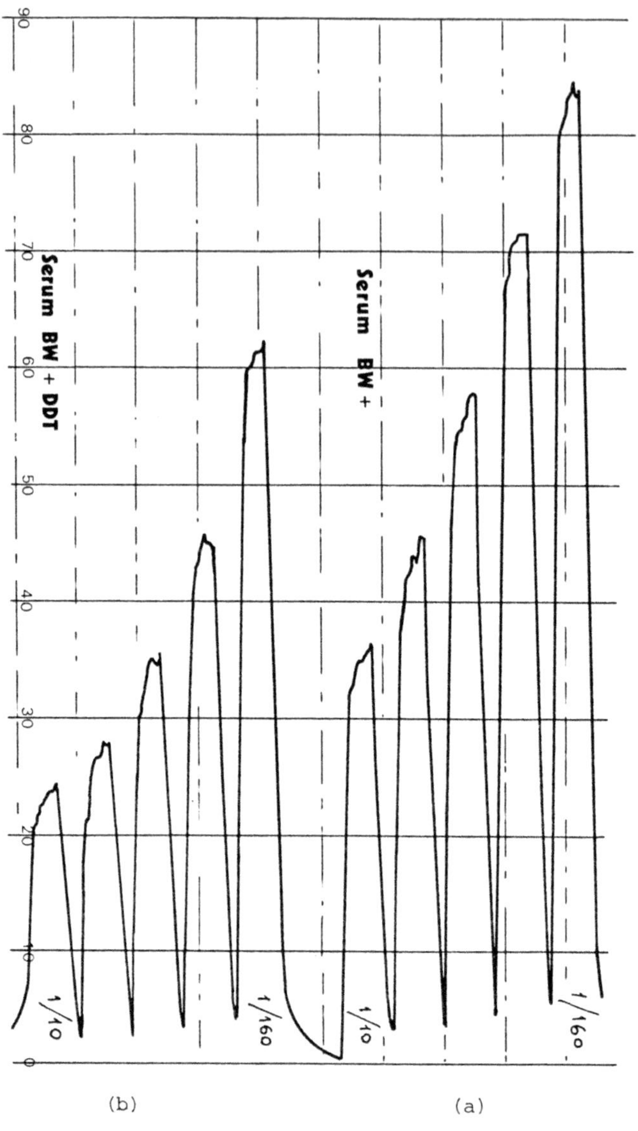

Fig. 18. Results of RF enhancement on the Behringwerke positive control serum.
(a) Without DTT treatment of samples.
(b) With DTT treatment of samples.

DISCUSSION

Interestingly and only in passing, the PACIA technique would suggest that both the negative control serum and serum 6, listed as negative, had some slight positive reaction. An examination of the ACFT trace is consistent with this observation as the peak height of both these sera is somewhat higher than the agreed negative sera 5, 7 and 8.

The very strong interference from anti-complementary activity of positive bovine leukosis sera has been a surprise to us. In spite of warnings that bovine sera tested for brucellosis antibody contained excessive anti-complementary activity, Te Punga (1971) reported that in 10 000 samples tested he had never observed a serious interference from anti-complementary activity, an observation confirmed subsequently on a programme running 300 000 sera/month (Timbs et al., 1977).

Possible sources of high anti-complementary activity could arise from bacterial contamination, endotoxins, DNA, some product of an inflammatory syndrome or most probably, circulating immune complexes. Inasmuch as bovine leukosis is a viral infection of leukocytes, whereas brucellosis is a bacterial infection localised to certain organs, the theory of high levels of circulating immune complexes is attractive. The use of complement to enhance the reaction would further indicate that immune complexes may be the cause of excessive anti-complementary activity. Miller (1975) has shown that C3 does dissociate immune complexes.

The very high peak recorded in ACFT with the Behringwerke control serum is shown to be due primarily to the anti-complementary activity of that serum. PACIA confirmed this conclusion by indicating that the Behringwerke control serum has a relatively low concentration of free antibodies. Finally, if only IgM agglutinating activity is destroyed by DTT, then, surprisingly two antisera are primarily IgM.

CONCLUSION

Based on our preliminary observations, automated complement fixation testing is probably an adequate screening technique, operating at 240 samples/hour.

PACIA, with its extreme potential sensitivity and currently operating at 60 samples/hour is undoubtedly an acceptable confirmatory test. Its proven sensitivity is probably 50 times greater at least than ACFT but such extreme sensitivity may prove an embarrassment unless the technique is used in a confirmatory role.

Apart from sensitivity, the major advantage of PACIA seems to be specificity. As far as we have been able to determine, no interferences are apparent. However, considerable work must still be done to establish this point.

In both assays commercial antigen and antisera are available.

REFERENCES

Cambiaso, C.L., Leek, A.E., De Steenwinkel, F., Billen, J. and Masson, P.L., 1977. Particle Counting Immunoassay (PACIA) I. A general method for the determination of antibodies, antigens and haptens. J. Immunological Methods, 18, 33-44.

Cambiaso, C.L., Sindic, D. and Masson, P.L., 1979. Particle Counting Immunoassay (PACIA) III. Automated determination of circulating immune complexes by inhibition of an agglutinating factor of mouse serum. J. Immunological Methods, 28, 13-23.

Collet-Cassart, D., Magnusson, C.G.M., Cambiaso, C.L. and Masson, P.L., (in press). A fully automated non radioisotopic assay for alpha-fetoprotein using the PACIA technique. Clinical Chemistry.

Eskildsen, M., 1975. Complement fixation with porcine serum antibodies enhancing effect of porcine Clq on complement fixation with IgG prepared from porcine pseudorabies immune serum. Acta Path. Microbiol. Scand., Sect. C., 83, 315-324.

Hoff-Jørgensen, R. and Eskildsen, M., 1977. Demonstration of antibodies against bovine leukosis virus in bovine sera by complement fixation. Use of homologous complement component Clq and concentrated antigen in a direct test. From: Bovine Leukosis. Various methods of molecular virology (Ed. A. Burne) EEC Communication.

Limet, J.N., Moussebois, C.H., Cambiaso, C.L., Vaerman, J.P. and Masson, P.L., 1979. Particle counting immunoassay. IV. The use of $F(ab')_2$ fragments and N^{ε}-chloracetyl lysine N-carboxy anhydride for their coupling to polystyrene latex particles. J. Immunological Methods, 28, 25-32.

Miller, G.N., Nussenzweig, V., 1975. A new complement function; solubilization of antigen-antibody aggregates. Proc. Nat. Acad. Sci. USA, 72, (2) 518-522.

Portetelle, D., Bruck, C., Burny, A., DeKegel, D., Mammerickx, M. and Urbain, J., 1978. Detection of complement dependent lytic antibodies in sera from bovine leukemia virus-infected animals. Ann. Rech. Vét., 9, (4) 667-674.

Sindic, C.J.M., Chalon, M.P., Cambiaso, C.L., Collet-Cassart, D. and Masson, P.L., (in press). Particle Counting Immunoassay (PACIA) VI. The determination of rabbit IgG antibodies against myelin basic protein using IgM rheumatoid factor. Mol. Immunol.

Technicon Method. Complement fixation test for brucellosis.

Technicon Operation Manual. Automated complement fixation testing.

Technicon PACIA System, Monograph 1: Instrumentation; Monograph 2: Reagents, 1979. Technicon International Division SA, Geneva, Switzerland.

Te Punga, W.A., 1971. An automated complement fixation test for the identification of cattle infected with *Brucella abortus*. Technicon Australia, Symposium, Feb. 1971.

Timbs, D.V., Moxham, J.W. and Liberona, H.E., 1977. The use of automated complement fixation techniques in the brucellosis eradication scheme. N.Z. Vet. J., 26, 52-56.

MICROPLATE ENZYME-LINKED IMMUNOSORBENT ASSAY FOR BOVINE LEUKAEMIA VIRUS ANTIBODY*

G. Poli[1], A. Balsari[1], A. Toniolo[1], W. Ponti[1] and G. Vacirca[2]

Istituto di Microbiologia e Immunologia Veterinaria[1] and Istituto di Patologia Speciale e Clinica Medica Veterinaria[2] Università di Milano, Milan, Italy.

ABSTRACT

A microplate enzyme-linked immunosorbent assay method was developed for the measurement of bovine immunoglobulin G antibody specific to the envelope antigen (glycoprotein 60) of bovine leukaemia virus. The test was then performed on 440 sera samples from dairy cows belonging to herds in which bovine leukaemia was suspected or which were leukaemia free and the results were compared with those obtained with the gel-diffusion technique.

* Paper in press on Journal Clinical Microbiology 13 no. 1

O.C. Straub (ed.), Fourth International Symposium on Bovine Leukosis

INTRODUCTION

Several immunological tests, such as the indirect immunofluorescence test (Ferrer et al., 1972), the Ouchterlony immunodiffusion technique (Baumgartener et al., 1975; Mammerickx et al., 1976), the complement fixation test (Miller and Van der Maaten, 1974), the radioimmunoassay (Lévy et al., 1977), and the early polykaryocytosis inhibition (Guillemain et al., 1977) are used at present for detection of antibodies against bovine leukaemia virus (BLV). None of these appears to be fully adequate for mass-screening purposes insofar as experimental ease, promptness of response, analytical reliability, and practicability are concerned.

Wc have recently proposed the use of counter-immunoelectrophoresis (Poli et al., 1980) to overcome some of the limitations of the agarose immunodiffusion technique which is, at present, the method of choice in screening herds for BLV.

This paper reports our evaluation of the enzyme-linked immunosorbent assay (ELISA) which has been shown to be a promising serodiagnostic test for other infectious diseases (Sever and Madden, 1977).

After developing a microplate ELISA technique to detect bovine immunoglobulin G antibody specific for the envelope glycoprotein 60 antigen of BLV, we performed the test first on 210 sera samples from leukaemia-free herds (as indicated by previous serological and clinical surveys) to define the upper limit for the negative population; then the ELISA was performed on 230 sera samples from dairy cows (3 to 5 years old) belonging to four different herds in which BLV infection was suspected. The same samples were tested by the Ouchterlony immunodiffusion technique, and results of the two tests were compared to determine the specificity and sensitivity of our ELISA method.

MATERIALS AND METHODS

Antigen

A purified preparation of the envelope glycoprotein 60 of BLV was supplied by Behringwerke, A.G., Marburg/Lahn, FR Germany. A working solution contained 45 µg of protein/ml in 0.1 M $NaHCO_3$, pH 9.4. The optimal concentration of antigen for the ELISA was determined by chess-board titration: twofold dilutions of the antigen were reacted with a 1 : 20 dilution of a pool of bovine sera which had been shown to be strongly positive for BLV antibody by the double-diffusion technique. The dilution of the antigen giving the highest absorbance reading, indicating saturation of binding sites on the solid phase, was chosen for performing the test.

The working solution of the antigen did not react in the ELISA with sera which were strongly positive for bovine viral diarrhoea antibody as detected by the serum neutralisation technique.

Sera

Bovine field sera and standard reference sera samples shown to be positive, weakly positive, or negative by the Ouchterlony double diffusion technique were tested. The sera were diluted 1 : 10 in phosphate-buffered saline containing 0.05% Tween 20 and 0.5% bovine serum albumin for examination by ELISA.

ELISA reagent and procedure

(i) Coating of the solid phase

Wells of Microelisa plates (Dynatech Laboratories, Inc. Alexandria, Va.) were sensitised by adding 0.2 ml of the working dilution of antigen per well. After incubation at 37°C for 3 h the wells were washed three times with a solution containing 0.05% Tween 20, 0.5% bovine serum albumin, and 0.15 M NaCl in de-ionised water (washing solution).

(ii) Enzyme-labelled anti-bovine immunoglobulins

Horseradish peroxidase (Boehringer, Mannheim) and rabbit immunoglobulin G fractions of anti-bovine immunoglobulin G, purified by diethylaminoethyl cellulose chromatography, were coupled by the periodate method of Nakane and Kawaoi (1974) which was slightly modified to obtain an approximate horseradish peroxidase/immunoglobulin G molar ratio of 2. The conjugate was purified by gel-filtration on Sephadex G 200 columns (Pharmacia, Sweden) and used in the assay at a concentration of approximately 4 μg/ml in the same diluent used for the test sera.

(iii) Substrate for the enzymatic reaction

o-Phenylenediamine dihydrochloride (2 mg) was added to 10 ml of 0.25 M phosphate-citrate buffer containing 0.02% H_2O_2, to obtain a final pH of 4.8; this solution, kept in the dark, was used within 30 minutes.

(iv) Procedure

The following scheme was used. To two wells of the microplate, coated with the antigen as described, was added 0.2 ml of a 1 : 10 dilution of each test serum. After 2 h of incubation at 37°C, the wells were washed three times with 0.35 ml/well of the washing solution. Then, 0.2 ml/well of the enzyme-labelled anti-bovine immunoglobulin was added. After 30 min of incubation at 37°C, washing occurred as just described. Next, 50 μl of the substrate/well was added. After 5 min of incubation at room temperature, 50 μl of 2 N H_2SO_4/well was added to stop the reaction. Absorbance at 492 nm was determined by Microelisa Reader AM 115 (Dynatech).

(v) Ouchterlony immunodiffusion technique

The procedure and the interpretation of the reactions were previously described (Poli et al., 1980).

RESULTS

Establishment of the working dilution of test sera for the microplate ELISA

The ideal ELISA should provide a quantitative answer derived from a single reading at a determined dilution of serum rather than from a titration curve. Besides advantages in terms of experimental ease, this could circumvent problems related to titre evaluation (measurement at levels close to the assay sensitivity limit).

We chose a working dilution of antigen at which both the high titre samples (bell-shaped curve) and the low titre samples (which influence the sensitivity and discriminating potency of the test) gave reliable results (Figure 1). In practical terms, any dilution in the range of 1 : 10 to 1 : 100 seemed suitable.

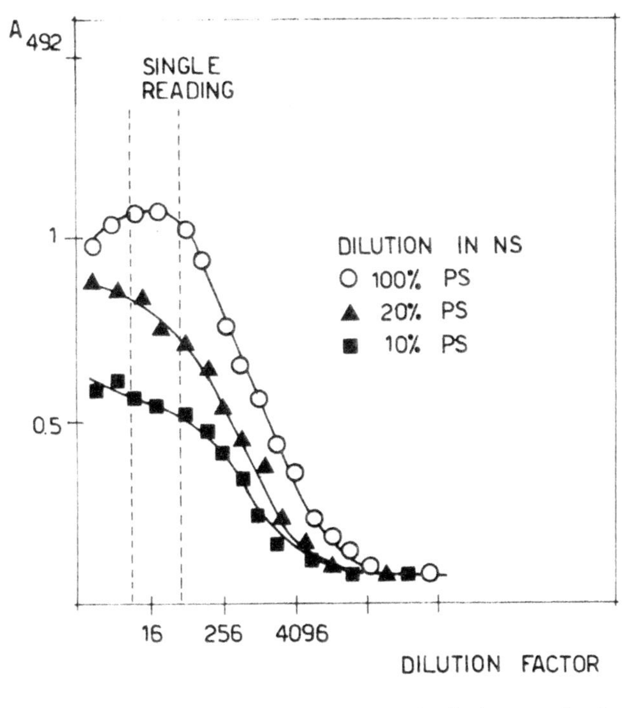

Fig. 1. Dilution curves of a positive sample (PS) increasingly diluted with a negative sample (NS) (immunoglobulin G, ELISA). Optimal dilution range is indicated by dotted lines.

Definition of negative ELISA optical density value

Two hundred and ten sera samples from leukaemia-free herds giving a negative reaction in the Ouchterlony immunodiffusion test were used to assess the normal range of ELISA values. In the ELISA system, this population gave a mean value and standard deviation (SD) of 136 ± 30 mU. Therefore, assuming a 1% probability of misclassification (i.e., $\bar{x}$ + 3 SD), the upper limit for the negative population is 224 mU.

Analysis of the sample population from herds with suspected BLV

From an analysis of the ELISA data of a test population from herds with suspected bovine leukaemia, 23 of the 230 sera samples gave negative results. The remaining 207 positive samples gave a mean value and a SD of 583 ± 172 mU in the ELISA system. This corresponds to a distribution ranging, at a 95% probability ($\bar{x}$ - 2 SD to $\bar{x}$ + 2 SD), from 237 to 927 mU, without any overlap with the previously defined negative class.

A comparison of the results with those obtained by the reference immunodiffusion technique demonstrated that (i) no ELISA-negative samples were classified as positive by the reference method, and (ii) eight ELISA-positive samples were classified as negative by the double diffusion technique. A further analysis of these eight samples gave an $\bar{x}$ and SD of 325 ± 45, with an experimental range from 254 to 380 mU and giving, at a 95% confidence limit, a range from 210 to 415 mU.

Assuming that the discrepancies with respect to the reference method are related to improved sensitivity of the ELISA method, we have tentatively assumed, for the borderline population (i.e., weakly positive), the interval reported in Table 1.

TABLE 1

CLASSIFICATION OF THE SAMPLES (n = 440) BY THE IMMUNODIFFUSION AND THE ELISA RESPONSE (mU)

Samples classification	Immunodiffusion[a]	ELISA[b]		
	No.	No.	Mean ± SD	Range
Negative	241	233	136 ± 30	<224
Borderline		8	325 ± 45	224-415
Positive	199	199	583 ± 172	>415

[a] Identity precipitation bands were classified as positive regardless of the type, intensity, or position of the band.

[b] Optical densities values; SD, standard deviation.

CONCLUSIONS

Two conclusions emerge from these results: (i) the ELISA method is valid for the detection of the BLV antibody, showing substantial agreement in terms of positive and negative samples with the immunodiffusion technique, and (ii) the data can be expressed as single readings which provide a quantitative answer. On the other hand, the immunodiffusion technique (which is the most widely used for BLV serodiagnosis) gives an all-or-nothing response. Moreover, despite the small number of samples examined, it is possible to assume tentatively a range of values for a borderline population so that the samples can be clearly classified by the ELISA method as either negative, weakly positive, or positive.

REFERENCES

Baumgartener, L.E., Olson, C., Miller, J.M. and Van der Maaten, M.J., 1975. Survey for antibodies to leukemia (C-type) virus in cattle. J. Amer. Vet. Med. Ass. 166: 249-251.

Ferrer, J.F., Avila, L. and Stock, N.D., 1972. Serological detection of type C viruses found in bovine cultures. Cancer Res. 32: 1864-1870.

Guillemain, B., Mamoun, R., Levy, D., Astier, T., Irgens, K. and Parodi, A.L., 1977. Early polykaryocytosis inhibition: a simple quantitative *in vitro* assay for the detection of bovine leukemia virus infection in cattle. Eur. J. Cancer 14: 811-827.

Lévy, D., Deshayes, L., Parodi, A.L., Lévy, J.P., Stephenson, J.R., Devare, S.G. and Gilden, R.V., 1977. Bovine leukemia virus specific antibodies among French cattle. II. Radioimmunoassay with the major structural protein (BLV p24). Int. J. Cancer 20: 543-550.

Mammerickx, M., Portelle, D., Kettmann, R., Ghysdael, J., Burny, A. and Dekegel, D., 1976. Diagnostic test of bovine leukemia. Comparison between a hematological test and the serological diagnosis. Eur. J. Cancer 12: 433-439.

Miller, J.M. and Van der Maaten, M.J., 1974. A complement fixation test for the bovine leukemia (C-type) virus. J. Natl. Cancer Inst. 53: 1699-1702.

Nakane, P.K. and Kawaoi, A., 1974. Peroxidase-labeled antibody: a new method of conjugation. J. Histochem. Cytochem. 22: 1084-1086.

Poli, G., Pozza, O., Ponti, W., Balsari, A. and Vacirca, G., 1980. Application of counterimmunoelectrophoresis for a rapid serodiagnosis of enzootic bovine leukosis. Br. Vet. J. 136: 51-55.

Sever, J.L. and Madden, D.L., 1977. Enzyme linked immunosorbent assay (ELISA) for infectious agents. J. Infect. Dis. 136 (Suppl.): S258-S340.

GENERAL DISCUSSION

R.J. Lorenz *(FRG)*

I would like to ask Dr. Behrens on what he bases his assertion that the ELISA technique is 100 times more sensitive than the IDT.

F. Behrens *(FRG)*

We made a quantitative assay of the ID test on 32 animals from one infected herd. We got titres in the ID test, the highest dilution which showed the specific precipitation line, and compared them with the titres we got in the ELISA technique. In the ELISA our titres were obtained by dilution, not as described by Dr. Poli.

R.J. Lorenz

I think the relative sensitivity of one method against another is still open to discussion.

B. Guillemain *(France)*

I would suggest that the value of a titre has nothing to do with the sensitivity; it is something which varies. You can have a value of 0.05 which will compare well with 10 000 in another system.

F. Behrens

That is right, but if you detect more positives, that is another way to differentiate between the different sensitivities, or where ELISA shows a superior sensitivity. There are two facts that show that ELISA is more sensitive. One is the higher titres; the second is that we detect more positive animals with the ELISA technique in comparison with the ID test.

R. Hoff-Jørgensen *(Denmark)*

The important question is how many more infected animals did you find using the ELISA technique?

F. Behrens

4.6% of infected herds were more positive in the ELISA technique in comparison with the immunodiffusion test.

J.F. Ferrer *(USA)*

How do we know that the animals that are positive in the ELISA test and negative in the ID test are not giving false positive results?

A.A. Ressang *(Netherlands)*

That is the crucial question - how do we prove the specificity of the ELISA.

F. Behrens

One way is the comparison with the anti-complement immunofluorescence test which also detects some positive sera where the ID is negative. We checked certain sera that were positive only in the ELISA technique and did a neutralisation with the pure p24 and gp antigens. We were then able to reduce the titre by this procedure of pre-incubation with pure antigen.

M. Mussgay *(FRG)*

I am coming back to this 4.6%. It is 4.6% more in July. If you go back to this herd now, will it be 4.6%, or zero? From my point of view what happens in four or six months is very important.

F. Behrens

We only have data on what happened after one month with this particular herd which was under survey for one year. There we saw that the ELISA positive animals all became positive in the ID test.

M. Mussgay

Therefore it is very sensitive.

G.H. Theilen *(USA)*

We did not have time to discuss Dr. Rutili's paper that dealt with sequential studies over a period of time. We have been doing this for years in the feline system and I think before you can analyse a test it has to be done sequentially over a period of years. I would like to corroborate what Dr. Mussgay has said because this is extremely important in analysing a test.

D.H. Roberts *(UK)*

There are times when even the agar gel immunodiffusion test is a little bit too sensitive. With at least one in a thousand you do get inconclusive results. What we want is not a sensitive test; we just want a reliable test in any circumstances.

A.A. Ressang

That's right. You hear about the big discrepancy between the ELISA and the AGID tests. The question arises, how do you perform the AGID, because the gel diffusion test is called insensitive but there are two exceptions - equine infectious anaemia and enzootic bovine leukosis. These are the two exceptions in which the AGID is very very sensitive.

SESSION V

Transmission (I)

Chairmen : M. Van der Maaten and C. Olson

FACTORS AFFECTING THE TRANSMISSION OF BOVINE LEUKAEMIA VIRUS FROM COWS TO THEIR OFFSPRING

M.J. Van Der Maaten, Janice M. Miller and M.J.F. Schmerr

National Animal Disease Center, Agricultural Research, Science and Education Administration, US Department of Agriculture, PO Box 70, Ames, Iowa 50010, USA

ABSTRACT

Bovine leukaemia virus (BLV) control programmes that do not involve the immediate removal of all infected cows from a herd tend to focus considerable attention on the potential for virus transmission from cows to their calves. Previous studies have indicated that in utero infections with BLV are relatively infrequent, but it was not always clear whether the calves had been kept in isolation for a sufficient time after birth to allow for the identification of latent infections or infections which may have been initiated late in gestation or during birth. We collected 18 calves from cows persistently infected with BLV and found all calves to be negative for BLV antibodies at birth. The first four calves were not carefully washed at birth and were reared in a building where BLV infected cattle were kept. Three of these calves subsequently became infected, probably as a result of contact infection. The other 14 calves were washed and removed to individual pens in a building where there were no BLV infected cattle and none became infected.

To determine the effect of a BLV infection initiated during gestation on the frequency of in utero transmission of BLV, 15 BLV free pregnant cows were inoculated with blood from a BLV infected donor. All cows became infected as a result of this inoculation. One cow aborted 38 days after inoculation, but there was no evidence that the abortion was BLV related. The other 14 cows carried their calves to term. One cow gave birth to twin calves, one dead and one live, both of which were BLV infected. The other 13 cows delivered calves that were not BLV infected at birth and did not become infected in one year. These results indicate that calves born to BLV infected cows:

1. *are only rarely infected in utero,*

O.C. Straub (ed.), Fourth International Symposium on Bovine Leukosis

2. *do not harbour latent BLV which is activated within 12 months after birth,*

3. *are not infected with BLV during the birth process,*

4. *can be successfully reared free of BLV infection if care is exercised at the time of birth and the animals are isolated from BLV infected cattle.*

Another matter to be considered if calves from BLV infected cows are to be retained in the herd is the advisability of feeding them colostrum from their dam. To test the effect of colostral antibody on infection of neonatal calves, 3 pairs of calves were fed BLV antibody positive colsotrum with 10^7, 10^8 *or* 10^9 *admixed BLV infected blood lymphocytes. None of these calves became infected. One pair of control calves was given* 10^6 *BLV infected lymphocytes suspended in colostrum which did not contain BLV antibodies and both became infected. One of a pair of newborn calves given an intradermal inoculation of BLV infected lymphocytes at the time of the first feeding of BLV antibody positive colostrum developed a persistent virus infection. These results indicate that there is a marked protective effect of colostral antibody in neonatal calves.*

In related studies, it was found that the pH of sour milk was sufffficient to prevent virus production by BLV infected lymphocytes. Thus, the practice of feeding pooled sour colostrum to young calves would not seem to constitute a potential source of BLV infection.

INTRODUCTION

A longstanding concern that calves born to bovine leukaemia virus (BLV) infected cows represent a serious problem in BLV control and eradication programmes is evidenced by requirements in some eradication programmes that the most recent offspring be removed from the herd along with the infected cow (Mitscherlich et al., 1976). Later, as reports appeared indicating that only a few of the calves born to infected cows were BLV infected (Ferrer et al., 1976; Piper et al., 1979), these requirements were dropped. These events occurred at a time when BLV control and eradication programmes required the immediate slaughter of infected cattle, thus limiting the number of potentially infected calves on any given farm. It now seems likely, however, that producers in the USA may enter into less drastic BLV control programmes in which infected herds are divided into isolated BLV negative and BLV positive groups of animals maintained on the same farm. Furthermore, in an effort to maintain genetic lines and provide additional BLV negative replacement animals, many producers may wish to rear BLV negative herd replacements using calves born to BLV infected cows. In such situations, there may be large groups of calves from BLV infected dams reared on some farms. It seemed worthwhile, therefore, to extend some of the previous studies of *in utero* transmission of BLV and evaluate other calf rearing practices in an effort to develop some general recommendations for calf rearing in such situations. Our investigations included:

1. Observations of calves born to cows with pre-existing persistent BLV infections or calves born to cows infected with BLV during gestation.
2. Evaluation of the effectiveness of colostral antibody in protecting newborn calves from BLV infection.
3. Studies of various factors which might influence the quantity of BLV infectivity present in the colostrum or milk from infected cows.

MATERIALS AND METHODS

Serological tests

The glycoprotein agar gel immunodiffusion (gpAGID) test was conducted as described by Miller and Van der Maaten (1977). The radioimmunoprecipitation assays for antibodies to BLV antigens were conducted as previously described (Miller et al., in press). Virus neutralisation tests were done as described by Van der Maaten et al.(in press).

Virological tests

Syncytium induction tests were done with bovine embryonic spleen indicator monolayers or F-81 indicator monolayers as previously described (Diglio et al., 1978; Van der Maaten et al., in press). A previously described water lysis technique (Stock and Ferrer, 1972) was used to prepare the large numbers of leukocytes for sheep inoculation to test for infectivity in blood. In this instance, 2.94×10^8 leukocytes were inoculated intraperitoneally into a sheep and the sheep was tested for BLV specific antibodies at monthly intervals with the gpAGID test to determine whether an infection had been initiated.

Inocula

For routine use as virus inocula, blood was collected from an isolation reared donor steer persistently infected with BLV and known to be free of bovine viral diarrhoea virus. In some of the milk studies, peripheral blood lymphocytes were also obtained from other donors persistently infected with BLV. Lymphocytes were separated from blood using a ficoll-hypaque technique (Van der Maaten et al., in press).

Experimental animals

The 18 calves born during the initial studies (Experiment 1) of *in utero* transmission of BLV came from Holstein cows infected with BLV prior to breeding. One of the four calves involved in the first year of this study was delivered by Caesarean section.

These 4 calves were removed from their dams at birth and placed in pens in a building where BLV infected cattle were kept. The calves were fed 500 ml of colostrum from BLV negative cows. The Caesarean derived calf was kept in an individual pen. The other three calves were penned together after they were about 2 weeks old and, when BLV specific antibodies were detected, the infected individual was removed from the pen. The 14 calves involved in the second year of the study were removed from their dams at birth, washed with warm water, dried and placed into individual isolation pens in a building where no BLV infected cattle were kept. They were fed 500 ml of colostrum from BLV negative cows. The calves were kept in these isolation pens for 1 year. One of the dams in this group had tumorous leukosis at the time she calved. In a subsequent study (Experiment 2), 15 pregnant BLV free Jersey cows were purchased from farm herds. The cows were selected so that 1/3 were in the first trimester, 1/3 in the second trimester and 1/3 in the third trimester of pregnancy. The cows were infected with BLV by the intravenous inoculation of 100 ml of whole blood from the BLV infected donor described above.

Calves used to test the potential protective effect of colostral antibody were obtained from BLV negative cows in a research herd at our institute.

Milk and colostrum

These were obtained from BLV infected or BLV free cows in a research herd at our institute or from selected cows in farm herds. Pasteurised whole milk was purchased from a commercial dairy. Milk and colostrum were soured by placing the fresh products into a $37^{o}C$ incubator for 24 hours. Whey was separated from milk products by centrifugation at 40 000 g for 60 min. The clarified whey was sterilised by passing it through a 0.22 μ membrane filter.

Pooled positive colostrum consisted of the first two milkings from 3 BLV infected cows. This was frozen and thawed twice and then frozen and stored until use. The presence of BLV specific antibodies in this material was confirmed by gpAGID tests. The pooled colostrum was fed to 2 calves to test for residual infectivity.

Infectivity tests

For oral infectivity tests (Experiment 3), the predetermined number of peripheral blood lymphocytes was suspended in 500 ml pooled colostrum and immediately fed to a 4 to 6 hour old calf that had been given no oral fluids since birth. Calves were fed an additional 500 ml of pooled colostrum, without admixed lymphocytes, 4 - 6 hours later. Two 4 to 6 hour old calves were given intradermal inoculations of 2.5×10^5 BLV infected blood lymphocytes and fed colostrum (without admixed lymphocytes) as described above.

Tests of effects of pH or freezing on BLV infectivity

Peripheral blood lymphocytes isolated by ficoll-hypaque flotation were suspended in fresh whey, soured whey or tissue culture media at pH 7.2 or 3.5 and held at ambient temperature for 24 hours. Lymphocyte suspensions in milk products or tissue culture media were frozen in a -30°C freezer and then allowed to thaw at ambient temperature. The infectivity of these preparations was tested using F-81 indicator cells as described above (Van der Maaten et al., in press).

RESULTS

None of the four calves born during the first year of the *in utero* infectivity study (Experiment 1) was BLV infected at birth, but only one of these animals remained BLV antibody negative throughout the 1 year of observation. The other 3 calves became seropositive at 2, 5 and 8 months of age, respectively, and all remained seropositive on subsequent monthly tests, indicating that they had persistent BLV infections. The calf that had BLV specific antibodies at 2 months of age had been delivered by Caesarean section. The 14 calves born to

BLV infected dams during the second year of the study were not infected with BLV at birth and monthly serological tests and syncytium induction tests of the 13 calves that survived for 1 year indicated that all remained uninfected.

All 15 pregnant Jersey cows inoculated with BLV in Experiment 2 became infected. Both serological and virological test results were positive for all cows before parturition with the exception of the first cow to calve. She was virus positive but not yet antibody positive at the time her calf was born 20 days after inoculation. One cow aborted on the 38th day after inoculation. BLV was not isolated from the foetus nor were BLV specific antibodies present in the foetal blood, so the abortion was not considered to be BLV related. The remaining 14 cows gave birth to single live calves except for one cow that delivered twin calves, one live and one dead, 188 days after she was inoculated with BLV. On the basis of serological tests, the twins were considered to be BLV infected at birth and the survivor remained positive in serological and virological tests conducted during the 1 year of observation. Three of the remaining 13 calves died during the observation period, but serological tests of these animals up to the time of death indicated that they were not BLV infected. The 10 calves that survived for 1 year were BLV free as determined by serological and virological tests.

In preliminary studies for Experiment 3, the two calves that were fed the frozen and thawed, pooled colostrum from BLV positive cows, did not become infected. Two other calves, fed 10^6 BLV infected lymphocytes suspended in colostrum devoid of BLV specific antibodies, both became infected.

In further studies (Experiment 3), pairs of calves were fed 10^7, 10^8 or 10^9 BLV infected lymphocytes that were suspended in BLV antibody positive colostrum. Passive antibody was detected by gpAGID tests in these calves for 2 to 4 months, but the animals were BLV antibody negative in gpAGID tests thereafter. All six calves were tested for BLV using a syncytium induction technique when they were 12 months old, and the results were negative. Sera collected from four of the six animals were tested for BLV specific antibodies using a glycoprotein radioimmunoprecipitation technique. Three of the four animals were negative in this test at 12 months of age, the fourth animal had a low level of BLV specific antibodies. Tests of other monthly samples from this animal indicated that the level of antibodies was constantly decreasing, so these were considered to be residual colostral antibodies. On the basis of the above findings, the calves were considered to be BLV free.

Only one of 2 calves that was given an intradermal inoculation of BLV and fed BLV antibody positive colostrum was protected from infection. Antibody levels in the non-protected calf decreased until about 4 months after birth and then increased markedly and remained positive through the rest of the year of observation (Table 1). Repeated attempts to isolate virus from this calf (8531) using syncytium induction tests gave negative results, but the inoculation of a large number of peripheral blood leukocytes from this calf into a sheep proved that the calf was persistently infected with BLV.

Results of gpAGID tests of colostrum and milk from two BLV infected cows indicate that significant quantities of BLV specific antibodies are present in mammary secretions for several days after parturition (Table 2).

The detrimental effect of freeze-thaw cycles on the infectivity of peripheral blood leukocytes suspended in tissue culture media or various milk products, with or without BLV specific antibody, is clearly indicated by results presented in Table 3. Other tests indicated that the exposure of peripheral blood leukocytes to the low pH of soured milk products for 24 hours at ambient temperature (65°F) is sufficient to destroy BLV infectivity (Table 4).

TABLE 1

COMPARISON OF GLYCOPROTEIN AGAR GEL IMMUNODIFFUSION (gpAGID) TEST RESULTS AND TITRES OBTAINED IN VIRUS NEUTRALISATION (VN) OR RADIOIMMUNOASSAYS (RIA) OF SERA FROM CALF 8531 AFTER THE INTRADERMAL INOCULATION OF BLV INFECTED LYMPHOCYTES AND INGESTION OF COLOSTRUM CONTAINING BLV SPECIFIC ANTIBODIES

Test method	Pre-colostral	Post-colostral	Test results (Months Post-inoculation)							
			1	2	3	4	5	6	7	12
VN	< 2*	16	4	4	4	16	≥ 64	≥ 64	32	...
RIA	0	300ϕ	120	80	40	20	3000	340	80	27
gpAGID	-	+ϕϕ	+	+	+	-	+	+	+	+

* Indicates the reciprocal of the serum dilution which completely inhibited syncytium formation by the test virus.

ϕ Indicates the reciprocal of the serum dilution that binds 20% of the labelled antigen

** Indicates a negative serological response

ϕϕ Indicates a positive serological response

TABLE 2

RESULTS OF GLYCOPROTEIN AGAR GEL IMMUNODIFFUSION (gpAGID) TESTS FOR BOVINE LEUKAEMIA VIRUS (BLV) ANTIBODIES IN MAMMARY SECRETIONS FROM BLV INFECTED COWS DURING THE POSTPARTUM PERIOD

Cow no.	Test results (days postpartum)								
	0	1	2	3	4	5	6	14	21
93	+*	+	+	+	+	+	-	-	-
1204	+	+	+	-	-	-	-	-	-

*+ indicates positive gpAGID test result

- indicates negative gpAGID test result

TABLE 3

TESTS FOR BOVINE LEUKAEMIA VIRUS (BLV) INFECTIVITY IN PERIPHERAL BLOOD LYMPHOCYTES (PBL)* THAT WERE SUSPENDED IN VARIOUS MEDIA AND FROZEN AND THAWED

Suspending medium	Number of freeze-thaw cycles	Syncytium-induction test result[Φ]
Whey from pasteurised commercial milk	1	-[ΦΦ]
Whey from 7445 BLV-P** milk	1	-
Whey from 7296 BLV-P colostrum	1	-
Whey from 463 BLV-N milk	1	-
Whey from 463 BLV-N milk	2	-
Whey from 463 BLV-N milk	3	-
Tissue culture medium	1	-

* In tests of doubling dilutions of the fresh unfrozen lymphocytes, syncytia were found in wells inoculated with 4 000 but not in wells inoculated with 2 000 lymphocytes.

Φ For syncytium-induction tests, 10^6, 5.0×10^5 or 2.5×10^5 PBL were inoculated into each of 3 test wells.

ΦΦ Indicates that no BLV specific syncytia were present.

** BLV-P indicates mammary secretions obtained from a BLV infected cow. BLV-N indicates mammary secretions obtained from a BLV free cow.

TABLE 4

TESTS FOR BOVINE LEUKAEMIA VIRUS (BLV) INFECTIVITY IN PERIPHERAL BLOOD LYMPHOCYTES (PBL) SUSPENDED AT A CONCENTRATION OF 10^7/ ml IN VARIOUS MEDIA AND KEPT AT AMBIENT TEMPERATURE FOR 24 HOURS

PBL donor animal	Suspending medium	pH	Syncytium-induction test result*
8549	Tissue culture medium	3.5	-**
8549	Tissue culture medium	7.2	+
8549	BLV-N$^{\phi}$ 1195 Whey (fresh)	6.9	+
8549	BLV-N 1195 Whey (sour)	3.8	-
8549	BLV-N 258 Whey (fresh)	6.7	+
8549	BLV-N 119 Whey (sour)	4.4	-
7290	Tissue culture medium	3.5	-
7290	Tissue culture medium	7.2	+
7290	BLV-N 1195 Whey (fresh)	6.9	+
7290	BLV-N 1195 Whey (sour)	3.8	-
7290	BLV-N 258 Whey (fresh)	6.7	+
7290	BLV-N 119 Whey (sour)	4.4	-
7826	Tissue culture medium	7.2	+
7826	Phosphate buffered saline	7.5	+
7826	BLV-N 1195 Whey (sour)	3.8	-
7826	BLV-N 258 Whey (fresh)	6.7	+
7826	BLV-N 119 Whey (sour)	4.4	-

* For syncytium-induction tests 10^6, 5.0×10^5 or 2.5×10^5 PBL were inoculated into each of 3 test wells.

** + indicates that BLV specific syncytia were present in all test wells.
- indicates that no BLV specific syncytia were present.

ϕ BLV-N indicates mammary secretions from a BLV free cow.

DISCUSSION

The identification of *in utero* BLV infections in fewer than 6% of the calves born to BLV infected dams is in close agreement with results reported for other studies of cattle in farm herds (Ferrer et al., 1976). There was no evidence that significant numbers of unavoidable infections occurred during parturition or immediately thereafter. It is apparent, however, from results obtained during the first year of the study, when 3 of 4 calves developed BLV infections, that considerable care must be used in the handling of newborn calves. In this group of calves, it is most likely that the Caesarean derived calf was infected by exposure to maternal blood during the surgery. The calf was not washed after birth, and the detection of a serological response when the calf was 2 months old indicates that infection occurred when the calf was quite young. The other two infected calves developed BLV antibodies at 5 and 8 months of age. It seems most likely that these animals were infected by contact with BLV in the barn where they were kept. However, we have not had a problem with contact transmissions among older cattle in this facility, so young animals may be particularly susceptible to contact infection. This is, therefore, an important factor to consider when attempts are made to devise practical programmes for use in farm herds. The indications that sanitation and isolation are important when attempting to rear calves from BLV infected dams is supported by observations during the second year of the study when a considerable effort was made to be certain that calves were promptly removed from their dams and the calves were washed to remove infective material from their skin. These procedures and the removal of the calves to individual pens in a barn where there were no BLV infected cattle seems to have prevented contact transmission.

Inoculation of pregnant cows with BLV provided proof that the initiation of a BLV infection during gestation did not greatly affect the prevalence of *in utero* BLV infections. It is also apparent that the BLV infection had little effect on the course of the pregnancy, thus agreeing with epidemiological studies (Langston et al., 1978) indicating that BLV infection did not influence reproductive efficiency. The year-long isolation and testing of the calves, with negative results, indicates that there were no latent BLV infections established *in utero* which were activated within 1 year.

The effectiveness of colostral antibody in protecting calves against oral exposure to BLV is evident from the results of our tests of colostrum with admixed BLV infected lymphocytes. Results of the preliminary studies in which 2 calves were infected by 10^6 BLV infected lymphocytes suspended in colostrum devoid of BLV antibodies indicate that the anti BLV activity is not due to some non-specific action of colostrum on lymphocytes. It should also be recognised that the inoculum of 10^6 lymphocytes was chosen arbitrarily and does not represent a minimal oral infectious dose of BLV. Nevertheless, the colostrum that contained BLV specific antibodies protected calves against oral doses of 10^7, 10^8 or 10^9 BLV infected lymphocytes. It is likely that any colostrum which contains sufficient antibody to be detected by gpAGID will have a protective effect far in excess of its infectivity, because it has been shown that only a very few lymphocytes are present in colostrum from normal cows (Lee et al., 1980; McDonald and Anderson, in press). Furthermore, the negative test results we obtained with 3 of 4 colostrum samples tested for BLV infectivity by sheep inoculation (Miller and Van der Maaten, 1979) would indicate that only limited infectivity was present. The failure of the frozen and thawed, pooled colostrum from BLV infected cows, to infect two test calves provides additional evidence that colostrum is probably not highly infectious for calves. The results of the above tests in calves and the demonstrated detrimental effect of freezing and thawing on peripheral blood lymphocytes suspended in various media indicates that there would be only minimal risk of infecting newborn calves by feeding frozen and thawed colostrum obtained from BLV infected cows. This feeding method could be exploited, therefore to provide passive antibodies to susceptible newborn calves. Our studies indicate that these antibodies would protect against oral exposures to BLV. The protective effect of passive antibody against other types of exposure to BLV was less complete, and a potential danger of creating latent BLV infections should also be recognised.

The inactivation of BLV infectivity by soured milk or colostrum, probably due to the low pH of these products, indicates that the practice of feeding pooled soured colostrum would not have a detrimental effect on calf rearing programmes designed to control and eradicate BLV infections. These findings contradict earlier conclusions, based on herd tests, that pooled soured colostrum might be a source of infective BLV (Seger and Morgan, 1976).

In conclusion, it seems that a variety of programmes, ranging from isolation rearing of calves to the intentional feeding of colostrum known to contain BLV specific antibodies, could be devised for use in specific farm situations where BLV eradication or control is desired. In all instances, appropriate serological, and in some instances virological, tests would also have to be used to identify infected calves. It should be clearly understood, however, that the possibility for success of such programmes applied in farm situations is still a matter of conjecture, at the present time, because the studies on which these recommendations are based have been conducted under closely controlled experimental conditions. It remains to be determined how successfully these laboratory findings can, or will, be applied to solve practical herd problems.

ACKNOWLEDGMENT

The technical assistance of Ms. Roberta Vegors, Ms. Katherine Goodwin, Mr. Stephen Hay and Mr. Kevin Raisch in conducting these studies is gratefully achnowledged.

REFERENCES

Diglio, C.A., Piper, C. and Ferrer, J.F., 1978. An improved syncytia infectivity assay for the bovine leukemia virus. In Vitro, 14: 502-505.

Ferrer, J.F., Piper, C.E., Abt, D.A., Marshak, R.R. and Bhatt, D.M., 1976. Natural mode of transmission of bovine C-type virus (BLV). Bibl. Haematol, 43: 235-237.

Langston, A., Ferdinand, G.A.A., Ruppanner, R., Theilen, G.H., Drlica, S. and Behmyer, D., 1978. Comparison of production variables of bovine leukemia virus antibody-negative and antibody-positive cows in two California dairy herds. Am. J. Vet. Res., 39: 1093-1098.

Lee, C.H., Wooding, F.B.P. and Kemp, P., 1980. Identification, properties, and differential counts of cell populations using electron microscopy of dry cow secretions, colostrum and milk from normal cows. J. Dairy Res., 47: 39-50.

McDonald, J.S. and Anderson, A.J., In press. Total and differential somatic cell counts in secretions from non-infected bovine mammary glands: The peripartum period. Am. J. Vet. Res.

Miller, J.M. and Van der Maaten, M.J., 1977. Use of glycoprotein antigen in the immunodiffusion test for bovine leukemia virus antibodies. Eur. J. Cancer, 13: 1369-1375.

Miller, J.M. and Van der Maaten, M.J., 1979. Infectivity tests of secretions and excretions from cattle infected with bovine leukemia virus. J. Natl. Cancer Inst., 62: 425-428.

Miller, J.M., Schmerr, M.J.F. and Van der Maaten, M.J., In press Comparison of four serologic tests for the detection of antibodies to bovine leukemia virus. Am. J. Vet. Res.

Mitscherlich, E., Plünnecke, A., Schmidt, F.W. and Albrecht, A., 1976. Techniques and results of immunodiffusion test in field trials. Vet. Microbiol., 1: 219-230; O.C. Straub (Ed.), Elsevier Scientific Publishing Company, Amsterdam and CEC, Luxembourg.

Piper, C.E., Ferrer, J.F., Abt, D.A. and Marshak, R.R., 1979. Postnatal and prenatal transmission of the bovine leukemia virus under natural conditions. J. Natl. Cancer Inst., 62: 165-168.

Seger, C.L. and Morgan, D., 1976. Differential incidence of bovine leukemia virus (BLV) antibody in yearling herdmates nursed on milk replacer or pooled sour colostrum. In: A. Burny (Editor), Bovine Leukosis: Various methods of molecular virology. Commission of the European Communities, Luxembourg, pp. 267-269.

Stock, N.D. and Ferrer, J.F., 1972. Replicating C-type virus in phytohemagglutinin-treated buffy-coat cultures of bovine origin. J. Natl. Cancer Inst., 48: 985-996.

Van der Maaten, M.J. and Miller, J.M., 1980. Use of a continuous feline cell line for virologic and serologic investigations of bovine leukemia virus infections. Am. J. Vet. Res. 41: 1785-1788.

DISCUSSION

F.-W. Schmidt *(FRG)*

What would you consider to be a safe separation of the groups of adult animals? Secondly, for how long did you observe the calves that received positive colostrum and, afterwards, inoculum of blood? Was it just for 12 months?

M.J. van der Maaten *(USA)*

At the end of the one year we terminated the experiment as far as the observation of calves was concerned. However, a number of those calves are still alive, a number are 18 months old now. We have run those through other experiments later on but when we went into those experiments those calves were still negative.

With regard to the separation of the cows, we are thinking in terms that if we are going to have negative and positive groups of cows on the same farm we would like to see about 60 ft between pens. Now, we realise that in a practical situation where they are milking in a milking parlour, they will run the negatives through the first and then the positives because they are not going to build two milking parlours.

B.S. Samagh *(Canada)*

At what age after birth were the calves treated?

M.J. van der Maaten

About 4 to 6 hours. They seemed to be born during the night. We wanted to give the entire 500 ml; we did not want to go in there 20 minutes after birth when the calves would only drink 100 ml and have to sit and wait with the suspension of lymphocytes. The lymphocytes were put in the positive colostrum and that was fed immediately. The calves drank that within 5 or 10 minutes. They were hand fed with a nipple actually.

F. Bürki *(Austria)*

I will be less optimistic in my report tomorrow. Under natural conditions we have a negative selection of cows which are positive and give birth to calves, and the outcome is not so favourable as yours. You have experimentally infected yours. Maybe there will be time to discuss this tomorrow.

D.R. Roberts *(UK)*

What do you regard as the minimal infective dose in terms of numbers of lymphocytes?

M.J. van der Maaten

We took 2 500 lymphocytes from the particular donor animal and got infection after intradermal application. That is really the only information I have got.

C. Olson *(USA)*

Do you have evidence of another donor having a different level of lymphocytes infective?

M.J. van der Maaten

No, that is the only BVD negative donor we have, so we use it all the time!

A.A. Ressang *(Netherlands)*

My question is related to the second question asked by Dr. Schmidt. If you are compelled to keep a calf from a leukotic cow for some reason, and you have the opportunity to follow up this calf serologically and virologically, for how long should you observe this calf before you can say it is in the clear?

M.J. van der Maaten

I don't think I can answer that question. We followed these animals for 12 months and they were negative but I have no proof that they would not have been positive at two years of age. I don't think they would be, but I have no proof of that.

G.H. Theilen *(USA)*

May I clear up one point? You mentioned putting the negative cows through the milking parlour first. Has that been done, in fact, or are you suggesting that it should be done?

M.J. van der Maaten

We did that with a herd in Kansas. Janice Miller reported on that a couple of years ago. We did not have a lot of transmission. The results have been published.

O.C. Straub *(FRG)*

We have kept some of our animals from positive dams for three years now; so far we had one that came out in the third year. It had been positive after the intake of colostrum until 7 months of age.

A STUDY OF THE NATURAL TRANSMISSION OF BOVINE LEUKAEMIA VIRUS: PRELIMINARY RESULTS*

M.C. Thurmond and M.J. Burridge
Department of Preventive Medicine,
College of Veterinary Medicine, University of Florida,
Gainesville, Florida 32610, USA.

ABSTRACT

A prospective observational study was undertaken to investigate possible factors associated with the natural transmission of bovine leukaemia virus (BLV) in calves. The study was initiated in July 1979 in a Florida dairy herd, which had a BLV antibody prevalence of over 75% in animals over 18 months of age. The BLV antibody status was determined precolostrally, postcolostrally, and at monthly intervals for every calf born and followed. Infection status was based upon seroconversion using the agar gel immunodiffusion test with a glycoprotein antigen. Factors examined for a possible association with BLV infection were age, breed, season of year, BLV status of the dam at birth, season of birth, and BLV antibody status of colostrum ingested. The results of 15 months of observations and 336 calvings are presented.

*Supported by United States Department of Agriculture cooperative agreement 58-519B-0-872.

O.C. Straub (ed.), Fourth International Symposium on Bovine Leukosis

INTRODUCTION

Bovine leukaemia virus (BLV) infection poses an important threat to the export of cattle and semen from the United States (Mix, 1979; Miller, 1980). It is necessary, therefore, that practical programmes for the control and/or eradication of BLV be created. A prerequisite to the establishment of such programmes is a clear understanding of the natural mode of transmission of BLV, which is presently lacking (Burny et al., 1980). Consequently, a detailed epidemiological investigation was designed to define the mode of natural transmission in a Florida dairy herd. This paper presents some preliminary results of that study.

MATERIALS AND METHODS

The animals studied included all calves born alive and retained in the 200 plus University of Florida Dairy Research Unit herd. In this herd, over 75% of animals over 18 months of age had antibodies to BLV (Burridge et al., 1979). Serum samples were collected from all dams at the time of parturition and from calves precolostrally, at 2 days of age, and at monthly intervals from 1 month of age. After the precolostral sample was taken, calves were fed 1 - 2 litres of colostrum from their own dam. No interventions were made in the routine management of calves.

Infection with BLV was based upon the presence of persisting antibodies to BLV, as determined by the agar gel immunodiffusion test, using a glycoprotein antigen (Leukassay-B, Pitman-Moore Inc., Washington Crossing, New Jersey). The test was performed as described by Burridge et al. (1979). Information recorded for each calf included the following: breed, birth date, parity of the dam, BLV antibody status of the dam, and BLV antibody status of the colostrum ingested. The BLV antibody status of colostrum was based upon seroconversion of the calf at 2 days of age. Incidence rates for BLV seroconversion were calculated as the number of animals seroconverting in a period divided by the average number of BLV negative animals during that period.

Associations of parity of the dam and season of year born to BLV infection of calves were tested using a chi-square procedure which calculated exact P values (Agresti et al., 1979). A chi-square procedure, which corrected for continuity (Snedecor and Cochran, 1967), was used to test for independence between BLV infected calves and BLV antibody status of colostrum ingested, BLV status of the dam, and breed.

RESULTS

From July 1979 through September 1980, 296 calves had been born alive. Of the 183 calves followed, one (0.5%) was infected precolostrally, and 15 seroconverted between birth and 6 months of age. There were 141 calves born to BLV positive cows and 42 born to BLV negative cows. At the end of September 1980, 63 calves had colostral antibodies to BLV and 104 calves were serologically negative.

No significant association was found between parity of the dam and BLV infection in the offspring ($P = 0.66$, Table 1) or between season born and BLV infection ($P = 0.8$, Table 2). No significant difference was found between the proportion of Jersey calves infected (4/30) and the proportion of Holstein calves infected (11/89) ($P = 1.0$), or between the proportion of infected calves from BLV positive dams (9/80) and the proportion from BLV negative dams (6/39) ($P = 0.73$), or between the proportion of calves consuming BLV positive colostrum (9/79) and the proportion consuming BLV negative colostrum (6/40) ($P = 79$).

The incidence rate of BLV seroconversion was greatest in the third month of life and declined to zero by the seventh month. Of the 7 calves seroconverting within 3 months of age, 6 had been born to BLV negative dams. No seroconversions were seen in animals over 6 months of age (Figure 1). The incidence rate was zero in the months from July to October, and highest in November and December (Figure 2).

TABLE 1

RELATIONSHIP OF BLV INFECTION STATUS OF CALVES TO PARITY OF DAM IN THE UNIVERSITY OF FLORIDA DAIRY RESEARCH UNIT HERD FROM JULY 1979 TO SEPTEMBER 1980

Parity of dam	BLV infection status of calves +	-	Total
1	5	42	47
2	6	25	31
3	2	18	20
4	2	19	21
Total	15	104	119

$\chi^2 = 1.75$ $(P = 0.66)$

TABLE 2

RELATIONSHIP OF BLV INFECTION STATUS OF CALVES TO SEASON BORN IN THE UNIVERSITY OF FLORIDA DAIRY RESEARCH UNIT HERD FROM JULY 1979 TO SEPTEMBER 1980.

Season born	BLV infection status of calves +	-	Total
Spring	1	7	8
Summer	4	32	36
Winter	8	41	49
Autumn	2	24	26
Total	15	104	119

$\chi^2 = 1.26$ $(P = 0.8)$

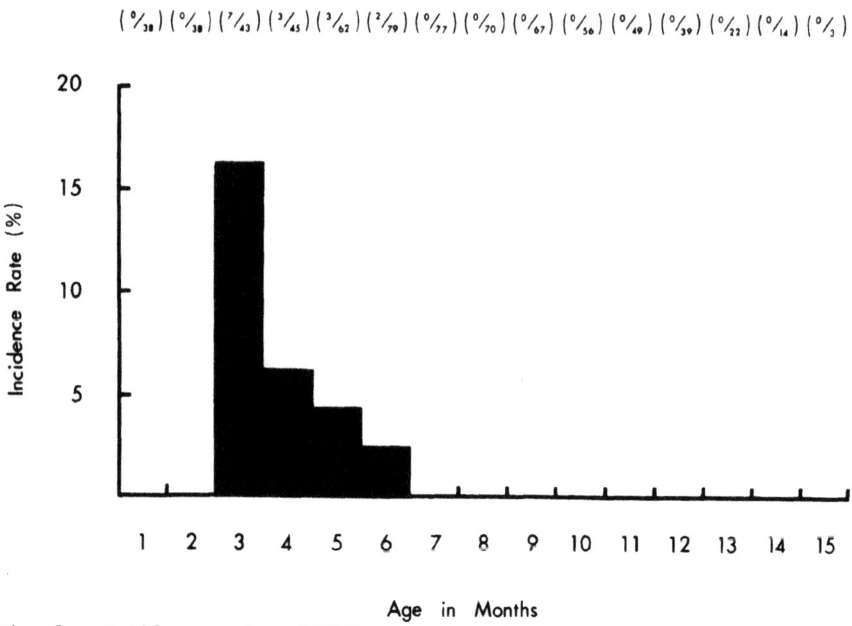

Fig. 1. Incidence rate of BLV seroconversion by month of age in calves at the University of Florida Dairy Research Unit, between July 1979 and September 1980 (numbers in parentheses are the number that seroconverted divided by the average seronegative).

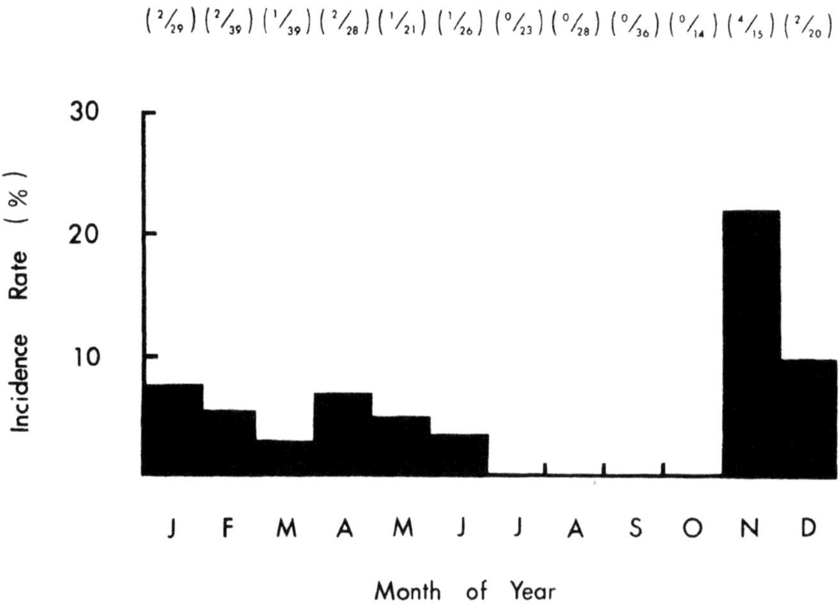

Fig. 2. Incidence rate of BLV seroconversion by month of year in calves at the University of Florida Dairy Research Unit, between July 1979 and September 1980 (numbers in parentheses are the number that seroconverted divided by the average number seronegative).

CONCLUSIONS

1. The preliminary data suggest no association between BLV transmission in calves < 16 months of age and the following factors:
   a. BLV status of dam;
   b. BLV antibody status of colostrum;
   c. breed (Jersey vs. Holstein);
   d. parity of dam;
   e. season of year born.
2. Monthly seroconversion rates do not support vectors as a major mode of transmission of BLV, since no seroconversions occurred during periods of high biting-fly activity.
3. Calves < 7 months of age experienced a greater risk of infection than did those 7 - 15 months of age.
4. The prenatal BLV infection rate (0.5%) was very low in this herd.
5. Antibodies to BLV can be found in calves within 3 months of natural infection.

REFERENCES

Agresti, A., Wackerly, D. and Boyett, J., 1979. Exact conditional tests for cross classification: Approximation of attained significance level. Psychometrika 44, 75-83.

Burny, A., Bruck, C., Chantrenne, H., Cleuter, Y., Dekegel, D., Ghysdael, J., Kettmann, R., Leclercq, M., Leunen, J., Mammerickx, M. and Portetelle, D., 1980. Bovine leukemia virus: Molecular biology and epidemiology. In: Viral Oncology, ed. G. Klein. Raven Press, New York, pp. 231-289.

Burridge, M.J., Wilcox, C.J. and Hennemann, J.M., 1979. Influence of genetic factors on the susceptibility of cattle to bovine leukemia virus infection. Europ. J. Cancer 15, 1395-1400.

Miller, L.D., 1980. Export testing for enzootic bovine leukosis. J. Amer. Vet. Med. Ass. 177, 620-622.

Mix, M.E., 1979. Export significance - industry observations. In: Proceedings of Bovine Leukosis Symposium. United States Department of Agriculture, Washington, pp. 183-186.

Snedecor, G.W. and Cochran, W.G., 1967. Statistical Methods. Iowa State University Press, Ames, pp. 213-214.

DISCUSSION

F. Bürki *(Austria)*

Do your cattle stay outside the year round?

M.C. Thurmond *(USA)*

No, the cattle stay in barns until they are three or four months of age. After that they are outside.

F. Bürki

It may be that the winter peak is related to closer crowding, or insects according to the incubation period, if they were outside.

M.C. Thurmond

Well, they are outside but I would not say that they are crowded.

F. Bürki

No, they are not crowded outside; if they were in a barn they would be crowded and this would explain this peak.

C. Olson *(USA)*

Explanations may not be clear at this point but in time they should be.

M.J. Burridge *(USA)*

Although there is an apparent peak in the winter we are talking about a very small number, perhaps 4. The important point is that we have about 175 calves at risk and very few infections have occurred. If there is vector transmission there is no evidence from our studies thus far that it is an important mode of transmission at this time. There has been very little infection - and we have a massively heavy fly population throughout the summer.

J.F. Ferrer

How many animals were there from which the flies could have transmitted the virus to the non-infected animals?

M.J. Burridge

About 75% of the adult animals in the animal population are infected. On the question of distance of transmission by mechanical means, how many infected calves do we have in the summer months, 15 to 20?

M.C. Thurmond

Not that many. But we have infected adults in adjacent fields, across the fence.

C. Olson

It may be of interest to tell you that in Japan, Dr. Oshima has transmitted leukosis by tabanids feeding on a cow. These were immediately removed from that cow and put on to a sheep whose skin was shaved and clipped. In the first year he had about 100 feedings to infect the sheep. In the second year he was able to do it with only 25 tabanid fly bites. This will be reported in the Japanese Journal of Veterinary Science. So it can be done experimentally.

EXPERIMENTAL TRANSMISSION OF ENZOOTIC BOVINE LEUKOSIS IN CALVES

M. Severini[1], D. Rutili[2], G. Fruganti[3], L. Rampichini[1] and G. Cenci[1].

[1] Istituto di Ispezione degli Alimenti di Origine Animale - Facoltà di Medicina Veterinaria - Perugia, Italy.

[2] Istituto Zooprofilattico Sperimentale dell'Umbria e delle Marche - Perugia, Italy.

[3] Istituto di Patologia e Clinica Medica Veterinaria - Facoltà di Medicina Veterinaria - Perugia, Italy.

ABSTRACT

Two newborn Chianina breed calves and one Friesian calf were infected experimentally with BLV (bovine leukosis virus). All three calves developed antibodies to BLV, 45 - 60 days post-infection. The results of this investigation show that the Chianina breed cattle are also experimentally susceptible to BLV.

O.C. Straub (ed.), Fourth International Symposium on Bovine Leukosis

INTRODUCTION

The Chianina is one of the most important Italian breeds. Chianina cattle are raised mainly in the central regions of Italy and are exported to many foreign countries for cross-breeding with local breeds. During the epidemiological investigations that we have carried out until now we have never found cattle of this breed which were serologically positive for BLV (Rutili et al., 1978). In the adults, moreover, cases of lymphosarcoma from BLV infection have never been found but on the other hand, calves have rather frequently shown the juvenile form of lymphosarcoma. In these calves with lymphosarcoma, and in other cattle belonging to the same stable it was never possible to detect the presence of BLV antibodies, even if in one case the presence of C type particles in tissue cultures co-cultivated with blood lymphocytes was suspected (Severini et al., 1978).

The present investigation was performed to study the susceptibility and response of Chianina calves to experimental BLV infection.

MATERIALS AND METHODS

Animals

Two Chianina calves (No. 1 and No. 2) and one Holstein-Friesian calf (No. 3) of 26 - 30 days of age and originating from BLV infection free herds, were involved in the experiment. The calves were held under observation in the stables of our Institute for 7 - 10 days and then inoculated intravenously at the 35th (No. 1), 37th (No. 2) and 34th (No. 3) day of age. The calves were held in isolation for the whole observation period.

Inoculation

Short-term lymphocyte cultures were prepared from a cow which had been under direct observation for three years. This cow showed a persistent lymphocytosis, BLV and antibodies to both glycoprotein and p24 antigens. The culture medium, rich in viral particles observed with the EM, was filtered through a 450 nm Millipore membrane and immediately inoculated intravenously into the calves as follows:

Calf No. 1 : 50 ml
Calf No. 2 : 100 ml
Calf No. 3 : 50 ml

Examinations

The calves were clinically observed each day. In each of the calves the behaviour of the following serological parameters was evaluated: urea and ureic nitrogen, glucose, serum glutamic-pyruvic-transaminase (SGPT) and serum glutanic-oxalacetic-transaminase (SGOT), alkaline phosphatase (AP), lactic dehydrogenase (LDH), bilirubin, total protein and protein fractions, sodium, potassium, calcium and inorganic phosphorus.

Blood samples were collected periodically from the jugular vein for lymphocyte counts, the preparation of short-term lymphocyte cultures and for the collection of serum. The lymphocyte cultures were collected after 72 hours and included in Epon 812 for the EM. The sera were used for the agar gel immunodiffusion (AGID) test.

AGID test

The test was run in 0.8 agarose in 0.05 M Tris-HCl buffer (pH 7.2) containing 8.5% NaCl. The agarose was placed in 85 mm Petri dishes (15 ml of agarose/plate). A central well 5 mm in diameter and six peripheral wells 6 mm in diameter were cut. The distance between the reactant wells was 2.5 mm. The antigen was placed in the central well and the reference positive serum in 3 peripheral wells alternating with 3 test sera. The plates were incubated at room temperature in a humidified chamber and examined after 24, 48 and 72 h.

Antigens

The glycoprotein (gp) antigen was obtained commercially (Pitman Moore, USA). The major internal BLV antigen (p24) was prepared in our Institute from medium of foetal lamb kidney cell cultures chronically infected with BLV. Culture fluid was clarified and the virus was pelleted by centrifugation at 60 000 g for 2 h. The pellet was resuspended in PBS containing 0.1% EDTA, at final concentration of 1% of the original volume and layered on to a 10 - 40% sucrose gradient and centrifuged at 90 000 g for 2 h. The opalescent virus band was recovered, dyalised against PBS, treated with an equal volume of ether and stored in small aliquots at -80°C until required. The molecular weight of the isolated antigen was determined with SDS polyacrylamide gel electrophoresis (Weber and Osborn, 1969). This antigen was constituted prevalently by a fraction with a molecular weight of 24 000 daltons.

Reference sera

The reference anti gp serum was obtained commercially (Pitman Moore, USA). For p24 we chose as reference the serum of cow SE-273 that showed persistent lymphocytosis, BLV in lymphocyte cultures and gp and p24 antibodies. Negative control serum SE-60 obtained from a cow in a leukosis-free herd was negative for antibodies to gp and p24.

RESULTS

The values of biochemical blood parameters observed in the experimentally inoculated calves ranged within physiological values (Rosenberger, 1979). During the observation period one calf (No. 1) showed a transient enlargement of the prescapular lymphnodes.

The results of the haematological and serological studies are reported in Tables 1, 2 and 3. Examination of these Tables shows that calf No. 1 (Chianina) presented a high lymphocyte increase immediately after the inoculation and subsequently the

TABLE 1

NUMBER OF LYMPHOCYTES PER μl: RESULTS OF IMMUNODIFFUSION TESTS CARRIED OUT WITH SERUM FROM CALF NO. 1 (CHIANINA).

Date	No. of lymphocytes	Antibodies against gp	p24
Before inoculation	4 816	-	-
1 day post inoculation	16 380	-	-
2 days " "	3 956	-	-
4 " " "	NC	-	-
11 " " "	3 774	-	-
16 " " "	6 160	-	-
25 " " "	4 042	-	-
32 " " "	8 064	-	-
39 " " "	7 480	1:1(*)	-
46 " " "	9 520	1:2	-
2 months" "	7 253	1:8	-
3 " " "	7 956	1:8	-
4 " " "	7 400	1:8	-
5 " " "	6 816	1:8	-
6 " " "	10 064	1:8	-
7 " " "	8 968	1:4	-
8 " " "	10 050	1:8	-
9 " " "	8 030	1:4	-
10 " " "	10 064	1:16	-

* Highest positive dilution NC Not counted

lymphocyte values were marginally above normal (according to the haematological EC key) on only three occasions (6th, 8th and 10th month). The AGID test demonstrated the presence of glycoprotein antibodies 39 days after the inoculation. The antibody titre was 1 : 1 and subsequently increased until a maximum value of 16 : 1 at 10 months post-inoculation.

Calf No. 2 (Chianina) constantly presented normal lymphocyte values. At the 46th day post-inoculation antibodies to both glycoprotein (1 : 8) and p24 (1 : 1) were demonstrated. The

TABLE 2

NUMBER OF LYMPHOCYTES PER µl: RESULTS OF IMMUNODIFFUSION TESTS CARRIED OUT WITH SERUM FROM CALF NO. 2 (CHIANINA)

Date	No. of lymphocytes	Antibodies against gp	p24
Before inoculation	6 810	-	-
1 day post inoculation	5 280	-	-
2 days " "	5 740	-	-
4 " " "	3 960	-	-
11 " " "	3 640	-	-
35 " " "	5 700	-	-
46 " " "	5 192	1:8(*)	1:1(*)
55 " " "	6 110	1:16	1:1
3 months" "	6 004	1:16	1:1
4 " " "	5 472	1:8	1:1
5 " " "	4 410	1:8	1:1

TABLE 3

NUMBER OF LYMPHOCYTES PER µl: RESULTS OF IMMUNODIFFUSION TESTS CARRIED OUT WITH SERUM FROM CALF NO. 3 (FRIESIAN)

Date	No. of lymphocytes	Antibodies against gp	p24
Before inoculation	4 144	-	-
1 day post inoculation	4 794	-	-
2 days " "	3 300	-	-
7 " " "	2 640	-	-
21 " " "	4 662	-	-
32 " " "	5 254	-	-
55 " " "	8 928	1:4(*)	-
3 months" "	5 390	1:4	-
4 " " "	7 776	1:8	-
5 " " "	7 344	1:4	-
6 " " "	8 932	1:8	-

* Highest positive dilution

titre of the glycoprotein antibodies increased during the following two months (1 : 16) and then again showed the initial values, while the antibody titre to p24 remained constant.

Calf No. 3 (Friesian) always presented normal lymphocyte values. In this animal glycoprotein antibodies were demonstrated 55 days after the inoculation. The initial antibody titre was 1 : 4 and it subsequently rose to a maximum value of 1 : 8.

In the short-term lymphocyte cultures prepared from the blood of these three calves, mature viral particles definitely related to BLV were never found but particles were observed with a morphology similar to incomplete C-type particles.

CONCLUSIONS

The results of our observations demonstrate that the intravenous inoculation of material containing cell-free C-type virus particles, produced BLV antibodies in all three calves. The seroconversion was detected with the AGID test within 39 - 55 days after the inoculation. Two calves (No. 1 Chianina and No. 3 Friesian) showed only antibodies to the BLV glycoprotein antigen, while calf No. 2 (Chianina) showed antibodies both to BLV glycoprotein and p24. In all three calves the antibody titre to glycoprotein increased after the initial seroconversion and it never dropped below the initial titre. On the other hand, the antibody titre to p24 in calf No. 2, remained constant. The appearance of the antibody response and the antibody titres attained indicate that a BLV infection, similar to that which can be reproduced in neonatal calves (Miller and Van der Maaten, 1976), was produced in these three calves. The response to this infection was characterised by the presence of antibodies to glycoprotein and, in one case, also by the presence of antibodies to p24. We are not able to explain the significance of this different immunological behaviour. We can only point out that the absence of the irregular presence of antibodies to p24 in infected animals represents a possible occurrence which is difficult to interpret (Baumgartener and Olson, 1978). It is necessary to emphasise, however, that calf No. 2, which showed antibodies to both antigens received twice the dose of the other two calves.

The persistence of the infection was not definitely confirmed e.g. the clear proof of mature C-type virus particles in the short-term lymphocyte cultures. The EM observations revealed only the presence of particles that, while presenting morphological characteristics similar to those of incomplete C-type particles, were of uncertain interpretation. Previous experiments by other workers have demonstrated that it is possible to find C-type particles in experimentally infected calves (Miller et al., 1972; Van der Maaten et al., 1974; Kukaine et al., 1978). However, when the inoculum consists of filtered lymphocyte culture the particles can be present in an extremely limited number (Schmidt et al., 1975). It is possible, moreover, that our findings will become clearer and more significant in the course of further observations.

In conclusion, from the results of our research it clearly emerges that the intravenous inoculation of cell-free material containing BLV induced in the two Chianina calves an antibody response comparable to that induced in the Friesian calf. This may indicate that cattle of the Chianina breed are susceptible to experimental infection with BLV. Since cattle of this breed, raised in Italy, seem to be free from EBL at present (Rutili et al., 1981), it would be opportune, as a precautionary measure, to avoid contact between them and cattle of different breeds, especially Friesian, in order to avoid the risk of a possible transmission under natural conditions.

Finally, we must point out that the response of the Chianina calves to experimental BLV infection did not present any characteristic sign that could resemble the calf form of leukosis.

ACKNOWLEDGEMENTS

The authors thank S. Canalicchio, P. Proietti and C. Furia for their technical assistance.

REFERENCES

Baumgartener, L.E. and Olson, C., 1978. Immunodiffusion antibodies to p24 and gp antigens in cattle. CEC Workshop Conference on the Serological diagnosis of Enzootic Bovine Leukosis, Ed. A.A. Ressang, pp. 148-155 (Rotterdam, The Netherlands).

Kukaine, R.A., Nagayeva, L.I., Chapenko, S.V., Kudeleva, G.V., Loza, V.P., Runcis, A.J., Glazere, M.A., Ose, L.A., Yakovleva, L.A., Dyatchenko, A.G. and Lapin, B.A., 1976. Induction of bovine leukemia C-type oncornaviruses. Archiv für Geschwulstforsch. 46, 253-260.

Miller, L.D., Miller, J.M. and Olson, C., 1972. Inoculation of calves with particles resembling C-type virus from cultures of bovine lymphosarcoma. J. Natl. Cancer Inst. 48, 423-427.

Miller, J.M. and Van der Maaten, M.J., 1976. Serologic response of cattle following inoculation with bovine leukemia virus. Comparative Leukemia Research 1975, Bibl. Haemat., No. 43, Ed. J. Clemmensen and D.S. Yohn, pp. 187-189 (Karger, Basel).

Rosenberger, G., 1979. L'esame clinico del Bovino. Ed. Essegivi (Piacenza)

Rutili, D., Severini, M., Rampichini, L. and Titoli, F., 1978. Epidemiologic study on enzootic bovine leukemia in Italy. Ann. Rech. Vét. 9, 761-764.

Rutili, D., Severini, M., Bertorotta, G. and Titoli, F., 1981. Large scale survey of bovine leukosis virus infection in central and southern Italy. IV International Symposium on Bovine Leukosis, Bologna, Nov. 5-7, 1980 (this publication).

Schmidt, F.W., Garcia de Lima, E., Mitscherlich, E., von Milczewski, K.E. and Lembke, A., 1975. Versuche zur Züchtung eines Agens der Rinderleukose in Leukozytenkulturen vom Rind. Zbl. Vet. Med. 22, 673-686.

Severini, M., Rutili, D., Rampichini, L., Titoli, F., Fruganti, G. and Di Felice, G., 1978. Ricerche sulla Leucosi Linfatica (Linfosarcoma) dei Vitelli. Arch. Vet. It. 29, 83-91.

Severini, M., Rutili, D., Titoli, F., Rampichini, L. and Vizzani, A., 1981. Development of bovine leukosis virus infection in cattle of an experimental station. IV International Symposium on Bovine Leukosis Bologna, Nov. 5-7, 1980 (this publication).

Van der Maaten, M.J., Miller, J.M. and Boothe, A.D., 1974. Replicating type-C virus particles in monolayers cell cultures of tissues from cattle with lymphosarcoma. J. Natl. Cancer Inst. 52, 491-497.

Weber, K. and Osborn, M., 1969. The reliability of molecular weight determinations by dodecyl sulfate-polyacrylamide gel electrophoresis. J. Biol. Chem. 244, 4406-4412.

TRANSMISSION OF BOVINE LEUKOSIS VIRUS (BLV)

M.H. Lucas and D.H. Roberts
Central Veterinary Laboratory,
New Haw, Weybridge, Surrey, UK.

ROLE OF TUBERCULIN (TB) TESTING IN THE SPREAD OF INFECTION

The double intradermal comparative test was made using avian and bovine tuberculin in two separate sites. A series of experiments was carried out using cattle and sheep. Three EBL infected cattle were used as a source of infection; BLV was consistently isolated from the peripheral blood leukocytes of these 3 animals. BLV positive animals and susceptible animals were TB tested alternately. Fifteen susceptible calves and 15 susceptible sheep were TB tested. A further 3 calves and 3 sheep were used as controls; the needles of the tuberculin syringes were deliberately contaminated with blood from the BLV infected cattle, before being used in the test. Whereas all 3 calves and 3 sheep inoculated intradermally with contaminated TB syringes developed BLV infections, all of the other 30 animals have remained serologically negative to BLV.

PERSISTENCE OF THE VIRUS IN IMMUNOLOGICAL PRODUCTS

The survival of BLV in blood containing anticoagulant and stored at 4°C was investigated. A BLV infected cow was used as the source of infected blood; BLV had been consistently isolated from its peripheral blood leukocytes. The cow was bled using 20 ml vacutainers containing potassium oxalate. Two sheep were inoculated intramuscularly one with 5 ml whole blood and the other with 5 ml plasma at 0, 1, 2, 4 and 8 weeks after storage. BLV has persisted so far in the blood for two weeks.

The survival of BLV infected blood cells in serum free of specific antibodies and stored at +4°C was investigated. A BLV infected cow was used as a source of infected blood cells; BLV had been consistently isolated from these blood cells. The

O.C. Straub (ed.), Fourth International Symposium on Bovine Leukosis

BLV infected cow was bled using potassium oxalate vacutainers and the blood cells washed twice in phosphate buffered saline. Serum without antibodies was obtained from BLV susceptible cows and the BLV infected blood cells added to the pooled serum. Two sheep were inoculated intramuscularly, one with 5 ml of blood mixture and the other with 5 ml serum after the blood mixture had been centrifuged; sheep were inoculated at 0, 1, 2, 4 and 8 weeks after storage. BLV has persisted so far in the blood mixture and serum for 3 weeks.

EFFECT OF PASTEURISATION ON BLV INFECTED LEUKOCYTES

The high temperature short time batch procedure simulated a commercial pasteurisation process. The apparatus which consisted of two parallel stainless steel plates enclosing a thin film of milk between them was kept at the test temperature in a large water bath. The temperature of the water was controlled at a temperature $1^{o}C$ higher than the required milk temperature treatment. 250 ml quantities were poured into the unit which was allowed to remain in the water at $72.5^{o}C$ for 70 seconds after which it was immediately transferred to an adjacent cold water bath for cooling. Pooled milk was obtained from serologically negative lactating cows and BLV infected lymphocytes added. A BLV infected cow was used as a source of infected lymphocytes; BLV has been consistently isolated from these cells. Ten sheep were allotted to 2 groups, one group of 5 received pasteurised milk and the other group of 5 received non pasteurised milk. Each animal was inoculated intraperitoneally with 50 ml milk and each animal received 2×10^{6} lymphocytes. The 5 sheep inoculated with non pasteurised milk became BLV infected; none of the sheep inoculated with pasteurised milk have developed antibodies.

NATURAL TRANSMISSION FROM SHEEP TO SHEEP AND CALVES

Two seronegative calves, 5 seronegative sheep and 5 seropositive sheep were penned together in April 1980. Six months later there has been no evidence of spread of the virus from the positive sheep.

TRANSMISSION FROM SEMEN

(a) Undiluted semen from a bull, previously found to be excreting BLV in the ejaculate (Vet. Rec., 1980. 106: 128), had been stored at -70°C for about two months. It was then used to inseminate 4 heifers and to inoculate 1 sheep. None of these animals developed BLV antibodies.

(b) Semen from the same bull had been processed and stored in straws at an AI Centre since 1972. Volumes ranging from 15 to 40 ml of this processed semen were available for each year from 1972 to 1978. One sheep was inoculated intraperitoneally with one volume from each year. None of the 7 sheep developed antibodies.

More straws have recently become available and it has been possible to inoculate a further 26 sheep each with 100 ml processed semen.

DISCUSSION

A.A. Ressang *(Netherlands)*

We had five heavily infected bulls in Rotterdam which were allowed to serve naturally five normal cows. Five calves were born and we were able to observe these calves for a period of two years. There was no seroconversion. We also tried to find antibodies or antigen in the ejaculate of these bulls but we didn't find any.

D.H. Roberts *(UK)*

What method did you use to look?

A.A. Ressang

We used the agar gel immunodiffusion test.

M.J. Burridge *(USA)*

On the basis of the work you have done thus far, including this, can you tell us what your feelings are on the importance of semen in this regard?

D.H. Roberts

Well, I think you will find the virus in any secretion or excretion where you find lymphocytes. However, I don't think it is of any importance if you use AI, for example; I am sure that just the preparation of straws would destroy the virus.

J.C. Flensburg *(Denmark)*

Your work on the TB testing is very interesting. Did I gather from your presentation that you think that under practical conditions TB testing plays no role in the transmission?

D.H. Roberts

Well, you very rarely get any blood. I don't know whether you have had any experience of TB testing but I particularly looked at the animals and you very rarely get blood at the time of doing the test, although sometimes you get it afterwards. Of course, we were using the double intradermal test.

EXPERIMENTAL TRANSMISSION OF BOVINE LEUKOSIS TO SHEEP
(Clinicopathological consideration)

Z. Horváth
Department of Medicine, University of Veterinary Sciences, H-1400 Budapest, Hungary.

ABSTRACT

For experimental infections lymphocyte suspensions from a case of bovine leukosis, whole blood of BLV infected sheep, as well as supernatants of BLV containing FLK cell cultures have been used.

The leukosis of the bovine donor involving a large number of haemolymphnodes and splenomegalia was classified as a centrocytic-centroblastic B cell subtype. The five sheep infected with the donor's leukocyte suspension Mls developed T cell lymphoblastoma. Two of the sheep were the offspring of the F_1 generation.

One offspring from the ewe with uterine tumour leukosis, developed a lymphoma while leukaemia occurred in the other one (at present still alive).

ID tests and ELISA confirmed the presence of BLV antibodies in all sheep with manifest (neoplastic) leukosis as well as in the majority of the other animals inoculated. A moderate lymphocytosis developed during the course of the developing sheep leukosis after the inoculation of culture and cell free material. The experiments are still in progress.

O.C. Straub (ed.), Fourth International Symposium on Bovine Leukosis

INTRODUCTION

Experimental infections are the most simple and persuasive means for verifying infectivity of some diseases. Since Wittman (1969) found that bovine leukosis was transmissible to sheep by injecting whole blood, the possibility of transmission by leukocyte suspension, tumour cell suspension, leukocyte cell culture and cell free BLV has been confirmed by several authors (Olson, 1972; Hoss et al., 1974; Van der Maaten, 1974; Paulsen, 1975; Ressang, 1976; Horváth, 1976 etc.).

However, the artificial transmission of bovine leukosis to sheep yielded different results. Blood picture, appearance of serological positivity, character and frequency of clinicopathological findings, number and quality of blood lymphocytes of the infected animals showed substantial differences. Only scarce data are available concerning the clinicopathological form of the disease in the progeny of the artificially infected sheep. Therefore, studies on the artificial transmission of EBL to sheep may give numerous and valuable data.

The aim of the present experiments was to find an answer to the following questions:

1. Which type and number of neoplastic (clinically manifest) leukosis can be induced in lambs infected with the leukocyte suspension of a single, clinically, haematologically, and histologically classified bovine donor?
2. Which findings did the infected sheep and their progeny supply during the extremely long (7 to 10 years) observation period?
3. Was EBL experimentally transmissible from sheep to sheep?
4. When do BLV antibodies, lymphocytosis and neoplastic leukosis in sheep appear after infection with material from BLV infected FLK cell cultures?

MATERIALS AND METHODS

Experiment No. I.

Inoculation with lymphocyte suspensions.

Between September 1973 and March 1974, 17 lambs and 9 young Cameroon goats were inoculated with lymphocyte suspensions from a lymphocytic cow. Clinically manifest neoplastic leukosis developed during the later observation period. Approximately 50 million lymphocytes were injected subcutaneously closely to the superficial cervical and subiliac lymph nodes of each of the experimental animals. Immunosuppression was induced by 8 intramuscular injections of 0.2 mg/kg body weight glycocortisone every other day.

Clinical and haematological examinations were carried out every 3rd or 6th month during the control period i.e. for 7 years.

The donor cow and the experimental lambs with clinically manifest leukosis have been checked by haematological, cytological and histological examinations. In addition to WBCs blood smears stained according to Pappenheim and Giemsa as well as lymph node and spleen imprint preparations were examined. Cytochemical reactions for the demonstration of α-naphthylacetate esterase (T cell specific according to Müller, 1974) and acid phosphatase have also been performed.

Histological examinations were performed on samples fixed in formalin and embedded in paraffin. Besides haematoxylin-eosin and Giemsa, PAS and reticulin stains were used. Short term cultures of leukocyte suspensions of sheep with experimentally induced tumorous leukosis have been studied by electron microscopy.

Experiment No. II

Transmission of sheep leukosis by whole blood injection.

In December 1979, 5 young sheep were infected with whole

blood from BLV antibody positive and lymphocytotic sheep from experiment No. I.

Experiment No. III.

Infection with FLK cell culture containing BLV.

The experiment was started at the beginning of 1980. Five approximately one year old sheep and 4 one week old lambs were used. The adult animals received 2 x 50 ml supernatant of the cell culture subcutaneously. Prior to the inoculation, 20 mg Deltacortil were injected intramuscularly for a period of 4 days.

Experiment No. IV.

Infection of lambs originating from BLV-seropositive mothers.

Ten ml supernatant of the BLV containing FLK cell culture were injected subcutaneously to each of 5 lambs after the intake of colostrum.

The presence of BLV specific antibodies was checked at 3 month intervals using the ID test and the ELISA.

RESULTS

Data on the donor cow.

The clinical examination revealed a large number of bean and walnut sized subcutaneous cervical and abdominal lymph nodes. It was also supposed that a splenomegaly was present. The animal died suddenly due to a rupture of the spleen. At the time when the samples for the inoculation of the sheep were taken, some of the cow's lymphocytes in the peripheral blood were of the blast type. Using the SpA rosette technique (Kearney, 1975) they qualified as B type. As a result of the examination the malignant lymphoma (ML) of the donor cow was classified as a centrocytic-centroblastic (follicular-germinocytic) type (Gerard-Marchant, 1974).

Data on the experimental sheep.

Experiment No. I.

During the 7 years observation period, distinct leukosis involving clinical and pathological symptoms was induced in 5 animals, of which 3 originated from the original experiment and 2 were progeny of those. One animal from the ewes infected on the first day of life died earlier than its dam, from neoplastic leukosis. Another offspring of this ewe shows lymphocyte counts as high as 25 000/mm^3 and positive reactions in the ID test and ELISA. Later, uterine tumorous proliferation characteristic of leukosis developed in this ewe. Clinical symptoms of leukosis appeared 19, 36 and 60 months after the infection. Two animals derived from the infected ewes developed tumours after 38 and 52 months.

A striking lymphocytosis was found in all cases before ML developed revealing blast type lymphocytes of various shape and size. Mitotic cell forms were seen in 2 tumour bearing sheep. T-specific α-naphthyl-acetate esterase and acid phosphatase tests yielded characteristic blood smear findings. Stained focal paranuclear granules were found in almost each lymphocyte. Paranuclear and focal reactions obtained with the stains mentioned as well as characteristic light and electron microscopic findings (convoluted nuclear surfaces, multiple nucleoli, irregular distribution of nuclear chromatin of immature lymphoid cells etc.) were considered to be characteristic for T-lymphocytes.

The clinicopathological pattern of leukosis developing in sheep corresponded with the findings in the bovine. Enlargement of regional and mesenteric lymph nodes developed in each case. An enormous thymus weighing 1 300 g was found in the first lymphomatous sheep and weights of 100 and 150 g respectively found in the other 2 sheep. Neoplastic lymphoid infiltrations of the perithymic tissues were found in one animal. Leukotic tissue was found in the heart muscle of 2 animals. Its existence had been assumed on the basis of ECG records.

Seventy five to 80% of the animals in groups II - IV showed a seroconversion within 2 to 5 months following the inoculations. Persistent lymphocytosis developed also in several animals; so far there is no evidence of clinical or pathological manifestations of leukosis. C-type virus was found in short term cultures of peripheral lymphocytes (buffy coat) of sheep with neoplastic leukosis by the electron microscopy. The morphological characteristics resembled those of BLV observed in bovine lymphocytes and FLK cultures.

DISCUSSION

Our studies suggest that terminal ML in cattle and sheep can be classified into sub-types based on the cytological and histological findings. The ML of the single bovine donor used in the experiment differed completely from that induced in the 5 sheep with its lymphocytes. B cell centrocytic-centroblastic ML was present in the bovine donor while ML in sheep was exclusively a T lymphoblastoma.

Electron microscopical examinations confirmed that an identical virus has been responsible for bovine and sheep leukosis. Nevertheless additional studies are required to determine whether the various sub-types of lymphocytes of the bovine donor and cell free BLV always induce T-type lymphoblastoma in sheep.

The current classification of spontaneous and experimental MLs in animals has little in common with that of human ML. The latter is based on the differentiation and functional aspects of lymphocytes, the former chiefly on the gross and microscopic morphology of the altered haemopoietic and lymphoid tissues. Classification of the neoplasma of haemopoietic tissues according to the nomenclature recommended by the World Health Organisation (Jarret and Mackey, 1974) may be objectionable. The classification scheme proposed by Koudriavtseva (1976) describes leukosis and reticulosis as the two main forms of bovine haemoblastosis: accordingly, lymphoid leukosis and

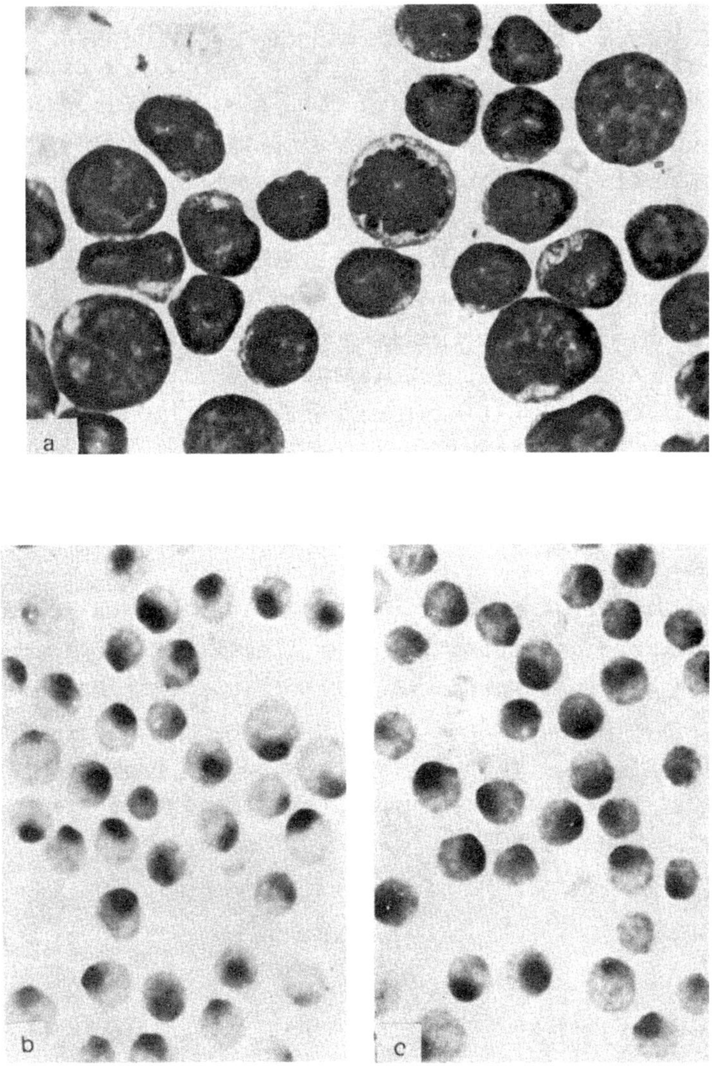

Fig. 1. Peripheral buffy coat smear.

(a) Immature cells x 675.

(b) Acid phosphates reaction.

(c) T cell specific acid naphthyl-acetate esterase reaction (focal, perinuclear).

haemocytoblastosis (immature cell leukosis) are classified as leukosis, while lymphosarcoma, reticulosarcoma, systemic reticulosis, and lymphogranulomatosis (Hodgkin's disease) are different forms of reticulosis. The MLs occurring in animals have often been typed on the basis of the morphological classification proposed by Anderson et al. (1968), who differentiate lymphosarcoma sub-types: 1. multicentric, 2. thymic, and 3. intestinal or cutaneous in manifestation. The identification of the ML sub-types has been hampered by the frequent use of certain non-informative terms, such as 'reticulosis', 'reticulosarcomatosis', 'lymphoreticular sarcomatosis' and 'lymphatic leukosis'. The classifications currently used in human pathology (Lukes and Collins, 1974; Gerrard-Marchant et al., 1974) have been based primarily on functional aspects and are fairly informative in respect of pathogenesis and prognosis.

The striking similarity between the changes found in our cases and those occurring in human T cell lymphoblastomas has led to the conclusion that the classification scheme used for human MLs may be practicable for the diagnostic differentiation of MLs in animals. The reclassification of experimental and spontaneous MLs in animals under the scheme used for human MLs is therefore proposed.

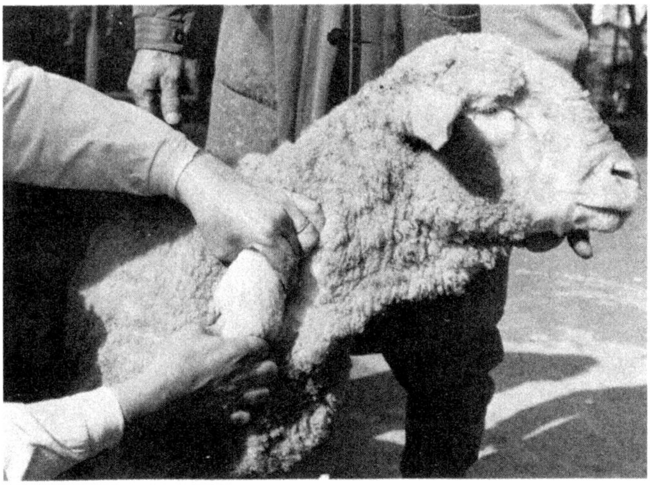

Fig. 2. Enormously enlarged praescapular lymphnode

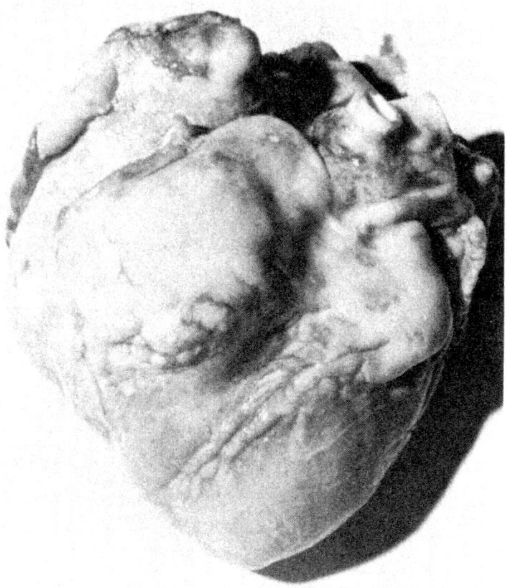

Fig. 3. Lymphoma in the heart muscle.

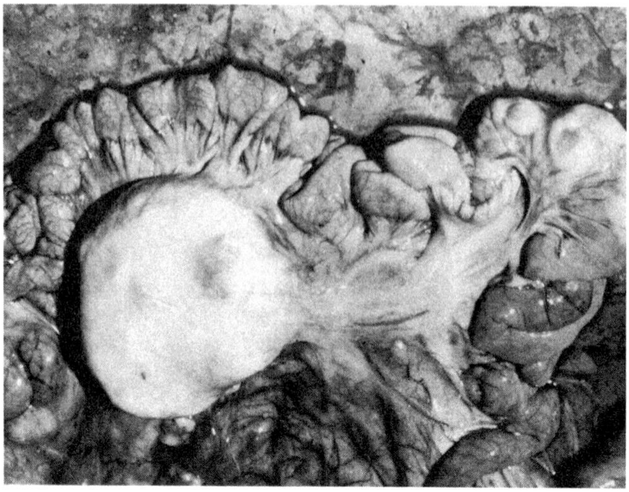

Fig. 4. Lymphnode conglomerate in the mesenterium.

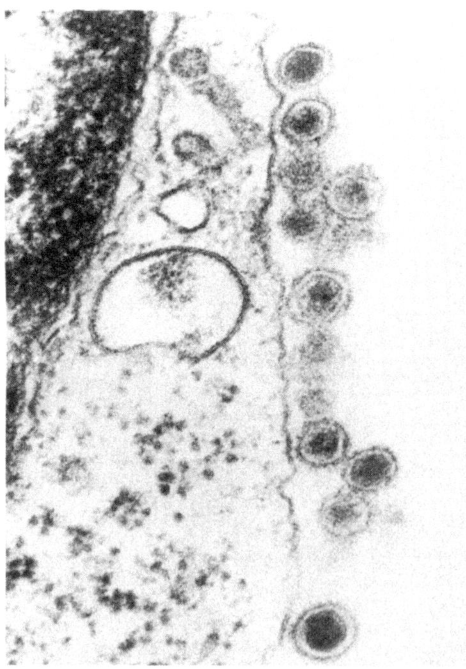

Fig. 5. C-type virions in the buffy coat cell of short term lymphocytes culture x 75 000.

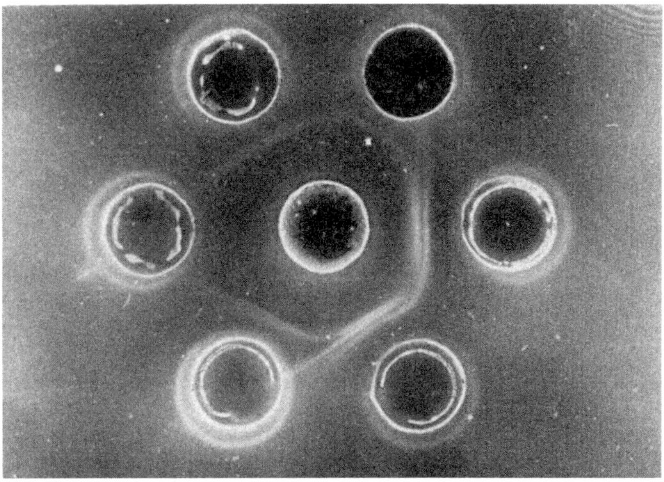

Fig. 6. Positive ID-test with double line.

REFERENCES

Anderson, L.J., Jarret, W.H. and Crighton, G.W., 1968. A classification of lymphoid neoplasms of domestic animals. Natl. Cancer Inst. Monograph. 32, 343-353.

Gerard, R., Marchant, I.H., Lenner, K., Rilke, F. and Stanfeld, E., 1974. Classification of non-Hodgkin's lymphomas. Lancet. 2, 405-409.

Horváth, Z., 1976. Experimental transfer of enzootic bovine leucosis to sheep. Acta Vet. Hung. 26, 31-32.

Hoss, H.W. and Olson, C., 1974. Infectivity of bovine C-type (Leukaemia) virus for sheep and goats. Am. J. Vet. Res. 35, 633-637.

Jarret, W.F. and Mackey, L.J., 1974. II. Neoplastic diseases of the haematopoietic and lymphoid tissues. Bull. World Health Org. 50, 21-34.

Kearney, R., Chic, E. and Basten, A., 1975. Detection of membrane-associated antigens on lymphoid cells by antibody coupled to staphylococcal protein. A. J. Immunology 114, 1143-1146.

Koudriavstseva, T.P., Simonian, G.A. and Petrovski, G.S., 1976. Les hemoblastoses des bovins, leur classification et leur diagnostique. Bull. Off. Int. Epiz. 85, 289-297.

Lukes, R.J. and Collins, R.D., 1974. A functional approach to the classification of malignant lymphomas. Rec. Results Canc. Res. 46, 18-31.

Müller, J., Brun, G., Bürki, H., Keller, H.U., Hess, M.W. and Cottier, H., 1974. Nonspecific acid esterase activity: a criterion for differentiation of T and B lymphocytes in mouse lymphnodes. Eur. J. Immunol. 5, 270-274.

Olson, C., Miller, J.M. and Hoss, H.E., 1972. Transmission of lymphosarcoma from cattle to sheep. J. Nat. Cancer Inst. 4, 1463-1467.

Paulsen, J., 1976. Comparative studies in bovine and ovine leukosis. Vet. Microbiol. 1, 211-218; O.C. Straub (Ed.), Elsevier Scientific Publishing Company Amsterdam and CEC, Luxembourg.

Ressang, A., Baars, J., Calafat, J., Martenbrock, N. and Quark, J., 1976. Studies on bovine leukaemia III. Zbl. Vet. Med. 23, 662-668.

Van der Maaten, M.J., 1976. Induction of lymphoid tumours in sheep with cell-free preparations of bovine leukaemia virus. Biblioth. Haemat. 43, 378-379.

Wittman, W., Urbanek, D., Seils, H. and Beyer, J., 1971. Untersuchungen zur Atiologie der Rinderleukose.Arch. exp. Vet. Med. 25, 587-595.

DISCUSSION

B.S. Samagh *(Canada)*

Are T type lymphoblastomas common in cows?

Z. Horvath *(Hungary)*

We have not seen any in cows.

C. Olson *(USA)*

I think this might be suggested in some of the sporadic types but not in the enzootic.

A.L. Parodi *(France)*

Perhaps we should discuss the problem of T cell lymphoma in cows, spontaneous tumours in cows, tomorrow morning. I would like to ask Dr. Horvath whether the tumorous sheep developed thymic tumours?

Z. Horvath

Three of them did. In the first the thymus weighed 1 300 g, in the second about 150 g, in the third about 120 g.

C. Olson

I have particularly enjoyed this report on the pathology; it illustrates just what a pathologist can do. I might also comment that this is the first time we have seen much on the histochemistry of these cells and those esterase positive cells are certainly used in human haematology.

EXPERIMENTAL TRANSMISSION OF BOVINE LEUKOSIS VIRUS INFECTION IN SHEEP

G. Gentile[1], D. Rutili[2] and G. Ferrari[1]

[1] Clinica Medica Veterinaria - Università degli Studi di Bologna, Italy.

[2] Istituto Zooprofilattico Sperimentale dell'Umbria e delle Marche - Perugia, Italy.

SHORT COMMUNICATION

This investigation follows our previous researches on the experimental transmission of EBL in cattle and sheep. In the present study the results obtained in an experiment concerning the sheep-to-sheep transmission of BLV are reported.

Two sheep, experimentally infected with BLV, were used as donors. Having received whole blood from leukotic calves intravenously, these two animals showed specific antibodies (2 - 3 months after inoculation) and BLV in short-term lymphocyte cultures (25 - 34 months after inoculation).

Cultures of lymphocytes from donor animals were prepared for inoculation of 8 lambs. Portions of cultures used for inoculation were processed by electron microscopy to verify the presence of BLV.

Four lambs were inoculated intraperitoneally with 25 ml lymphocyte suspension (2×10^8 cells). The cell suspension was kept at -70^oC for 3 days.

Four lambs were inoculated intravenously with 20 ml of lymphocyte culture medium filtered through 450 nm Millipore membrane.

All subjects found negative for precipitating antibodies to BLV were inoculated at 4 - 5 days of age. Two lambs were used as controls and inoculated with lymphocyte culture material

O.C. Straub (ed.), Fourth International Symposium on Bovine Leukosis

prepared from blood of normal sheep.

Blood samples were collected monthly from inoculated lambs for haematological and serological examinations. The virological examinations were performed every 6 months beginning 3 months after inoculation, by examining the lymphocyte cultures with an electron microscope.

The results of this investigation refer to an observation period of 27 months and concern 7 lambs, including one lamb (4 weeks old) which died from bacterial infection.

Two lambs out of 7 never showed any haematological change and were always serologically and virologically negative. Five lambs showed a seroconversion 30 to 60 days after inoculation. After that the antibody titre increased until the fifth month in all lambs. BLV was found in the lymphocyte cultures of only 2 lambs. One of these, inoculated with cell free material, showed the virus 27 months after inoculation. The other one, inoculated with cell suspension, was virologically positive 21 months after inoculation.

On the basis of the results obtained, it can be concluded that BLV infection was passaged in sheep as shown by the serological reaction and by the proof of virus in the infected lambs.

Evidence of infection was found both in lambs inoculated with lymphocyte suspension and with filtered culture medium.

Freezing of the infective cultured lymphocytes did not destroy their infectivity.

DISCUSSION

G.H. Theilen (*USA*)

What buffers are you using in the virus preparation?

D. Rutili (*Italy*)

Only the culture media. Starting from the buffy coat cultures, we collect the cells to prepare the cell suspension in tissue culture medium. We used two lots of control animals inoculated with buffy coat culture media from normal sheep.

B.S. Samagh (*Canada*)

What is the effect of freezing on infected lymphocytes? How long do they remain infective?

D. Rutili

Three days at -80°C in the freezing box.

M.J. van der Maaten (*USA*)

We have frozen lymphocytes in DMSO plus cell culture fluid and you can maintain infectivity for an indefinite period of time that way.

A.A. Ressang (*Netherlands*)

It does not hold for whole blood. As soon as you freeze whole blood you cannot use it anymore for experimental purposes.

C. Olson (*USA*)

Is that because the red cells are breaking up?

A.A. Ressang

Yes, something happens. If you freeze it and thaw it and inject it into sheep you won't get any results.

C. Olson

At what temperature are you freezing it?

A.A. Ressang

At -70°C. But if you store lymphocytes in liquid nitrogen then they retain their infectivity.

C. Olson

So it is just like a tissue culture that is stored in liquid nitrogen.

SESSION VI

Transmission (II)

Chairmen : D.H. Roberts and F.-W. Schmidt

PRESENCE OF THE BOVINE LEUKAEMIA VIRUS (BLV) IN MILK OF NATURALLY INFECTED COWS

S.J. Kenyon, P. Gupta and J.F. Ferrer
School of Veterinary Medicine, University of Pennsylvania, New Bolton Center, Kennett Square, Pa 19348, USA.

ABSTRACT

A sheep bioassay was applied to study the frequency with which BLV and/or BLV infected cells can be detected in milk from cows naturally infected with the virus. Milk or milk cells were inoculated into sheep which were then monitored for the presence of BLV by applying a serological test and two direct virus assays.

BLV was detected in whole milk samples collected at 10, 30 and/or 50 days of lactation from 7 of 14 cows naturally infected with BLV. Milk cells obtained at 1, 4 - 6 and/or 10 - 13 days of lactation from 7 naturally infected cows were also positive for BLV in the sheep bioassay. The milk cell inoculum induced BLV infection in the recipient sheep more efficiently and rapidly than the whole milk inoculum. There were no significant differences in the frequency with which BLV and/or BLV infected cells were released into milk at the various sampling times used. Of the 20 different donor cows examined, 13 (65%) released BLV or BLV-infected cells in milk at one or more of the sampling times used.

O.C. Straub (ed.), Fourth International Symposium on Bovine Leukosis

INTRODUCTION

The presence of BLV in milk of BLV-infected cows has been examined by injecting milk samples into lambs which were subsequently monitored for the development of viral antibodies and infection. Using this sheep bioassay, BLV was detected in colostrum and/or milk from 4 of 6 infected cows (Miller and Van der Maaten, 1979). Since 3 of the 4 cows whose milk was positive in the sheep bioassay had been infected experimentally, this study did not answer the question of the frequency with which BLV is released into colostrum and/or milk of naturally infected cows. The purpose of the study reported here was to answer this question and to determine if the release of the virus and/or virus-infected cells into milk varies during the lactation period.

MATERIALS AND METHODS

Colostrum and milk were collected from cows naturally infected with BLV in a Jersey and a Holstein dairy herd. All of the cows were positive in the radioimmunoassay using the internal p25 virion antigen (RIAp25) (Gupta and Ferrer, 1978).

Recipient lambs were born at our facility to Shropshire ewes purchased from a commercial flock. None of the lambs was positive for BLV antibodies at birth, as determined by the agar gel immunodiffusion test using the virion glycoprotein antigen (IDgp) (Gupta and Ferrer, 1978). All of the ewes which were retained for further breeding remained negative for BLV antibodies for at least one year.

Samples of whole milk or milk cells were injected into lambs that were less than one week of age. In virtually all cases each sample was injected into two recipient lambs. Each recipient lamb received either 100 ml of whole milk intraperitoneally or 1 x 10^8 viable milk cells subcutaneously. The milk cells were washed twice prior to inoculation.

The inoculated sheep and non-inoculated controls were kept in the same facilities and monitored at regular intervals for the presence of BLV antibodies applying the IDgp test. In addition, the presence of BLV was examined in the blood leukocytes of the sheep by the competitive RIA (Gupta and Ferrer, 1979) and/or the syncytia infectivity assay (SIA) using indicator CC81 cells (Ferrer and Cabradilla, 1978). The extracts tested in the competitive RIA were prepared from 48 h blood leukocyte cultures seeded with 5 x 10^6 cells/ml of Eagles' minimum essential medium supplemented with 5% heat-inactivated foetal calf serum and phytohaemagglutinin (0.02 ml/ml). Each extract was prepared from both the cell pellet (1 000 g x 20 min) and virus pellet (100 000 g x 60 min) of 2 ml leukocyte culture, and then sonicated and treated with NP40.

RESULTS

In the first experiment whole milk samples obtained at 10, 30 and/or 50 days of lactation from 14 naturally infected cows were assayed. The milk of only 6 cows could be assayed at two of the sampling times. The results of the bioassay were evaluated 12 months after injection. At that time the number of recipient sheep that were positive for BLV antibodies in the IDgp test was higher than 4 or 8 months after injection. Moreover, an antibody response that persists for 12 months after injection is more likely to be due to infection rather than just to immunisation by virion antigens contained in the milk inoculum.

As shown in Table 1, BLV was present in milk samples from 7 of the 14 donor cows examined in the sheep bioassay. There were no significant differences in the frequency of positive milk samples at the three sampling times used. Of the 6 cows whose milk was assayed at two sampling times, 4 were positive in the sheep bioassay, but none of these was positive at both times. Nine of the recipient sheep that reacted in the IDgp test 12 months after injection were tested for infectious BLV in the SIA. Six of them were positive. None of the 7 non-inoculated control lambs nor the 7 lambs inoculated with milk samples of a non-infected cow in a BLV-free herd became positive in the IDgp test during the 12 months' observation period.

TABLE 1

DETECTION OF BLV IN MILK OF COWS NATURALLY INFECTED WITH BLV APPLYING THE SHEEP BIOASSAY[a]

Milk donor	Day of lactation at which milk was collected		
	10	30	50
G-245	+[b]	−	
BF-157	+	−	
BF-138	+	−	
G-142	−	+	
G-266	−		
BF-269	−		
BF-291		+	
G-255		−	
G-189		−	
G-43		−	+
G-257		−	−
G-263			−
G-24			+
G-265			−
No. Positive[b]	3/6	2/9	2/5

[a] Each milk sample was injected intraperitoneally into one or two lambs (100 ml of milk/lamb).

[b] + = one or both recipient sheep positive in the syncytia infectivity assay, and/or the IDgp test 12 or more months after injection.

In another experiment, the sheep bioassay was applied to examine the presence of BLV in cells obtained from colostrum and milk of 7 naturally infected cows. (Only 1 of these 7 cows had been used as a donor in the previous experiment). Most of

TABLE 2

DETECTION OF BLV IN MILK CELLS OF COWS NATURALLY INFECTED WITH BLV APPLYING THE SHEEP BIOASSAY[a]

Milk cell donor	Day of lactation at which milk cells were collected					
	1 day		4-6 days		10-13 days	
	Ab[b]	Virus[c]	Ab	Virus	Ab	Virus
G-4182	+	+	+	+		
G-314	-	+				
	-	-				
BF-138	+	+	+	+	+	+
	+	+			+	+
BF-283	+	+	+	+	+	-
	+	-	+	+	+	+
G-149	+	+	+	+	+	+
	+	-	+	+	+	+
G-312	+	+	+	+	+	+
	+	+			+	+
G-281	-	-	+	+		
	-	-	+	+		

a Each milk cell preparation was injected subcutaneously into one or two lambs (1×10^8 viable cells/lamb).

b Ab = antibody against BLV as determined by the IDgp test.

c Virus = presence of BLV as determined by the syncytia infectivity assay and/or the competitive radioimmunoassay in blood leukocytes collected 8 - 9 months after injection.

the recipient sheep inoculated with the milk cells from these donors became positive for BLV, as determined by the SIA and/or competitive RIA, and for BLV antibodies, as determined by the IDgp test, within only 12 weeks after inoculation. Nevertheless, for a more accurate evaluation of the results, all recipient sheep were tested again at 33 - 38 weeks after inoculation. The results (Table 2) show that BLV-infected cells were present in the milk of the 7 donors at one or more of the three sampling times used. There were no differences in the frequency with which infected cells were present in the milk at these times. None of the 8 non-inoculated control sheep that were continuously kept in the same barn and pasture with the inoculated sheep became positive in the SIA, RIA or IDgp test during the 8 - 9 months' observation period.

CONCLUSIONS

In the present study, whole milk or milk cells from 13 of 20 cows naturally infected with BLV were positive in the sheep bioassay for this virus.

In the first experiment, BLV was detected in whole milk samples collected from 7 of 14 donor cows at 10, 30 or 50 days of lactation. The frequency with which the virus was detected did not seem to differ between these 3 sampling times. Since in most cases only one of a pair of recipient lambs inoculated with a given whole milk sample developed BLV antibodies, it appears that the quantity of BLV or BLV-infected lymphocytes in 100 ml of milk is close to the limit of sensitivity of the sheep bioassay. If this is the case, it is not possible to determine whether the failure to detect BLV at successive sampling periods in a given positive cow is due to intermittent release or constant release of BLV at low levels.

In cattle BLV seems to infect only the lymphocytes (Ferrer et al., 1980). BLV infected lymphocytes do not usually replicate BLV *in vivo* but they do so a few hours after *in vitro* culture (Baliga and Ferrer, 1977). These findings suggest that in the BLV-infected animals there is an inhibitor that blocks the expression of BLV. On the basis of this information, it seems most likely that infection of the recipient sheep after milk inoculation is due mainly to the transfer of BLV-infected lymphocytes. Once in the sheep these cells, in the absence of the inhibitor, may release the virus until they are rejected by the xenograft response. The results of our second experiment showed that BLV-infected cells can indeed be readily detected in colostrum and milk of BLV-infected cows using the sheep bioassay.

In virtually all instances, both sheep inoculated with a given milk cell sample became infected. In contrast, only half of the whole milk samples that were positive in the sheep bioassay induced infection in both recipient sheep. Moreover, while the majority of the sheep inoculated with milk cells became infected within 3 months, in most of the sheep inoculated with whole milk, BLV infection was detected only after 8 to 12 months. Thus, using 1×10^8 viable milk cells, rather than 100 ml whole milk as the inoculum per recipient sheep, greatly increased the sensitivity of the sheep bioassay for the detection of BLV.

The present results are in contrast with those of Straub (this publication), who, with one exception, failed to induce BLV infection in sheep with milk of infected cows. Among other possibilities, Straub's failure may be due to the fact that he administered the milk to the sheep by the oral route rather than parenterally, as was the case in our study and in that of Miller and Van der Maaten (1979).

Despite the frequency with which BLV and/or BLV-infected lymphocytes are present in colostrum and milk of infected cows, milk-borne transmission of BLV seems to be relatively infrequent (Ferrer et al., 1976; Ferrer and Piper, 1978). This is probably due to the virus neutralising antibodies that all calves born to BLV-infected dams acquire through colostrum (Ferrer et al., 1977; Ferrer and Piper, 1978).

It has been estimated that at least 20% of the adult dairy cattle population in the United States is infected with BLV. From the present study, it seems that most of the infected cattle release BLV-infected lymphocytes in milk and therefore that humans, particularly children, are frequently exposed to the virus. On the other hand, extensive serological surveys have failed to detect BLV antibodies in humans (for a review see Caldwell, 1979).

REFERENCES

Baliga, V. and Ferrer, J.F., 1977. Expression of the bovine leukemia virus and its internal antigen in blood lymphocytes. Proc. Soc. Exp. Biol. Med. 156: 388-391.

Caldwell, G.G., 1979. Bovine Leukemia Virus, Public Health Serologic Studies. Proc. Bovine Leukosis Symposium. College Park, MD. pp. 143-159.

Ferrer, J.F. and Cabradilla, C.D., 1978. The phenomenon of polykaryocytosis induced by BLV in mixed cultures: specificity, mechanism, and application to the diagnosis of BLV infection in cattle. Ann. Rech. Vét. 9: 721-728.

Ferrer, J.F. and Piper, C.E., 1978. An evaluation of the role of milk in the natural transmission of the bovine leukemia virus. Ann. Rech. Vét. 9: 803-807.

Ferrer, J.F., Cabradilla, C.D. and Gupta, P., 1980. Bovine leukosis: a model for viral carcinogenesis. In: Viruses in naturally occurring cancers. Cold Spring Harbor Conferences on Cell Proliferation. Vol. 7. Ed. M. Essex, G. Tardaro, and ZurHausen, H., pp. 887-899 (Cold Spring Harbor Laboratory).

Ferrer, J.F., Piper, C.E., Abt, D.A. and Marshak, R.R., 1977. Diagnosis of bovine leukemia virus infection; evaluation of serological and hematological tests by means of a direct infectivity assay. Am. J. Vet. Res. 38: 1977-1981.

Ferrer, J.F., Piper, C.E., Abt, D.A., Marshak, R.R. and Bhatt, D.M., 1976. Natural mode of transmission of the bovine C type leukemia virus (BLV). Comparative leukemia disease 1975, Bibl. Haemat., No. 43. Ed. J. Clemmesen and D.S. Yohn, pp. 235-237 (Karger, Basel).

Gupta, P. and Ferrer, J.F., 1978. A critical comparison of the virus neutralization, radioimmunoprecipitation, and immunodiffusion tests for the serological diagnosis of BLV infection. Ann. Rech. Vét. 9: 683-688.

Gupta, O. and Ferrer, J.F., 1980. Detection of a precursor-like protein of bovine leukaemia virus structural polypeptides in purified virions. J. Gen. Virol. 47: 311-322.

Miller, J.M. and Van der Maaten, M.J., 1979. Infectivity tests of secretions and excretions from cattle infected with bovine leukemia virus. J. Natl. Cancer Inst. 62: 425-428.

Straub, O.C., 1981. Transmission studies from leukotic cattle to sheep using secretions, excretions, breath, and skin scrapings. Proceedings of the Fourth International Symposium on Bovine Leukosis, CEC, Bologna - Italy, 1980 (this publication).

DISCUSSION

O.C. Straub *(FRG)*

Did you exclude mastitis and increased cell counts due to handling and so on, in your results?

J.F. Ferrer *(USA)*

The herds from which we obtained the milk samples do not have mastitis that I know of.

C. Olson *(USA)*

Were cell counts done on the milk?

J.F. Ferrer

No. We injected known numbers of cells but we do not know what the original concentration of cells was in the milk.

A.A. Ressang *(Netherlands)*

You have provided another proof that BLV is cell bound. You injected whole milk; it is a pity that you did not inject milk without cells, in relation to your first slide.

J.F. Ferrer

I agree with you. Our experiments show that there are infected cells in colostrum and milk but do not exclude the possibility that free virus may be present in milk. This is not probable in colostrum because of the antibodies, but in milk it is possible that free virus is present.

TRANSMISSION STUDIES FROM LEUKOTIC CATTLE TO SHEEP USING SECRETIONS, EXCRETIONS, BREATH AND SKIN SCRAPINGS

O.C. Straub
Federal Research Institute for Animal Virus Diseases
D 7400 Tübingen, Federal Republic of Germany.

ABSTRACT

Oral mucus, nasal mucus, saliva, breath (minimum of 6 h/day for 3 days), skin scrapings, urine, semen, colostrum and/or milk from seropositive cattle - some of which were at the same time used in successful bovine transmission studies - were given to newborn lambs and to older sheep by oral, intranasal, intraperitoneal and/or intravenous routes. A seropositive reaction in the immunodiffusion test using both gp and p24 antigens was shown by only one sheep; this had received colostrum and milk from the first day post partum The observation periods range from 2 to 30 months.

O.C. Straub (ed.), Fourth International Symposium on Bovine Leukosis

INTRODUCTION

Earlier studies (Wittmann and Urbaneck, 1969; Mammerickx, 1970) confirmed later by Olson and Baumgartener (1976) showed that sheep are the ideal host other than the bovine for transmission experiments.

The importance of horizontal transmission has also been pointed out by a number of authors (Straub, 1971 and 1978; Straub et al., 1978; Ferrer, 1979; Piper et al., 1979). It was quite natural then to investigate by which means this horizontal transmission occurs using sheep for infectivity tests. Results obtained by Ressang (1980) and Miller and Van der Maaten, (1979) showed that a transmission occurred via milk from infected cattle and saliva after treatment of the infected animal by an anaesthetic drug. It was also demonstrated that a transmission is possible by mechanical means (Wilesmith et al., 1978). A possible transmission by insects was indicated by Bech-Nielsen et al. (1978). The possible role played by semen was investigated by Lucas et al. (1980). The latest news comes from Kaaden et al. (1980) who report in this publication a transmission obtained by ticks.

In the studies to be reported various excretions, secretions, breath and skin scrapings from infected cattle were used to prove the presence or absence of infectious virus by inoculating sheep of different ages by various routes. Most of the cattle were at the same time used for horizontal transmission studies to cattle which proved successful.

MATERIALS AND METHODS

Infected donors

Two groups of donors were used: one which was only gp-seropositive, and another one which was antigen (AG) and seropositive, in general containing antibodies against the glycoprotein (gp) and the internal protein (p24) as indicated in the Tables.

Material

Nasal and mouth swabs were taken and the mucus eluted by adding tissue culture medium (MEM). Then the samples were shaken for 30 min at $4^{o}C$ and the gauze squeezed. Next the fluid was centrifuged at 2 200 g for 10 min and the supernatant used as inoculum. Details may be taken from Table 1.

Saliva

The donors were stanchioned, the front part of the head put into a plastic bag at the open other end of which a box was placed which allowed air to pass through. The lambs were kept inside the box. The saliva was collected at the lowest point of the bag and given to the lambs as indicated in Table 1.

Breath

The lambs were kept in the box as described above. They could not come into direct contact with the bovines in whose air flow they were for various periods of time as shown in Table 2.

Skin scrapings

They were obtained by first shearing the hair and then using a razor blade for the superficial layer of the epidermis. In no case was there any visible blood involved. The scrapings were then mixed with skimmed milk powder and immediately given orally to the sheep as described in Table 3.

Urine

The urine was not taken by artificial means but by collecting it during normal urination. It was injected or given orally together with skimmed milk as given in Table 3.

Semen

Three ejaculates from each of three bulls were collected and the whole ejaculate except a small amount for laboratory

TABLE 1

RESULTS OF TRANSMISSION STUDIES FROM BLV-INFECTED CATTLE TO SHEEP USING NASAL OR ORAL SWAB MATERIAL AND SALIVA

Material	No. of animals	Age	Route of inoculation	Duration of observation period (in months)	Result of IDT
Nasal swabs mixture from 6 donors gp + p24 + AG +	2	newborn	i.v. and/or i.p.	30	-
Nasal swabs mixture from 4 donors gp +	4	newborn	i.v. and/or i.p.	29 or 30	-
Oral mucus mixture from 6 donors gp + p24 + AG +	2	newborn	i.v.	32	-
Oral mucus mixture from 4 donors gp +	2	newborn	1 - i.v. 1 - i.v. (10 ml) + i.p. (20 ml)	29	-
Saliva mixture from 3 donors gp + p24 + AG +	4	newborn to day 3	oral 1) 380 ml 2) 830 ml 3) 500 ml 4) 570 ml	21 20 21 20	- - - -
Saliva mixture from 3 donors gp +	1	newborn to day 3	oral	29	-
Saliva from one donor gp + p24 + AG +	2	newborn to 6 months of age (daily)	oral (minimum of 20 l)	10	-

TABLE 2

RESULTS OF TRANSMISSION STUDIES FROM BLV-INFECTED CATTLE TO SHEEP USING BREATH

Material	No. of animals	Duration	Duration of observation period (in months)	Result of IDT
Breath from 3 donors gp + p24 + AG +	3	3 x 6 hours	21	-
Breath from 3 donors gp +	3	3 x 6 hours	20	-
Breath from 1 donor gp + p24 + AG +	2	6 hours daily for 6 months	10	-

experiments used as inoculum as shown in Table 3. In the laboratory the semen was tested for the presence of blood constituents, antigen and antibodies (in the immunodiffusion test).

Colostrum and milk

The amounts given from which type of donor at which time after parturition may be taken from Table 4. All samples were administered orally, because it was the object to simulate the possible natural transmission from dam to offspring.

Conduct of the experiment

After the inoculations or administration of the various material the recipients were tested first at short intervals then monthly for the presence of antibodies against both major antigens in the immunodiffusion test as described before (Straub, 1978). At the same time the WBC and a differential were determined. The observation periods varied as shown in Tables 1 - 4.

TABLE 3

RESULTS OF TRANSMISSION STUDIES FROM BLV-INFECTED CATTLE TO SHEEP USING SKIN-SCRAPINGS, URINE AND SEMEN

Material	No. of animals	Age	Route of inoculation	Duration of observation period (in months)	Result of IDT
Skin scrapings from 3 donors gp + p24 + AG +	4	newborn	oral	22 or 24	-
Urine mixture from 6 donors gp + p24 + AG +	2	newborn	1) 20 ml i.v. + 20 ml i.p. 2) 20 ml i.p. for 2 days	30 30	- -
Urine mixture from 4 donors gp +	2	newborn	1) 30 ml i.p. 2) 400 ml for 3 days	30 20	- -
Semen from 1 bull gp + p24 + AG +	3	approx. 6 months	half of 1 ejaculate each oral and intraperitoneal	7 - 8	-
Semen from 1 bull gp + AG +	3	approx. 6 months	half of 1 ejaculate each oral and intraperitoneal	6 - 8	-
Semen from 1 bull gp +	3	approx. 6 months	half of 1 ejaculate each oral and intraperitoneal	6 - 8	-

TABLE 4

RESULTS OF TRANSMISSION STUDIES FROM BLV-INFECTED CATTLE TO SHEEP USING COLOSTRUM AND/OR MILK AT VARIOUS DATES

Material	No. of animals	Amount in ml	Observation period (months)	Result of IDT
Colostrum donor gp +	3	250 - 500	2 - 10	-
Colostrum & milk from day 1 p.p. donor gp + p24 + AG +	1	2 x 1000	3	+ (after 5 weeks)
donor gp +	1	500 & 1000	6	-
Milk from day 1 p.p. donor gp +	1	600	10	-
Milk from day 2 p.p. 3 donors gp +	3	700 - 1500	2 - 10	-
1 donor gp + p24 + AG +	1	2800	3	-
Milk day 3 p.p. same 3 donors	3	700 - 1500	2 - 10	-
same 1 donor	1	2500	3	-
Milk day 4 p.p. same 3 donors	3	1000 - 2500	2 - 10	-
same 1 donor	1	3500	3	-
Milk day 5 p.p. 2 donors gp +	3	1000 - 1400	2 - 10	-
Milk day 6 p.p. 2 donors gp +	3	700 - 1400	2 - 10	-
Milk day 7 p.p. 2 donors gp +	3	1500	2	-
Milk 2 months p.p. donor gp + p24 + AG +	5	750 - 2000	10	-
Milk 3 months p.p. donor gp +	4	2000	10	-
Milk 4 months p.p. donor gp +	2	1000 & 2000	10	-

RESULTS

Up to the present, only one sheep has become seropositive (Table 4). It had received colostrum and first day milk from an animal that had become seropositive and antigen positive during pregnancy. From all the animals tested in another experiment for the presence of the different amounts of globulins and of classes of immunoglobulin this animal had the sharpest drop in those constituents within the first 24 hours p.p. (Matthaeus and Straub, 1980). No antibodies nor antigen could be found in the 9 semen samples tested. In one, some blood constituents were found.

DISCUSSION

Those negative results cannot demonstrate that a transmission via those materials tested will never occur, but it rates them as a rather rare event. This statement appears possible because the horizontal transmission experiment carried out at the same time proved successful. Insects as vectors can be excluded too, since the experiments were conducted in completely or semi-isolated stalls. Mechanical transmission by the bleeding-needle can also be excluded. Therefore, unless other results are obtained later, the conclusion must be drawn that the horizontal transmission occurs via minor amounts of blood. Neighbouring animals, especially when tied, seem to fight quite a bit. It is realised that this is a poor answer, but no other can be offered at present.

REFERENCES

Bech-Nielsen, S., Piper, C.E. and Ferrer, J.F., 1978. Natural mode of transmission of the bovine leukemia virus: Role of bloodsucking insects. Am. J. Vet. Res. 39: 1089-1092.

Ferrer, J.F., 1979. Bovine Leukosis: Natural transmission and principles of control. J. Am. Vet. Med. Ass. 175: 1281-1286.

Kaaden, O-R., Fischer, W., Meerman, A. and Liebisch, A., 1981. Transmission of BLV by *Ixodes ricinus* Ticks. 4th International Symposium on Bovine Leukosis, CEC, Bologna, November, 1980 (this publication).

Lucas, M.H., Dawson, M., Chasey, D., Wibberley, G., Roberts, D.H., 1980. Enzootic bovine leukosis virus in semen. Vet. Rec. 106: 128.

Mammerickx, M., 1970. Sur l'utilisation du mouton pour les expériences sur la leucose bovine. Expérimentation Animal 3: 285-293.

Matthaeus, W. and Straub, O.C., 1981. Immunoglobulin levels of serum, colostrum and milk during the periparturient period of dams and their offspring during the first days of life. 4th International Symposium on Bovine Leukosis, CEC, Bologna, November, 1980 (this publication).

Miller, J.M. and Van der Maaten, M.J., 1979. Infectivity test of secretions and excretions from cattle infected with bovine leukosis virus. J. Nat. Cancer Inst. 62: 425-428.

Olsen, C. and Baumgartener, L.E., 1976. Pathology of lymphosarcoma in sheep induced with bovine leukemia virus. Cancer Res. 36: 2365-2373.

Piper, C.E., Ferrer, J.F., Abt, D.A. and Marshak, R.R., 1979. Postnatal and prenatal transmission of the bovine leukemia virus under natural conditions. J. Nat. Cancer Inst. 62: 165-168.

Ressang, A.A. CEC Scientific workshop on Bovine Leukosis, 1979, (Ed. Markson, L.M.) Discussion remark p 43.

Straub, O.C., 1971. Studies on horizontal transmission of bovine leukosis. Arch. Virusforsch. 33: 145-150.

Straub, O.C., 1978. Horizontal transmission studies on enzootic bovine leukosis. In: Ann. Rech. Vét. 9, (Ed. Parodi, A.L.), Institut National de la Recherche Agronomique, Paris and CEC, Luxembourg: 809-813.

Straub, O.C., Fischer, W. and Frerking, H., 1978. Über die Zunahme leukose-seropositiver Reagenten in einem hämatologisch negativen Rinderbestand. Tierärztl. Umschau 33: 657-661.

Wilesmith, J.W., Straub, O.C. and Lorenz, R.J., 1978. Untersuchungen zur iatrogenen Übertragung des Virus der Rinderleukose. Tierärztl.Umschau 33: 519-523.

Wittman, W. and Urbanek, D., 1969. Untersuchungen sur Ätiologie der Rinderleukose 8. Übertragungsversuche mit Blut leukosekranker Rinder auf Schaflämmer. Arch. Exp. Vet.-med. 23: 709-713.

DISCUSSION

A.A. Ressang *(Netherlands)*

We announced in Paris that we have started infectivity experiments using newborn lambs in which we applied, as infective material, saliva after injection of the cows with urine and faecal extracts. We have been luckier than you because out of 25 infected lambs, with saliva, five turned out to be positive. This was not the case with the urine and the faecal extracts. My question is, there is one point that I cannot understand, that is your philosophy of using skin scrapings as infective material. Do you really expect the virus to be excreted through the skin?

O.C. Straub *(FRG)*

You have to exclude everything. Think of Marek's disease; there infectious material is contained in the follicle of the feather. We know that BLV is transmitted if the animals are in close contact but not if the distance between animals is 2 m or more. So, I decided to check the upper layer of the skin. Animals do have close contact with skin, they rub each other all the time. I think it was worth trying.

HUMORAL SPONTANEOUS RESPONSE TO BOVINE LEUKAEMIA VIRUS INFECTION IN ZEBU, SHEEP, BUFFALO AND CAPYBARA

C. Marín, N. de López
L. de Alvarez, H. Castaños, W. España, A. León and A. Bello
Instituto de Investigaciones Veterinarias, Apdo. 70,
Maracay-Venezuela.

ABSTRACT

The participation of species other than bovine (Bos taurus) in the epidemiological chain of bovine leukaemia has not previously been reported. Ecological factors in tropical areas seem to influence the behaviour of the bovine leukaemia virus (BLV) according to an investigation we carried out in which it was demonstrated that infection by the virus is not exclusive to Bos taurus but that it is also capable of inducing the formation of specific antibodies, haematological changes of the lymphocyte fraction (persistent lymphocytosis), and development of multicentral lymphosarcomas in Bos indicus. Furthermore, it has been proven for the first time ever that there is spontaneous transmission of the infectious agent to the ovine species, while in the water buffalo (Bubalis bubalis) precipitating antibodies to BLV were detected. In the case of Capybara (Hydrochoerus hydrochaeris), it is considered that it could act as an amplifier by inducing seroconversion in the same way that BLV does in the species mentioned above.

O.C. Straub (ed.), Fourth International Symposium on Bovine Leukosis

INTRODUCTION

In spite of developments in the research into bovine leukaemia during the last ten years, there are many aspects of its natural history which are still not clear. However, it is accepted that BLV is the aetiological agent responsible for the known clinical symptoms such as persistent lymphocytosis and lymphosarcoma. This virus has morphological (Calafat and Ressang, 1977), biophysical and biochemical characteristics common to oncongenic viruses type C of other species (MacDonald and Ferrer, 1976), but it differs from these in its antigenic properties, which has made possible the detection of sero-specific antibodies used in its diagnosis. On the other hand, several investigators (Piper et al., 1975; Nielsen et al., 1978) have carried out studies to try to find its transmission mechanisms and to explore the possibility that there could be natural reservoirs of the virus other than the *Bos taurus*. Olson and Baumgartener (1975) did not detect precipitating antibodies in 2 321 domestic and wild animals. These two authors experimentally inoculated 179 mammals of 12 different species, and 23 fowl, also of different species, in which no serological response or tumoral development was found. Sheep and goats have been used in the experimental inoculation of BLV, inducing formation of generalised lymphosarcoma (Olson et al., 1972; Van der Maaten, 1975; Bex et al., 1979). However, natural transmission in these species has not so far been reported.

The occurrence of lymphosarcoma lesions in Indian buffaloes, the origin of which does not seem to be related to BLV, has been reported (Singh,1967). In 1977, Van der Maaten, examining serum of buffaloes in India, did not obtain a positive response in the agar gel immunodiffusion (AGID) test using p24 as antigen.

In this paper we report the detection of specific antibodies in animal species, other than *Bos taurus*, infected naturally with BLV: zebu *(Bos indicus)*, ovines *(Ovis ovis)*, buffaloes *(Bubalis bubalis)* and capybara *(Hydrochoerus hydrochaeris)*.

MATERIALS AND METHODS

Zebu

Eleven thousand, seven hundred and eleven bovines of various zebu-type breeds and their crosses, from different regions of the country, were examined with the purpose of demonstrating the susceptibility of *Bos indicus* to infection by BLV. The animals studied were classified by age, breed, sex, and different management practices. In the same way, cytological and histopathological studies were made of generalised lymphosarcoma lesions using conventional as well as special techniques. Blood samples were collected for haematological evaluation in order to find qualitative and quantitative changes of the lymphocyte fraction.

Buffaloes

One thousand and seventy two sera of Indian and Australian type buffaloes, aged 1 to 9 years, from eastern and southern regions of the country, which had been raised in extensive systems in open fields, were examined for the detection of BLV antibodies. The samples were classified by age, breed and sex.

Sheep

One hundred and seventy nine sheep of various breeds and ages were examined serologically, kept in separate lots on a farm with a herd of 450 Holstein and Brown Swiss bovines, to a high percentage infected with BLV, with signs of persistent lymphocytosis and development of frequent tumours at a high incidence rate. Three samplings of sera were taken at intervals of six months.

Capybaras

Studies were carried out on 124 wild animals of different sex and ages. These large rodents are generally found in lagoons and rivers, living with nomad bovines in lowlands (Figure 1).

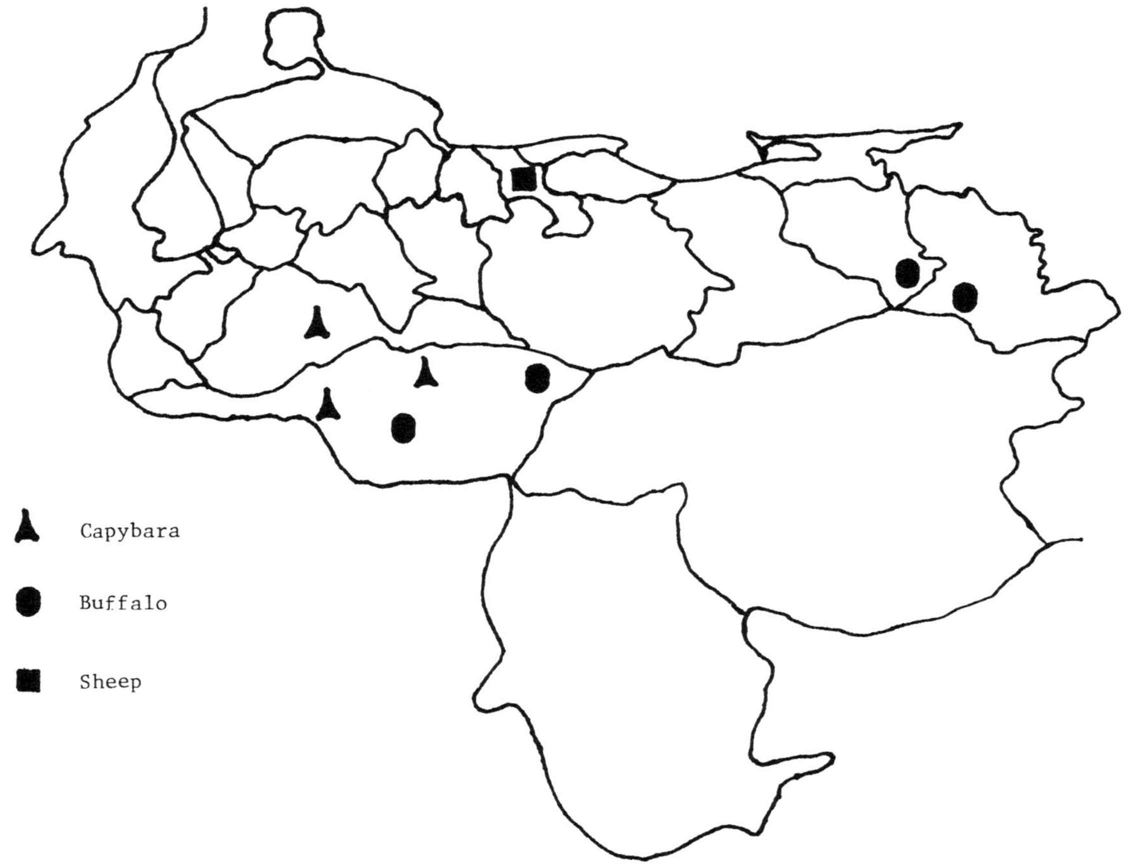

Fig. 1. Survey for detection of BLV infection in buffalo, sheep and capybara in Venezuela.

Agar gel immunodiffusion test

Tests for the detection of specific antibodies were made using the AGID test. It was run in 0.8% agarose, 0.05 M tris-HCl buffer (pH 7.2), containing 8.5% NaCl. The agarose was placed in 90 mm petri dishes and 7 wells of 5 mm diameter were made at a distance of 2.5 mm from each other. The antigen glycoprotein 60 was placed in the central well. The sera to be tested were placed alternately with positive reference sera in the peripheral wells.

The plates were incubated at room temperature in a humidified chamber and examined 24 and 48 hours later.

RESULTS

The presence of BLV antibodies in the sera of zebu, sheep, buffalo and capybara, was evaluated by the detection of a precipitation line similar to the one formed with the relevant reference serum, which indicates complete identity and specificity to the reaction of antigen and antibody.

In the trial for the detection of BLV antibodies performed on 11 711 sera of zebu, 2 174 (18.5%) were positive (Table 1). The results of the cytological and histopathological studies showed characteristic changes of the multicentral lymphosarcoma, indicating that the zebu, like *Bos taurus*, is capable of developing multiple tumoral cases.

By WBC and differentiation of the leukocytes, we were able to find in some animals, a noticeable increase in the number of lymphocytes, and alterations in their morphology.

In the first examination of the sheep flock, 8 were found to be positive at an age between 5 and 6 years; the second time 7 new positive animals were found, also 5 and 6 years of age; and the third time, only one, 5 years of age. In the sera from the 1 072 buffaloes, there were 85 positive reactors (7.9%).

TABLE 1

PREVALENCE OF BLV INFECTION IN VENEZUELAN ZEBU CATTLE

Breed	Number of animals	Negative	Positive	%
Gyr	1 932	1 408	524	27.12
Brahman	1 295	868	427	32.97
Nellore	1 123	1 000	123	10.95
Guzerat	271	233	38	14.02
Indu Brazil	175	115	60	32.28
Sta. Gertrudis	19	5	14	93.68
Zebu hybrid	6 896	5 908	988	14.33
	11 711	9 537	2 174	18.56

TABLE 2

HUMORAL SPONTANEOUS REACTION TO BLV INFECTION IN VENEZUELAN BUFFALOES

Age (years)	Number of animals	Negative	Positive	%
1	82	78	4	4.88
1 - 2	96	91	5	5.21
2 - 3	62	56	6	9.68
3 - 4	64	60	4	6.25
4 - 5	139	133	6	4.32
5 - 6	140	129	11	7.86
6 - 7	124	113	11	8.93
7 - 8	112	102	10	8.93
8 - 9	142	124	18	12.68
9	111	101	10	9.93
	1 072	987	85	7.93

A sero-conversion capacity was registered in all the age groups with a greater prevalence in the group over 5 years of age, and especially in the group which was between 8 and 9 years of age. The highest infection index was obtained in the herds of the southern region in proportion to the number of buffaloes studied (Table 2). Of the 120 capybara sera examined, 9 (7%) were found to be positive; they were three females and six males of 2 and 3 years of age.

DISCUSSION

Various investigations have been devoted to research into animal species, and even man, as possible natural reservoirs or receptors of bovine leukosis virus. The studies and experimental trials carried out have been unsuccessful in the investigation of infection and inoculation of mammals and fowls. The natural occurrence of tumours of the lymphosarcoma type in a flock of sheep has been reported in Rhodesia (Boyt et al., 1976), but the authors did not establish a connection between these lesions and BLV. These facts made us accept that BLV was exclusive to *Bos taurus*. However, in analysing our results we have found that zebu-type breeds *(Bos indicus)* are not only capable of inducing specific sero-conversion, but also of presenting persistent lymphocytosis and of developing generalised lymphosarcoma lesions such as are found in breeds of European origin.

The humoral response detected in ovines placed in a leukotic herd allowed us to demonstrate that spontaneous infection can occur in a ruminant species which has proven to be very susceptible to experimental inoculation. In considering how the ovines were infected, we can discard the possibility of the virus passing from bovines to ovines by simple contact, especially when the distance and isolation between the two species on the farms in question is taken into consideration. This fact made us consider the role of sucking insects (especially ticks) in the transmission of BLV.

Water buffaloes seem to be very efficient in their capacity

to respond immunologically to this virus, but not in the development of lymphosarcoma.

Capybara, a species which is zoologically separate from bovines, is also identified as being susceptible to serological conversion after infection by BLV, which seems possible because bovines and capybara both live in tropical ecological systems, highly populated by insects which may have acted as transmitters. This opens a new perspective on the epidemiological knowledge of the disease.

REFERENCES

Bendixen, H.J., 1963. Leukosis enzootica bovis: diagnostik, epidemiologi; Bekaemgelse thesis; Copenhagen.

Bex, F., Bruck, C.M., Mammerickx, M., Portetelle, D., Ghysdael, J., Cleuter, Y., Leclercq, M., Dekegel, D. and Burny, A., 1979. Humoral antibody response to bovine leukemia virus infection in cattle and sheep. Cancer Res. 39, 1118-1123.

Boyt, W.P., MacKenzie, P.K. and Emslie, V.W., 1976. Enzootic leukosis in a flock of sheep in Rhodesia. Vet. Rec. 98 (6), 112-115.

Calafat, J. and Ressang, A.A., 1977. Morphogenesis of bovine leukemia virus. Virology 80, 42-53.

Marín, C. and Medina de López, N., 1977. Abstr. 1st Int. Symp. on Bovine Leukosis, April 18-20, Caracas, 83-86.

Marín, C., Medina de López, N., P. de Alvarez, L., Lozano, O., España, W., Castaños, H. and León, A., 1978. Epidemiology of bovine leukemia in Venezuela. Ann. Rech. Vét. 9, 743-746.

MacDonald, H.C. and Ferrer, J.F., 1976. Detection, quantitation and characterization of the major internal virion antigen of the bovine leukemia virus by radioimmunoassay. J. Nat. Cancer Inst. 57, 875-882.

Miller, J.M. and Van der Maaten, M.J., 1975. Serology detection of bovine leukemia virus infection. CEC Workshop Conf. on Bovine Leukosis, Copenhagen, 17-18 Oct.

Nielsen, S., Piper, C. and Ferrer, J., 1978. Natural mode of transmission of the bovine leukemia virus: Role of bloodsucking insects. Am. J. Vet. Res. 39(7), 1089-1092.

Olson, C., Miller, L.D., Miller, J.M. and Hoss, H.E., 1972. Transmission of lymphosarcoma from cattle to sheep. J. Nat. Cancer Inst. 49, 1463-1467.

Olson, C. and Baumgartener, L., 1975. Lymphosarcoma (Leukemia) of Cattle. Bov. Pract. (Nov.).

Piper, C.E., Abt, D.A., Ferrer, J.F. and Marshack, R.R., 1975. Seroepidemiological evidence for horizontal transmission of bovine C type virus. Cancer Res. 35, 1714-1716.

Singh, C.M., 1967. Lymphosarcoma in Indian Buffaloes. Proc. 3rd. Int. Symp. Comp. Leukemia Res. Paris.

Van der Maaten, M.J., 1975. Induction of lymphoid tumors in sheep with cell-free preparations of bovine leukemia virus. Comp. Leuk. Res. Bibl. Haemat. No.13, Ed. J. Clemmesen and D.S. Yohn (Karger, Basel 1976), 377-379.

Van der Maaten, M.J., 1977. Cited by J. Miller. Proc. 1st Int. Symp. on Bovine Leukosis, Caracas, 102.

DISCUSSION

M. Mussgay *(FRG)*

Did you try to collect mosquitos or flies to isolate the virus?

C. Marin *(Venezuela)*

No, we did not.

M.J. Burridge *(USA)*

Have you got evidence that the flies you are talking about are feeding both on cattle and capybara?

C. Marin

I am not able to say whether the insects went from one animal to the other.

EXPERIMENTAL CROSS TRANSMISSIONS OF BOVINE LEUKAEMIA VIRUS (BLV) BETWEEN SEVERAL ANIMAL SPECIES

M. Mammerickx[1], D. Portetelle[2] and A. Burny[2]

[1]Institut National de Recherches Vétérinaires
Groeselenberg 99, B-1180 Brussels, Belgium.

[2]Faculté des Sciences Agronomiques de l'Etat
B-5800 Gembloux, Belgium

and Departement de Biologie Moléculaire
Université Libre de Bruxelles
B-1640 Rhode-Saint-Genèse, Belgium.

ABSTRACT

Sheep and goats were inoculated with BLV positive blood from a cow donor and were observed over a long period of time (1969 - 1980). Comparing the reactions of sheep and goats to an experimental infection by BLV from a bovine donor we can say:

1. *both species were receptive to the virus;*
2. *practically all BLV positive sheep developed tumours before the age of 7 years whereas in the same period, BLV positive goats were resistant to this phenomenon;*
3. *haematological changes (leukaemia and anaemia) were observed in sheep only and were linked to the tumoral transformation. The sheep is the most suitable experimental animal for the study of the tumoral effect of BLV.*

Cross transmission experiments taught us that BLV remains infectious for cow, sheep, goat and pig whatever the donor species (cow, sheep and goat). An interesting new fact is that BLV from bovine, ovine or caprine donors can pass to pig, and from this species back to sheep. This experiment with BLV positive porcine donors failed in two cows and in three of six sheep. This observation perhaps indicates that the infectious properties of the virus passed to swine are attenuated. We need a longer period of observation to appreciate better the biological effects of those viruses passed to several animal species.

O.C. Straub (ed.), Fourth International Symposium on Bovine Leukosis

INTRODUCTION

The problem of transmission of BLV to species other than cattle has been reviewed in a recent work (Burny et al., 1980). Some partial results of our experiments on interspecific transmissions have already been published (Bex et al., 1979; Burny et al., 1980; Mammerickx, 1969 - 1980, 1970; Mammerickx et al., 1976; Mammerickx et al., 1980). From them it appeared that BLV was infectious for some animal species, but differences appeared in the oncogenic activity.

To find an economical justification to combat an infectious disease, economists are interested by symptoms and lesions that produce economic losses in the animal breeding industry. For enzootic bovine leukaemia (EBL), lesions and symptoms to be considered are:

- tumoral development,
- persistent lymphocytosis,
- leukaemia,
- anaemia,
- immunosuppressive effects.

These manifestations are either observed in cattle naturally BLV infected, or in other animal species (human, murine, feline, etc.) infected by viruses classified in the 'retrovirus' group, or affected by a leukaemic disease of unknown aetiology.

Results obtained by transmission of a virus from one animal species to another are likely to allow differentiation between the role of the virus itself and the role of other factors which could influence the clinical aspect of the disease.

In Belgium, natural cases of enzootic bovine leukosis (EBL) induced by bovine leukaemia virus (BLV) occurred only in the bovine species. Our first interspecies transmission trials were done with a BLV infected cow as donor, and sheep or goats as recipients. More recently we added the species swine to our series of experimental animals.

The first results obtained taught us that experimental infection of a recipient animal, starting from a serologically BLV positive donor, can give several results, namely:

1. development of a persistent humoral reaction to BLV antigens, detected by agar gel immunodiffusion (AGID) or radio-immunoassay (RIA)-tests, and progressive rise of antibody titres; such animals, observed over a long period, can sometimes develop haematological disorders, and die naturally of a tumoral disease, or from another disease, or by accident.

2. no humoral response to BLV antigens; such animals never die of lymphosarcoma. Three mechanisms could explain such a situation:
   a. a case of natural resistance (interferon, intercurrent infection or other unknown reasons);
   b. recipient animal harbours maternal antibodies of colostral origin when infected with BLV;
   c. recipient animal dies very soon (before the development of a humoral response).

In order to study the biological effects of BLV on several animal species, we performed cross transmission trials starting from cows, sheep, goat and pigs as donors infecting the same series of animal species.

MATERIALS AND METHODS

Experimental animals

Experimental animals were housed in our barns in Uccle. They were born at the Institute or bought at birth from leukosis free herds. These animals were continuously surveyed by clinical, haematological and serological methods. At death, patho-anatomical and patho-histological examinations were performed.

Sheep and goats were kept untied in separate flocks where inoculated and non-inoculated control animals were housed together. After birth, sheep and goats fed naturally. Cattle were kept tied. Calves were fed with milk substitutes. Pigs were kept together untied. Newborn piglets were fed by their mother.

Cattle, sheep and goats can be kept under observation for a long period. Pigs were killed at the age of ten months; it was not practical to keep them for a longer period, considering the rapidity of growth in this species.

Laboratory tests

Agar gel immunodiffusion tests (AGID) and radio-immunoassay tests (RIA) for the detection of the BLVgp antibodies, haematological analysis, patho-anatomical and patho-histological findings were performed as previously described (Lorenz et al., 1978; Mammerickx et al., 1978a,b; Mammerickx et al., 1980; Portetelle et al., 1980; Straub et al., 1978).

Experimental inoculations

The starting material was whole blood collected in sodium citrate. This blood was:

- either inoculated by the oral route (forced feeding with a syringe - 20 ml of blood, once a day - for 5 to 6 weeks);
- or inoculated once by the intradermal route (0.5 to 1 ml of blood injected at several sites with a tuberculin needle);
- or inoculated once by intraperitoneal and intravenous routes (10 ml of a lymphocyte short-term culture each).

RESULTS

The results are reported in Tables 1 to 3.

Table 1 gives the results of a transmission trial from an EBL cow naturally infected (BLV +) to sheep and goats. Lambs were derived from four healthy BLV negative sheep and kids from a healthy BLV negative goat. Experimental inoculations took place between 1969 and 1973. Inoculated and control animals

TABLE 1

HUMORAL ANTIBODY REACTIONS TO BLV, AND TUMORAL TRANSFORMATIONS INDUCED BY EXPERIMENTAL INOCULATIONS OF SHEEP AND GOATS. ONE BLV POSITIVE COW WAS DONOR, AND THE OBSERVATION PERIOD RAN FROM 1969 TO 1980.

Observation period	Trials	Total number of animals		Animals still alive		Animals dead of lympho-sarcoma		Animals dead of other diseases	
		BLV +	BLV -	BLV +	BLV -	BLV +	BLV -	BLV +	BLV -
Sheep									
1969 - 1980	Infected**	33		7		19		7	
		24	9	1	6	19	0	4	3
1969 - 1978*	Controls	27		20		0		7	
		0	27	0	20	0	0	0	7
Goats									
1970 - 1980	Infected***	8		5		0		7	
		8	0	5	0	0	0	3	0
1970 - 1980	Controls	4		2		0		2	
		0	4	0	2	0	0	0	2

+ Positive; - negative;
* Since 1978 controls were used for other trials.
** Orally at birth (29 animals), or at the age of 4 - 5 months (4 animals).
*** Orally at birth (6 animals), or by intraperitoneal and intravenous routes at birth (2 animals)

TABLE 2

AGE AND HAEMATOLOGICAL DISORDERS IN INFECTED SHEEP DYING FROM LYMPHOSARCOMA. Y = YEAR, M = MONTH

Sheep number	Age at inoculation	Age at death due to lymphosarcoma	Haematological disorders			
			Lymphocytes		Erythrocytes	
			Number of lymphoid cells/mm^3 of blood at death, x 10^3	Age at the beginning of the leukaemia	Number of erythrocytes/mm^3 of blood at death, x 10^6	Age at the beginning of the anaemia
M.350	birth	10 M.	1.6	no change	12.2	no change
M.346	birth	1 Y.	36.2	1 Y.	9.5	no change
M.302	5 M.	1 Y. 5 M.	101.8	1 Y. 4 M.	7.5	1 Y. 5 M.
M.377	birth	2 Y. 3 M.	8.1	2 Y.	8.9	no change
M.338	birth	2 Y. 8 M.	37.3	1 Y. 9 M.	7.5	2 Y. 8 M.
M.319	birth	3 Y. 2 M.	4.6	no change	10.4	no change
M.344	birth	3 Y. 4 M.	925.9	2 Y. 9 M.	4.7	3 Y. 4 M.
M.373	birth	3 Y. 4 M.	11.7	2 Y. 7 M.	5.2	3 Y. 2 M.
M.359	4 M.	3 Y. 6 M.	3.2	no change	12.2	no change
M.303	5 M.	3 Y.10 M.	1.2	no change	6.3	3 Y. 8 M.
M.376	birth	3 Y.10 M.	2.1	no change	8.4	no change
M.340	birth	4 Y.10 M.	7.8	4 Y. 8 M.	8.3	no change
M.348	birth	4 Y.10 M.	232.0	3 Y.10 M.	4.5	4 Y. 3 M.
M.347	birth	5 Y. 4 M.	11.4	4 Y. 5 M.	9.4	no change
M.372	birth	6 Y. 1 M.	1.7	no change	8.7	no change
M.370	birth	6 Y. 2 M.	10.2	6 Y. 2 M.	8.3	no change
M.334	birth	6 Y. 4 M.	60.5	6 Y. 4 M.	5.1	6 Y. 4 M.
M.328	birth	6 Y. 6 M.	49.4	6 Y. 5 M.	9.0	no change
M.345	birth	6 Y. 7 M.	3.8	no change	7.0	6 Y. 7 M.

TABLE 3

HUMORAL ANTIBODY REACTIONS TO BLV, INDUCED BY EXPERIMENTAL INOCULATIONS TO SEVERAL ANIMAL SPECIES, ALL ANIMALS WERE INFECTED INTRADERMALLY WITH BLV+ BLOOD, AND THE OBSERVATION PERIOD RAN FROM 1979 TO 1980.

Donor species \ Recipient species	Bovine		Ovine		Caprine		Porcine	
	Total number of animals		Total number of animals		Total number of animals		Total number of animals	
	BLV +	BLV -	BLV +	BLV -	BLV +	BLV -	BLV +	BLV -
Bovine	1		1		1		2	
	1	0	1	0	1	0	2	0
Ovine	3		5		2		2	
	3	0	4	1	2	0	2	0
Caprine	2		5		3		1	
	2	0	5	0	3	0	1	0
Porcine	2		6		ND		ND	
	0	2	3	3	ND	ND	ND	ND

were observed over a period of eleven years (1969 - 1980). All animals, except four, were infected at birth; four sheep (M.302, M.303, M.358 and M.359) were 4 - 5 months old when infected.

During the observation period, 19 of 33 sheep inoculated died of lymphosarcoma. BLV infection was not proven in nine sheep (four harboured maternal antibodies from colostral origin when infected with BLV; three could be classified as naturally resistent to BLV for an unknown reason; two died before the development of a humoral response). One sheep serologically BLV positive is still alive; it was born in 1973. All the other serologically BLV positive sheep died from lymphosarcoma or another disease. The ages of the nineteen sheep which died from lymphosarcoma are listed in Table 2.

The eight goats inoculated developed signs of a BLV infection, but none of them died from lymphosarcoma. The five goats serologically BLV positive and still alive were born in 1970 (Burny et al., 1980), 1972 (Bex et al., 1979) and 1973 (Burny et al., 1980). They are thus all more than 7 years old.

In both species control animals remained serologically negative and none of them died from a tumoral disease.

Table 2 gives the results of the haematological changes in sheep dying from lymphosarcoma. The haematological disorders were:

- a true leukaemia (the level of lymphoid cells increased progressively and many blastic tumoral cells could be observed; the changes appeared towards the end of the disease, one year or less before death in the tumour phase. Circulating lymphocytes increased to leukaemia levels were present in twelve of nineteen sheep; at death the number of lymphoid cells/mm^3 of blood varied widely (from 7.8×10^3 to $925.9 \times 10^3/mm^3$ of blood).
- an anaemia; this change appeared also at the terminal phase of the disease. Decreased erythrocyte levels were found in eight sheep.

No haematological changes were observed in infected goats (except one) and in control animals of both species. One goat BLV positive (Chr.335) died of a severe anaemia, but no tumour or leukaemia was observed in this animal.

Table 3 gives results of cross transmission trials between several animal species. The observation period (1979 - 1980) is too short to permit conclusions on tumoral transformation; indeed, none of the animals of this series died of lymphosarcoma. We can only present the results concerning the humoral reactions to BLV antigens. The bovine donor is an animal naturally infected by BLV; ovine, caprine and porcine donors are animals experimentally infected with blood from a naturally infected cow.

Donor cow, sheep and goat were able to induce a BLV positiv serological reaction to recipient cows, sheep, goats and pigs. Only one of five lambs infected by an ovine donor did not take BLV infection. The results of the inoculations from porcine donors were quite different: none of the two cows inoculated and only three of the six sheep inoculated appeared to be infected.

CONCLUSIONS

Leukaemia viruses from a number of animal species (mice, chickens, cats, cattle, etc.) have been described. Considering their similarities they all belong to the group which has been given the name of 'retroviruses'. Nevertheless, differences remain between those viruses: morphology, size, antigenicity and biochemical characteristics of the proteins including reverse transcriptase. All of those viruses are able to induce haematological disorders, serological changes and tumoral diseases in the species of origin. Transmission of a leukaemia virus from one species to another, as was done in the present study, could differentiate the biological effects of the virus itself and the factors linked with the recipient animal (immune system, genetic or other unknown factors).

A cow naturally or experimentally infected by BLV originating from another cow generally reacts with a persistent humoral antibody response to the viral antigens. Such animals do, or do not, develop a persistent lymphocytosis and die:

- at the slaughterhouse,
- of any disease,
- by accident,
- of lymphosarcoma which may, or may not, be accompanied by a leukaemia.

Considering the relatively rare occurrence of lymphosarcoma in cattle and the high incidence of BLV infection in some countries, one can be tempted to conclude that BLV has a weak oncogenic effect. Economical limitations often prohibit keeping cattle alive for a long period of time. The number of cows aged 7 years or more decreases rapidly in normal breeding herds. We, and many other authors, have observed very old cows with BLV infection and no development of lymphosarcoma. There are practical and financial limitations which prohibit experiments of sufficient size and duration to establish clearly the oncogenic effect of BLV. One can only say that until the age of 7 years, tumour transformation in BLV infected cattle is low; a reasonable estimation is one lymphosarcoma per 500 infected cows (Ferrer, 1979; Sorensen and Beal, 1979; Van der Maaten, 1979).

BLV from a donor cow, experimentally inoculated to sheep resulted in persistent humoral antibody level to BLV antigens in 90% of the animals. Except for one animal, still under observation, all the BLV positive sheep died of lymphosarcoma before the age of 7 years if another cause of mortality did not interfere. Lambs inoculated at 4 - 5 months were as susceptible as newborn lambs to BLV infection. Terminal leukaemia appeared in 65% of infected sheep. This haematological disorder is not a persistent lymphocytosis because the level of lymphoid cells increased progressively until death during a time period of one year or less, and many blastic tumoral cells could be observed in blood smears. Anaemia, observed in 40% of sheep, was also a terminal phenomenon preceding death. Anaemia seemed to be linked to tumorous development. This anaemia was indirectly related to BLV infection and was correlated to the infiltration of bone marrow by tumoral lymphoid cells. Indeed, the most severe anaemias were observed in animals with the highest leukaemia level. In sheep, BLV infection did not weaken the animals' body defence mechanisms (immunosuppressive effects observed in human, mouse and feline leukaemias). Indeed, sheep killed by a non-tumorous disease were in the same proportion in the control group or in the BLV group and in the infected group. We can conclude that in sheep, the main, if not the only, effect of BLV infection is induction of lymphosarcoma in practically all infected animals before the age of 7 years.

Goats inoculated with BLV from a donor cow all gave positive humoral antibody response to BLV antigens. No goat died of lymphosarcoma during the time period which had seen the death of practically all the BLV positive sheep.

Comparing the reactions of sheep and goats to an experimental infection of BLV from a cow donor, we can state.

1. both species were receptive to the virus, particularly goat species in which no resistance was observed; on the other hand, natural resistance was observed in sheep, but rarely (10%);

2. concerning the tumoral transformation, goats and sheep did not react alike; all sheep developed tumours whereas in the same period goats were resistent to this phenomenon; leukaemia and anaemia were observed in sheep, and seemed to be linked to tumoral transformation.

From the experimental viewpoint, sheep appear to be the most suitable experimental animal for the study of the tumoral effect of BLV. Use of this species during a period of 7 years will allow the elucidation of some ill-defined aspects of the disease. We are thinking in particular of our present experiments on vaccination; the main question is: do the vaccines induce resistance to viral infection and/or to tumour development?

At the present time the duration of our cross transmission experiments is too short to draw more clear cut conclusions. We can only state that BLV remains infectious for cow, sheep, goat and pig no matter to which species the donor belongs. Indeed, we are confident that the infection in all those species was definitely established. Humoral responses to BLV antigens showed in many animals progressively rising antibody titres. We need a longer period of observation to appreciate better the biological effects of those viruses passed to different species. An interesting new fact in the study of bovine leukosis is that BLV from bovine, ovine or caprine donors can pass to swine, and, from this species, back to sheep. Nevertheless the experiment with porcine donors failed in two cows and in three out of six sheep. We must consider the possibility of an attenuation of the infectious properties of this virus. This observation perhaps indicates that pigs could be used to obtain a BLV strain suitable for vaccination.

The fact that BLV given to sheep induces tumours in practically all animals in a relative short time indicates that this virus is more dangerous than generally accepted considering the situation in cattle. In sheep at least, we are certain that BLV is directly responsible for a fatal tumoral disease. The situation is not so clear cut in the other species, but nobody could appear (by selection for example) and change the oncogenic power of BLV for cattle. Eradication of all BLV carriers or protection of all animal species against BLV infection is not an unrealistic idea of laboratory investigators. This view seems to be a logical attitude which must be considered by all authorities responsible concerned with animal health problems.

ACKNOWLEDGEMENTS

This study was performed with the financial support of the Belgian Ministry of Agriculture and the 'Fonds cancérologique de la Caisse Générale d'Epargne et de Retraite'.

The skilful assistance of P. Ridremont, J. Severs, G. Vandendaele and Y. Cleuter is most appreciated. D.P. is Chargé de Recherches du Fonds National de la Recherche Scientifique.

REFERENCES

Bex, F., Bruck, C., Mammerickx, M., Portetelle, D., Ghysdael, J., Cleuter, Y., Leclercq, M., Dekegel, D. and Burny, A., 1979. Humoral antibody response to bovine leukemia virus infection in cattle and sheep. Cancer Res., 39: 1118-1123.

Burny, A., Bruck, C., Chantrenne, H., Cleuter, Y., Dekegel, D., Ghysdael, J., Kettmann, R., Leclercq, M., Leunen, J., Mammerickx, M. and Portetelle, D., 1980. Bovine leukemia virus (BLV): molecular biology and epidemiology. In: Viral Oncology (G. Klein, ed.), Raven Press, New York, 1980, 231-289.

Ferrer, J.F., 1979. Diagnosis of bovine leukosis: basic concepts and methodology. Proceedings of Bovine Leukosis Symposium, College Park, Maryland (May 22-23, 1979), 77-92.

Lorenz, R.J., Straub, O.C., Donnelly, W.J.C., Flensburg, J.C., Gentile, G., Mammerickx, M., Markson, L.M., Ressang, A.A. and Taylor, S.M., 1978. Bovine hematology. II. Comparative breed studies on the leukocyte parameters of several European cattle breeds as determined in national laboratories. Zbl. Vet. Med. B 25, 245-256.

Mammerickx, M., 1969-1980. "Rapports d'Activité" Institut National de Recherches Vétérinaires, Bruxelles, Ministry of Agriculture,

Mammerickx, M., 1970. Sur l'utilisation du mouton pour les expériences sur la leucose bovine. Expér. anim., 3, 285-293.

Mammerickx, M., Dekegel, D., Burny, A. and Portetelle, D., 1976. Study on the oral transmission of Bovine Leukosis to sheep. Vet. Microbiol., 1, 347-350.

Mammerickx, M., Lorenz, R.J., Straub, O.C., Donnelly, W.J.C., Flensburg, J.C., Gentile, G., Markson, L.M., Ressang, A.A. and Taylor, S.M., 1978a. Bovine hematology, III. Comparative breed studies on the leukocyte parameters of several European cattle breeds as determined in the common reference laboratory. Zbl. Vet. Med. B 25, 257-267.

Mammerickx, M., Lorenz, R.J., Straub, O.C., Donnelly, W.J.C., Flensburg, J.C., Gentile, G., Markson, L.M., Ressang, A.A. and Taylor, S.M., 1978b. Bovine hematology. IV. Comparative breed studies on the erythrocyte parameters of 16 European cattle breeds as determined in the common reference laboratory. Zbl. Vet. Med. B 25, 484-498.

Mammerickx, M., Portetelle, D., Burny, A. and Leunen, J., 1980. Detection by immunodiffusion- and radio-immunoassay-tests of antibodies to bovine leukemia virus antigens in sera of experimentally infected sheep and cattle. Zbl. Vet. Med. B 27, 291-303.

Portetelle, D., Bruck, C., Mammerickx, M. and Burny, A., 1980. In animal infected by bovine leukemia virus (BLV) antibodies to envelope glycoprotein gp51 are directed against the carbohydrate moiety. Virology, 105, 223-233.

Sorensen, D.K. and Beal, V.C., 1979. Prevalence and economics of bovine leukosis in the United States. Proceeding of Bovine Leukosis Symposium, College Park, Maryland (May 22-23, 1979), 33-50.

Straub, O.C., Lorenz, R.J., Chevrier, L., Donnelly, W.J.C., Flensburg, F.C., Gentile, G., Mammerickx, M., Markson, L.M. and Ressang, A.A., 1978. Bovine hematology. I. Technical problems in the counting of leukocytes. Zbl. Vet. Med. B 25: 14-28.

Van der Maaten, M.J., 1979. Characteristics of bovine leukemia virus and its tumor inducing activity. Proceedings of Bovine Leukosis Symposium, College Park, Maryland (May 22-23, 1979), 119-133.

DISCUSSION

O.-R. Kaaden *(FRG)*

Have you ever seen naturally occurring BLV, or specific antibodies, in pigs?

M. Mammerickx *(Belgium)*

No, never.

M. Mussgay *(FRG)*

Do you have any evidence of multiplication of BLV in pigs?

M. Mammerickx

Yes, eight months after inoculation we recovered infectious particles.

B.S. Samagh *(Canada)*

I believe Danish workers have found tumours in goats after inoculation of BLV. Is that right?

M. Mammerickx

No.

R. Schön *(DDR)*

You told us that sheep do not develop PL. So, have you any evidence that goats might develop any haematological signs resembling PL?

M. Mammerickx

No, but the normal values of the lymphocyte numbers in sheep, goats and cows, are different. Goats normally have a very high number of lymphocytes and sheep a very low one. The lymphocyte number of normal cattle is between the two.

<u>O.C. Straub</u> *(FRG)*

I would just like to confirm Dr. Mammerickx' report as far as goats are concerned. Experiments at Tübingen showed that goats can stay seropositive for periods up to five years without any change in the blood picture or tumour formation.

HOST RANGE OF BOVINE LEUKOSIS VIRUS: PRELIMINARY REPORT

Lois E. Baumgartener* and C. Olson**[1]
*Norden Laboratories, Lincoln, Nebraska 68501, USA
**Department of Veterinary Science, University of Wisconsin
Madison, Wisconsin 53706, USA

ABSTRACT

Feral, domestic and laboratory animals (14 species) were inoculated with bovine leukosis virus (BLV) infective materials.

Species represented were chicken, chipmunk, coturnix, gray squirrel, ground squirrel, mouse, whitetail deer, pig, domestic rabbit, cat, dog, cottontail rabbit, guinea pig, and Sprague-Dawley rat.

The animals were observed from ½ to 54 months. Periodic blood counts and antibody tests were done. Persistent BLV gp antibody was found by agar gel immunodiffusion tests in the whitetail deer, pig, domestic rabbit and cat although dog, cottontail rabbit and rat had positive BLV gp antibody once.

No lymphoid tumours were found. Tissues taken for primary tissue culture included lymphnodes, spleen and kidney. Antigen preparations were made for p24 viral antigen from tissue culture fluid at periodic intervals. Pig, domestic rabbit, dog, cottontail rabbit, guinea pig and rat primary cell cultures had at least one passage positive for p24 BLV antigen.

Tissue culture cells from BLV inoculated rat, guinea pig, cottontail rabbit, domestic rabbit, dog and cat were inoculated into lambs. Twelve months after inoculation there was no evidence of BLV infection in these lambs as judged by absence of BLV gp antibody.

1 Research supported by College of Agricultural and Life Sciences, University of Wisconsin-Madison, Wisconsin, USA.

O.C. Straub (ed.), Fourth International Symposium on Bovine Leukosis

INTRODUCTION

Bovine leukosis virus (BLV), an exogenous virus (Kettman et al., 1976) will infect not only cattle but sheep and goats and will produce tumour in cattle and sheep. Sera from these animals contain antibody against p24 and gp BLV antigens (Onuma et al., 1976) and BLV can be cultured from cells and tissue of infected animals (Miller et al., 1969). Few reports record attempts to produce infection and/or tumour formation in laboratory animals with BLV (Barthold et al., 1976; Mammerickx, 1970, 1971, 1972; Ressang et al., 1976).

In this study laboratory animals were inoculated with BLV in an attempt to find a smaller animal susceptible to the virus. In addition, feral and domestic animals were inoculated with BLV to determine if these animals could be infected with the virus and transmit BLV to cattle. The feral animals chosen were those most likely to inhabit pastures or nearby areas where cattle are kept. The domestic animals chosen were those most likely to be found on a farm in contact with cattle.

Serum antibody tests against p24 and gp antigens were done as well as attempts to culture the virus from lymphocytes and tissues of these BLV inoculated animal species. In addition, tissue culture cells were inoculated into sheep to determine if infectious virus was present.

MATERIALS AND METHODS

BLV Source

Short-term lymphocyte cultures from two cattle known to be good BLV producers, two cattle with persistent lymphocytosis and one cow with the adult form of lymphosarcoma were used as the source of BLV. Lymphocyte cultures were prepared as described by Olson et al. (1973). In addition, culture fluid from a BLV producing cell line (A77th) was used as a virus source.

A tumour cell suspension extract made from prescapular lymphnodes of one cow with the adult form of lymphosarcoma was also used for inoculation.

Species Inoculated

Two chicken (white leghorn), 2 chipmunks *(tamia striatus)*, 15 coturnix (Japanese quail), 2 gray squirrels *(sciurus carolinensis)*, 11 13-lined ground squirrels *(spermorphilus tridecemlineatus)*, 3 whitetail deer *(odocoileus virginianus)*, 10 porcines *(sus scrofa)*, 4 canines *(canis familiaris)*, 4 cottontail rabbits *(sylvilagus floridanus)*, 8 domestic rabbits *(oryoctalagus cuniculus)*, 6 felines *(felis domestica)*, 23 guinea pigs *(cavia porcellus)*, 24 Sprague-Dawley rats, 22 mice (outbred white mice), and 12 sheep *(ovis aries)* were inoculated with BLV or tissue culture material.

After inoculation with BLV containing materials, periodic blood counts and serum antibody tests were done to find evidence of BLV infection. The agar gel double immunodiffusion test (Olson et al., 1973) was done on serum samples using both p24 and gp BLV antigen.

Necropsies were done. Tissues for primary tissue culture were taken aseptically and placed in sterile, cool, Eagle's minimum essential medium (MEM). Selected tissues were placed in 10% buffered formalin and processed for histopathological examination.

Primary Tissue Culture

Lymphnodes, spleen, kidney, and other selected organs from each animal were collected for culture. The tissues were minced into tiny fragments, transferred to small (25 cm^3) culture flasks with 10 - 12 ml of MEM with Hanks salts (20% foetal calf serum) and incubated at 37°C. After a period of growth, cells were removed from the flask and passaged to a larger culture flask. Cells were cultured until 10 passages were accomplished or until the cells would no longer grow. At the times of cell passage culture fluid was saved and prepared for the detection of p24 BLV antigen by the SRID test (Onuma et al., 1975).

Tissue culture cells for lamb inoculation

Primary tissue culture cells at a passage of good growth and from selected species were divided at the time of passage. Part of the cells were centrifuged and resuspended in 1 - 2 ml MEM (10% FCS), placed in a sterile vial and inoculated into lambs by the intradermal or intraperitoneal route without freezing or refrigeration of the cells.

RESULTS

No abnormalities were observed in the blood counts.

The only animals which were positive for p24 antibody were 2 pigs which had p24 antibody appear 16 months after inoculation.

Persistent gp antibody was found in 3 whitetail deer, 7 pigs, 3 cats, and 2 domestic rabbits. A summary of persistent antibody reactions is found in Table 1. Antibody to gp antigen appeared first in the whitetail deer as early as 3 months, in the pig as early as 5 months and as late as 17 months, in the domestic rabbit and cat as early as 3 months and as late as 23 months.

Cottontail rabbit, dog and rat were gp antibody positive once after inoculation (Table 2). Antibody appeared in the cottontail rabbit 10 months after inoculation, in the dog 11 months after inoculation and in the rat 3 to 19 months after inoculation.

Animals which had no gp antibody after inoculation were guinea pig, mouse, coturnix, ground squirrel, gray squirrel, chipmunk and chicken (Table 3). However, one guinea pig, otherwise negative, had spleen and lymph node primary tissue cultures positive for p24 antigen at passage 10 and 7 respectively.

TABLE 1

ANIMALS WITH PERSISTENT ANTIBODIES FOLLOWING BLV INOCULATION

	Number inoculated	Serum antibodies	BLV antigen	Time (months)
Domestic rabbits	8	4/8*	2/7	9 to 48
Cats	6	4/6	0/5	8 to 46
Pigs	10	9/10	1/6	14 to 17
Deer	3	3/3	0/1	8 to 12

* 4/8 = four of eight positive

TABLE 2

ANIMALS WITH ANTIBODIES ONCE FOLLOWING BLV INOCULATION

	Number inoculated	Serum antibodies	BLV antigen	Time (months)
Rat	24	8/22*	1/20	3 to 19
Guinea pig	23	0/21	1/18	3 to 30
Dog	4	2/4	2/4	11 to 35
Cottontail rabbit	4	2/4	3/4	21 to 23

* 8/22 = eight of twenty-two positive

TABLE 3

ANIMALS WITH NO ANTIBODIES FOLLOWING BLV INOCULATION

	Number inoculated	Serum antibodies	BLV antigen	Time (months)
Mouse	22	0/22*	-	2
Coturnix	15	0/15	-	1 to 12
Ground squirrel	11	0/11	-	9 to 54
Gray squirrel	2	0/2	-	2 to 39
Chipmunk	2	0/2	-	½ to 8
Chicken	2	0/2	-	10½

* 0/22 = none of twenty-two tested

At necropsy no lymphoid tumours were found. Tissues examined histopathologically contained no lymphoid tumour lesions. These tissues included lymphnodes, thymus, tonsils, spleen, lung, liver, small and large intestine, kidney, urinary bladder, adrenal gland, pancreas and heart.

Primary tissue cultures from 6 species were positive for BLV p24 antigen. One pig with persistent antibody had a kidney culture positive at passage 7. A domestic rabbit had a kidney culture positive at passage 8 and 11. In another domestic rabbit, spleen and lymphnode cultures were positive at passage 2 and 4 respectively. Two dogs had lymphnode cultures positive at passage 2. A cottontail rabbit had a kidney culture positive at passage 4. In another cottontail rabbit, a kidney culture was positive at passage 5 and 6 and a lymphnode culture was positive at passage 6. The third cottontail rabbit had a kidney culture positive at passages 9, 10, and 11. A guinea pig had a spleen and lymphnode culture positive at passage 11 and 7 respectively. A rat had a spleen and lymphnode culture positive at passage 8 and 6 respectively.

Selected primary tissue culture passages from 6 species were inoculated into lambs (Table 4). Twelve months after inoculation there was no evidence of BLV infection in these lambs as judged by absence of BLV gp antibody.

TABLE 4

SEARCH FOR BLV IN VARIOUS ANIMALS BY INOCULATION INTO LAMBS OF LYMPHOCYTES OR TISSUE CULTURES OF LYMPH NODES, SPLEEN AND KIDNEY AFTER SERIAL PASSAGE. ALL LAMBS REMAINED NEGATIVE FOR BLV ANTIBODIES BY AGID.

Animal	Serum antibody	BLV antigen	Tissue culture No. cultured	Tissue culture Passage inoculated
Rabbit	4/8*	0/3	1	5,6
Cat	4/6	0/5	3	3 to 7
Dog	2/4	2/4	2	2
Cottontail rabbit	2/4	3/4	1	6,8,9
Rat	8/22	2/21	7	4 to 10
Guinea pig	0/21	1/18	1	8,9

* 4/8 = four of eight positive

DISCUSSION

BLV did not produce abnormal blood changes or lymphoid tumours in any animal. It did not appear to induce any other virus to produce tumours or other related diseases. For example, three of six cats were positive for feline leukemia virus.

Antibody against gp BLV antigen was identified in several species and persisted for years after its first appearance. This was also found by Ressang et al.(1976, personal communication) in a study where a rabbit had persisting antibody after BLV inoculation. In addition some animals did not have detectable gp antibody for nearly two years, which after antibody was identified, persisted to the end of the study.

The identification of p24 BLV antigen in primary tissue culture fluid was infrequent and after several passages of cells.

Not all animals which had antibody, even persistent antibody, had cells which produced detectable p24 antigen. Van der Maaten and Miller (1976) report similar findings with chimpanzees. Several animals which had no detectable gp antibody had tissue culture cells produce p24 antigen. This may be a matter of antibody concentration, or the type of test done as well as the type of cell growth. Primary cell cultures do not grow well after many passages and it will be noted that p24 antigen was found most often after the 4th or 5th cell passage.

BLV antigen producing tissue culture cells inoculated into sheep, a very reliable indicator of infectious BLV, did not produce gp antibody, indicating that although the viral antigen was found in tissue culture, the virus was either partially expressed or defective and thus non-infectious.

Although animals of various species might be infected with BLV, the shedding of virus does not occur. Uninoculated contact control pigs and cats did not develop antibody or have tissue cultures produce BLV antigen.

There was no consistent evidence to establish BLV infectivity for all species. For example, BLV which infects cattle, sheep, and goats can be re-isolated from lymphocytes, persisting antibody against two BLV antigens is produced and tumour occurs. This did not occur in the present study. However, the persistent antibody found in the domestic rabbits without p24 antigen in tissue culture or infectivity in sheep indicates that further work is necessary.

REFERENCES

Barthold, S.W., Baumgartener, L.E. and Olson, C., 1976. Brief communication. Lack of infectivity of bovine leukemia (C-type) virus to rats. J. Natl. Cancer Inst., 56: 643-644.

Kettmann, R., Portetelle, D., Mammerickx, M., Cleuter, Y., Dekegel, D., Galoux, M., Ghysdael, J., Burny, A. and Chantrenne, H., 1976. Bovine leukemia virus: An exogenous RNA oncogenic virus. Proc. Nat. Acad. Sci., 73: 1014-1018.

Mammerickx, M., 1970, 1971, 1972. Report of activities, National Institute of Veterinary Research, Brussels.

Miller, J.M., Miller, L.D., Olson, C. and Gillette, K., 1969. Virus-like particles in phytohemagglutinin stimulated lymphocyte cultures with reference to bovine lymphosarcoma. J. Natl. Cancer Inst., 43: 1297-1305.

Olson, C., Hoss, H.E., Miller, J.M. and Baumgartener, L.E., 1973. Evidence of bovine C-type (leukemia) virus in dairy cattle. J. Amer. Vet. Med. Ass., 163: 355-357.

Onuma, M., Olson, C. and Baumgartener, L.E., 1975. Inhibition of bovine leukemia virus release. J. Natl. Cancer Inst., 54: 1199-1202.

Onuma, M., Olson, C. and Driscoll, D.M., 1976. Properties of two isolated antigens associated with bovine leukemia virus infection. J. Natl. Cancer Inst., 57: 571-578.

Ressang, A.A., Ellens, D.J., Mastenbroek, N., Quak, J., Miller, J.M. and Van der Maaten, 1976. Studies on bovine leukemia II. Hematological, serological, virological and electron microscopical diagnosis. Zbl. Vet. Med. B., 23: 566-579.

Van der Maaten, M.J. and Miller, J.M., 1976. Serologic evidence of transmission of bovine leukemia virus to chimpanzees. Vet. Microbiol., 1: 351-357. Straub, O.C. (ed.) Elsevier Publishing Company, Amsterdam and CEC, Luxembourg.

DISCUSSION

R. Hoff-Jørgensen *(Denmark)*

Do I understand you correctly that when you are looking for antigens you do it in peripheral lymphocyte cultures, and that this is the only source of antigen you are looking at?

C. Olson *(USA)*

No, we are looking for antigen also in some of the tissue culture fluids. I don't think we could do this much in the lymphocytes because you can't get much of this out of a guinea pig.

R. Hoff-Jørgensen

Which tissue are you cultivating then?

C. Olson

The tissues that are cultured are many of the internal organs, lymphnodes, spleen, sometimes pancreas, kidney.

M. Mussgay *(FRG)*

How did you store the material, at what temperature?

C. Olson

At -65 to -70°.

M. Mussgay

Could it happen that this material became inactivated during storage?

C. Olson

It is possible but some of these were fresh and we have stored other materials at that temperature and they retained infectivity.

TRANSMISSION OF BLV BY *Ixodes ricinus* TICKS

O.-R. Kaaden[1], W. Fischer[2], A. Meermann[2] and A. Liebisch[3]

[1] Institute of Virology,
[2] Clinic for Diseases of Cattle,
[3] Institute of Parasitology,
Veterinary School, D-3000 Hannover, Federal Republic of Germany.

ABSTRACT

Starved nymphae and adult ticks (Ixodes ricinus, Linné), collected from several parts of Lower Saxony and randomly tested to be free of BLV, were allowed to feed on cattle positive for BLV and BLV-gp antibodies. By competition radioimmunoassays and co-cultivation methods, BLV-p24 antigen and infectious virus were demonstrated in fully engorged ticks. For the transstadial transmission engorged nymphae harvested from BLV-positive cattle moulted in culture to starved adults were allowed to feed a second time on 4 bulls with negative records and tests for BLV. During the observation period of 10 months the tick-borne-infected bulls developed a transient viraemia for 3 - 4 months.

By immunofluorescence and ELISA tests, BLV-specific antibodies up to serum dilutions 1 : 256 were detected as temporary up to 5 months p.i. but did not give rise to positive reactions in the immunodiffusion test. Furthermore, none of the bulls developed lymphocytosis nor lympho-proliferative tumours of EBL.

The experimental findings and epizootiological observations suggest that Ixodes ricinus ticks may transmit BLV under natural conditions.

O.C. Straub (ed.), Fourth International Symposium on Bovine Leukosis

INTRODUCTION

Research on bovine leukaemia virus (BLV) and consequently the eradication of enzootic bovine leukosis (EBL) on the basis of a serological diagnosis has made great progress during the last ten years (for review see Burny et al., 1980). As far as the spread of EBL under natural conditions is concerned, both vertical and horizontal transmission modes have been considered. Biochemical experiments using molecular hybridisation studies, however, showed that BLV did not enter the germ line and truly vertical transmission can therefore be excluded. Furthermore, recent epizootiological data and controlled transmission experiments have demonstrated that the horizontal spread is the most important factor for the distribution of EBL. Amongst others, iatrogenic factors and biting insects were suspected to act as vectors for BLV in nature (Nielsen et al., 1978).

In a collaborative study performed by the Clinic for Diseases of Cattle and the Institutes of Parasitology and Virology, we have investigated the possible role of *Ixodes ricinus* ticks in the horizontal transmission of EBL in northern Germany. Here we report about transient BLV-infections and temporary induction of specific antibodies following a transstadial tick-borne infection of bulls.

MATERIALS AND METHODS

Experimental design

Starved nymphae and adults of *Ixodes ricinus* ticks were collected by dragging on the vegetation in different forest areas of Lower Saxony. Out of these, a total of 30 nymphae and adults were randomly selected, dipped in 70% alcohol followed by washing in a 1% aqueous solution of NaN_3 and homogenised with a pestle grinder in PBS. The homogenate was allowed to extract for 16 hours at 4^oC and then clarified by low-speed centrifugation at 3 000 x g for 10 min. The extract was tested for BLV by co-cultivation with foetal lamb kidney cells (Kaaden and Frenzel, 1980). To infect ticks during the 1st feeding

400 nymphae, 80 males and 80 females were allowed to feed on 4 cattle positive for BLV and specific antibodies. After 5 - 7 days, the engorged nymphae and adults were harvested, and the nymphae allowed to moult to adults under laboratory conditions. Adult starved ticks moulted in culture were then allowed to feed for a second time on 4 bulls with negative records of EBL and proved to be free of BLV and specific antibodies. The tick-borne-infected animals were kept in quarantine for 10 months in fly-proof cages. Samples to be tested for BLV and infectious virus were taken at fortnightly and four-weekly intervals respectively. The scheme of the experimental design of the tick-borne transmission experiments is presented in Table 1.

TADLE 1

SCHEME OF EXPERIMENTAL DESIGN

Sampling of nymphae and adult ticks *(Ixodes ricinus,* Linné) from vegetation

Nymphae and adults randomly tested for BLV in tissue culture

Nymphae, females and males fed on 4 BLV-positive cattle

Engorged nymphae harvested — Engorged females tested for BLV

Moulted to adults in 8 - 14 days

Feeding on 4 BLV negative bulls (sequential tests for BLV and antibodies)

Serological tests

Agar gel immunodiffusion (AGID) tests using BLV glycoprotein preparations as antigen, and a positive reference serum were performed according to the recommended CEC standard procedure for EBL.

The anti- (C'3) complementary immunofluorescence (ACIF) was done in FBL cells infected with BLV, kindly provided by Dr. A.A. Ressang, CDI Rotterdam as described by Frenzel et al. (1975).

ELISA for BLV-specific antibodies was performed with BLV-antigen-coated microtitre plates and alkaline-phosphatase-labelled anti-bovine IgG (Behrens et al., 1979). The enzymatic reaction was optically determined in an ELISA reader at 405 nm. Extinction figures exceeding the double-value of the negative control serum were considered to be positive. For the determination of BLV-p24-antigen in tick extracts, a competition radioimmunoassay was applied. The test was carried out as a solid-phase reaction in Immulon[R] caps coated with rabbit antibodies against BLV-p24. Serial dilutions of the tick extracts were tested for their competing activity against a constant amount of 125-iodinated BLV-p24. The radioactivity of the RIA samples specifically bound was determined in a PRIAS[R] automatic gammacounter (Packard Instruments, Frankfurt/M.).

Isolated blood lymphocytes from the bulls were tested for BLV by co-cultivation with BLV-susceptible foetal lamb kidney cells (Kaaden and Frenzel, 1980).

Protein determination

The protein content of the tick extracts was determined by the method of Schaffner and Weissman (1973), using bovine serum albumin as a standard.

RESULTS

Detection of BLV in tick-borne-infected bulls

Two pools each of 10 nymphae and adults collected from the vegetation were tested for naturally occurring BLV. By co-cultivation with lamb kidney cells after 3 culture passages no infectious virus was detected by applying the immunofluorescence method (results not shown).

Subsequently, 4 cattle with a known positive status of BLV were chosen for the 1st feeding of the ticks. Both adults and nymphae were brought into contact with BLV-carriers and were allowed to feed for several days. The feeding period varied between 5 and 7 days. The sequence of the feedings of the ticks and the tick-borne infection of bulls is represented in Table 2.

Control experiments with engorged ticks performed after the 1st feeding demonstrated that 3 out of 4 groups of adults harboured infectious BLV if tested by the co-cultivation method.

The engorged nymphae were then allowed to moult to adults in culture under controlled conditions in 8 - 14 days. A representative pool of adults moulted from engorged nymphae was homogenised and tested in the competition RIA using ^{125}-iodinated BLV-p24. Quantities between 5 - 7 µg p24-competing activity per ml were detected in the homogenate of the fully engorged ticks (protein content 34 mg/ml) (Figure 1).

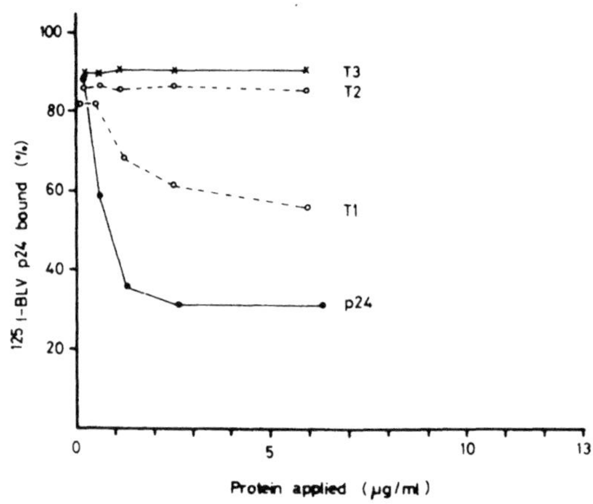

Fig. 1. Competition RIA using ^{125}-BLV-24 and tick extracts (T1 - T3).

For the tick-borne infection of bulls, starved adults (females and males) were allowed to feed a second time at the scrotum of BLV-negative animals. The sucking period was for 3 - 5 days. The experimental numbers are outlined in Table 2.

The tick borne infected bulls were kept in quarantine for 10 months in fly-proof cages. BLV was first detected 8 weeks after exposure in bull No. 39 followed by No. 37, 91737

TABLE 2

INFECTION OF BULLS BY *Ixodes ricinus* TICKS

BLV donors	1st feeding of ticks	Harvest of engorged ticks	Moulted adults (starved)	2nd feeding on ticks harvested BLV-negative bulls	fully engorged
No. 675 ♂	100 SNN	82 NN	56 AA	No. 39	5 ♀♀
	20 ♂♂	13 ♀♀	20 ♀♀		
	20 ♀♀	-----	36 ♂♂		
No. 688 ♂	100 SNN	35 NN	20 AA	No. 37	1 ♀
	20 ♂♂	6 ♀♀	12 ♀♀		
	20 ♀♀	-----	8 ♂♂		
No. 399 ♂	100 SNN	41 NN	30 AA	No. 91737	2 ♀♀
	20 ♂♂	9 ♀♀	14 ♀♀		
	20 ♀♀	-----	16 ♂♂		
No. 403 ♂	100 SNN	68 NN	57 AA	No. 91738	1 ♀
	20 ♂♂	17 ♀♀	23 ♀♀		
	20 ♀♀	3 ♂♂	34 ♂♂		

NN nymphae; SNN starved nymphae; AA adult ticks;
♂♂ males; ♀♀ females.

and 91738 between the 10th and 12th week p.i. The minimum and maximum total periods of BLV detection in tick-borne-infected bulls were 3 and 4 months, respectively.

In tissue culture experiments BLV was grown in *Dermacentor variabilis* cells and was detected by the immunofluorescence method (results not shown).

Detection of BLV-specific antibodies

Besides the detection of infectious BLV, the appearance of specific antibodies was also monitored by the immunodiffusion, immunofluorescence and ELISA tests. Low antibody titres were first detected 6 weeks post exposure by ACIF in bull No. 39 (Table 3). All bulls developed positive antibody titres till 12 weeks p.i. and remained positive up to 9 months p.i. (bull No. 39).

The specificity of the BLV-antibodies of the tick-borne-infected bulls was ascertained by at least two different methods. Furthermore, a set of serum samples from bull No. 91738, including the pre-exposure serum sample, were sent to Dr. Behrens, Behringwerke Marburg, to control our findings. By applying the ELISA technique, an increase of the BLV-specific antibodies up to the serum dilution 1 : 256 was found 5 months p.i. while the pre-exposure serum gave a negative result (Table 3). All serum samples from the 4 bulls, however, remained constantly negative in the immunodiffusion test during the observation period of 10 months. The specific antibodies disappeared 9 months p.i. Neither of the bulls developed tumours nor pathological findings of EBL during the quarantine.

TABLE 3

TIME COURSE OF TEST/RESULTS FOR BLV AND SPECIFIC ANTIBODIES IN TICK-BORNE-INFECTED BULLS

	Months p.i.								
Bull no.	2	3	4	5	6	7	8	9	10
37	negative	BLV+ ACIF 5	BLV+ ACIF+	BLV+ ACIF+	BLV+ ACIF+	BLV- ACIF+	BLV- ACIF-	BLV- ACIF-	BLV- ACIF-
39	BLV+ ACIF 5	BLV+ ACIF+	BLV+ ACIF+	BLV- ACIF+	BLV+ ACIF+	BLV+ ACIF+	BLV- ACIF+	BLV- ACIF 5	BLV- ACIF-
91737	negative	BLV+ ACIF+ ELISA 16	BLV+ ACIF+ ELISA 8	BLV+ ACIF+ ELISA-	BLV- ACIF+ ELISA-	BLV- ACIF 5 ELISA-	BLV- ACIF 5 ELISA-	BLV- ACIF- ELISA-	BLV- ACIF- ELISA-
91738	negative	BLV+ ACIF+ ELISA 8	BLV+ ACIF+ ELISA 32	BLV+ ACIF+ ELISA 256	BLV+ ACIF+ ELISA 128	BLV- ACIF+ ELISA-	BLV- ACIF+ ELISA-	BLV- ACIF- ELISA-	BLV- ACIF- ELISA-

Titres are expressed as reciprocal serum dilutions

CIF titres $\geq$ 1 : 10 considered positive

CONCLUSIONS

The transmission experiments were designed to investigate the possible role of *Ixodes ricinus* ticks for the horizontal spread of EBL under controlled conditions. Amongst other blood-sucking arthropods, ticks have long been considered as possible factors for the spread of BLV on pastures (for review see Wittmann and Urbaneck, 1969). Our attempts to isolate infectious BLV from a limited number of naturally occurring ticks (nymphae and adults) provided negative results. However, it could be demonstrated by detection of BLV and BLV-p24-antigen that *Ixodes ricinus* ticks fed on BLV-positive cattle harboured the virus for at least two weeks and spread it by transstadial transmission to BLV-negative animals. Engorged nymphae from BLV-positive cattle were able to infect BLV-negative bulls when moulted to adults and allowed to feed a second time (Table 3). In all 4 experimental animals, both BLV and specific antibodies were shown following the tick-borne infection. However, the BLV-infection was only transiently found for 4 - 6 months and neither bull developed a clinically overt form of EBL involving lymphocytosis or lymphoproliferative tumours.

The infectious dose applied to the cattle does certainly influence the onset of the BLV replication *in vivo* and possibly the length of the infection. No experimental data concerning the relationship between the infectious dose/animal and the incubation period are so far available for EBL. With regard to the numbers of ticks harvested fully engorged after the 2nd feeding (Table 2), one can assume a small dose of infectious BLV per animal in our study. It is likely, however, that more ticks had blood-meals than were harvested. Under European conditions of cattle breeding, massive infestations of cattle by ticks have no serious hygienic impact.

The experimental data of the study suggest the role which *Ixodes ricinus* ticks may play in the horizontal spread of BLV in northern Germany. The observation that low dose infected animals may undergo only a transient BLV-infection and antibody production has to be further studied.

ACKNOWLEDGEMENTS

Part of the work was supported by the Tierseuchenkasse des Niedersächsischen Landesverwaltungsamtes Hannover. We are especially grateful to Dr. C.E. Yunker, Rocky Mountain Laboratory Hamilton, Montana, for providing several samples of *Dermacentor variabilis* cells and for his continuous help to ensure the cultivation of the line.

We also thank Miss Regine Neth for her patient skill in cultivating the *Dermacentor* cells.

REFERENCES

Burny, A., Bruck, C., Chantrenne, H., Cleuter, Y., Dekegel, D., Ghysdael, J., Kettmann, R., Leclercq, M., Leunen, J., Mammerickx, M. and Portetelle, D., 1980. Bovine leukemia virus: Molecular biology and epidemiolgy. In: Viral oncology, ed. by G. Klein, Raven Press NY, pp. 231-289.

Behrens, F., 1979. Rinderleukosediagnostik: ELISA- ein neues Verfahren. Berl. Münch. Tierärztl. Wschr. 92, 429-432.

Frenzel, B., Mussgay, M., Schneider, L.G. and Straub, O.C., 1975. Immunofluorescence test for bovine-leukosis associated complement-fixing antibodies. Zbl. Vet. Med. B, 22, 519-523.

Nielsen, St. B., Piper, Ch. E. and Ferrer, J.F., 1978. Natural mode of transmission of the bovine leukemia virus: Role of blood-sucking insects. Am. J. Vet. Res. 39, 1089-1092.

Kaaden, O.R. and Frenzel, B., 1980. Eine Methode zum Direktnachweis von Rinderleukosevirus. Fortschritte Veterinärmed. 30, 184-187.

Schaffner, W. and Weissmann, C., 1973. A rapid, sensitive and specific method for the determination of protein in dilute solution. Anal. Biochem. 56, 502.

Wittmann, W. and Urbaneck, D., 1969. Leukose des Rindes, In: Handbuch der Virusinfektionen bei Tieren, Vol.V/1, Ed. H. Röhrer, pp.42-174 (Fischer, Jena 1969).

DISCUSSION

A.A. Ressang *(Netherlands)*

Your last statement is very curious in that you say that you found a transient viraemia. Do you think that this could be attributed to the passage in the pigs? What mechanism is underlying this situation?

O.-R. Kaaden *(FRG)*

We thought that there is a possibility that the dose of BLV is related to the onset of the virus production and also to the length of time that the infection persists. I cannot explain the mechanism, I can only say that we could demonstrate the presence of virus for several months. In some other experiments we observed animals from a negative herd (it was stated to be negative); the bulls were observed for several months, they developed infectious virus, they were completely negative in the immunodiffusion test, and we were able to infect sheep by using blood samples from those bulls. These bulls were kept under natural conditions. There is some indication that latent infections of BLV in cattle may appear, under certain circumstances, after several months.

J.F. Ferrer *(USA)*

Your data suggest that transmission was biological rather than mechanical. Have you tested the ticks for the presence of BLV, have you made cultures from the ticks?

O.-R. Kaaden

No, we did not succeed in cultivating ticks cells. We wanted to demonstrate specific antigens in the cellular components of the ticks because they are metabolically very active but we never succeeded.

J.F. Ferrer

Would you agree that your experiments indicate that transmission is biological rather than mechanical, because of the time lapse?

O.-R. Kaaden

All I can say is that 14 days after feeding we were able to transmit BLV infection under those experimental conditions. I have no idea whether this is mechanical or whether the BLV has actively promulgated in the ticks.

M.J. Burridge *(USA)*

The point here is that ticks feed on only one host at each stage. So it can only be from one stage to the next.

O.-R. Kaaden

That's right.

EMBRYO TRANSPLANTATION AND BOVINE LEUKOSIS VIRUS PRELIMINARY REPORT

C. Olson, R.F. Rowe and R. Kaja
Department of Veterinary Science, University of Wisconsin, Madison, Wisconsin 53706, USA.

ABSTRACT

Seven embryos were nonsurgically transferred from BLV infected donor cows, which had been artificially inseminated with semen from a BLV positive bull, to BLV negative recipients. These 7 embryos developed into calves which have remained negative for BLV antibodies for more than a year. This would indicate that such embryo transfers can be done without risk of BLV transmission.

Research supported by the College of Agricultural and Life Sciences, University of Wisconsin, Madison, Wisconsin.

O.C. Straub (ed.), Fourth International Symposium on Bovine Leukosis

INTRODUCTION

The methods for spread of bovine leukosis virus (BLV) infection are not entirely known. It has now been demonstrated that the infection can be controlled and eliminated by serological testing and removal of reactors from a herd (Bause et al., 1978; Mammerickx et al., 1978; Straub, 1978; Olson, 1979; Forschner, 1979). A herd with no BLV infection must be maintained with no contact with infected cattle. New genetic stock can apparently be safely introduced by artificial insemination (AI) with semen as prepared by commercial bull studs (Baumgartener et al., 1978) in which semen is routinely collected by use of an artificial vagina and only rarely by electroejaculation. Semen from 8 BLV infected bulls of a bull stud did not infect sheep into which it was experimentally inoculated (Miller and Van der Maaten, 1979). In a recent report (Lucas et al., 1980) semen from an 8 year old bull had been collected by rectal massage of its genital tract. Six collections were inoculated into 11 sheep and 3 sheep had become infected from three collections. The authors indicated that there was a large proportion of seminal fluid. Therefore it seems important that semen used in AI be examined for freedom from leukocytes, then properly diluted. Lymphocytes of BLV infected animals appear to be the cells producing BLV and as few as 2 500 (0.0005 ml blood) have transmitted the infection to experimental calves (Van der Maaten and Miller, 1978). Any means of transferring material containing blood or tissue from a BLV infected animal to other cattle is a potential hazard. This can include instruments, needles, transfusions, feeding of mastitis milk, etc.

Theoretically, spermatazoa and ova should not contain BLV in their genome since it is an exogenous viral infection in cattle (Burny et al., 1980). This seems to have been answered with respect to spermatozoa. This preliminary report on embryo transplant experiments concerns the question with respect to ova.

MATERIALS AND METHODS

Holstein-Friesian heifers were used in all the trials. Heifers serving as donors were inseminated with semen prepared for artificial insemination from a bull who had antibodies to BLV and therefore was infected with bovine leukosis virus. When BLV antibodies are found, the animal providing the serum can be called a reactor to the rest and BLV can be cultured from the animal's lymphocytes. The presence or absence of antibodies to bovine leukosis virus was an index of persistent infection with the virus (Burny et al., 1980) and was tested by the accepted agar gel immunodiffusion (AGID) test using antigen containing viral glycoprotein (Forschner, 1979; Baumgartener et al., 1978). Sera from both the donor and recipient of embryos were tested for BLV antibodies prior to embryo transplantation and again at the time of calving for recipients. The initial colostrum of recipients of embryos was also tested and sera from most of the calves was obtained prior to nursing their dam. The calves nursed their dams on the day they were born then were removed and fed a commercial calf starting ration. The calves were then kept in semi-isolation facilities with a separate record for calves born from BLV negative dams. Sequential sera were obtained from the calves until they were 10 to 17 months old.

Donor heifers were superovulated and submitted for non-surgical uterine flushing (Rowe et al., 1980a) 6 - 9 days after superovulatory oestrus (day 0). Embryos that were classified morphologically normal for their age were washed once and stored in fresh flushing medium until the time of transfer. Recipient animals which were within ± 24 hours of oestrus synchrony with the donors were used. A single embryo was transferred nonsurgically to the uterine horn ipsilateral to the corpus luteum bearing ovary (Rowe et al., 1980b). Pregnancy diagnosis was made by rectal palpation at day 40.

RESULTS

Seven calves were born from embryos transplanted from a BLV infected donor to a BLV negative cow (Table 1). The serum of all and colostrum from the 5 tested recipient cows were BLV negative at time of calving. Prenursing serum was obtained from 5 calves, postnursing serum from all 7 calves and all tested negative. One calf (6239, Table 1) died at 9 days of age. Six of the 7 calves lived for at least 12 and up to 16 months, during which time they have remained negative.

Four calves were born from embryos transplanted from a BLV reactor donor to BLV reactor recipients. The prenursing sera from 3 of these calves were negative and postnursing sera of 3 surviving calves had BLV antibodies indicating they were of maternal origin from colostrum. One of these calves (6241, Table 1) died at 15 days of age. In the other 3 calves, colostral antibodies were gone in sera taken at 4, 5 and 7 months and remained absent up to the last tests when 12 to 17 months of age.

Two calves came from embryos transplanted from BLV negative to BLV reactor cows. Prenursing negative serum was obtained from 1 of the calves. Postnursing sera from the 2 calves contained BLV antibodies. One calf (6238, Table 1) died at 3 days of age. The other calf (6248, Table 1) became negative after 3 months and remained so 12 months later.

TABLE 1

THIRTEEN CALVES BORN FROM EMBRYOS TRANSPLANTED FROM 11 DONORS WITH BLV INFECTION AND 2 DONORS WITH NO BLV INFECTION. SEVEN OF THE DAMS (RECIPIENTS OF OVA) WERE BLV NEGATIVE AND 6 WERE BLV INFECTED. ALL CALVES WERE SIRED BY THE SAME BLV INFECTED BULL. THE SEVEN CALVES FROM DAMS WITH NO BLV INFECTION HAVE REMAINED NEGATIVE FOR BLV ANTIBODIES.

Embryo donor		Recipient dam			Calves			
						Serum		
Cow	Serum	Cow	Serum	Colostrum	Number	Pre-nursing	From colostrum	Negative at months
167	+*	416	-		6237	-	-	16**
251	+	425	-		6239	-	-	died
420	+	433	-	-	6240	-	-	15
420	+	435	-	-	6243	-	-	15
223	+	417	-	-	6244	-	-	15
173	+	406	-	-	6247		-	12
429	+	441	-	-	6249		-	13
192	+	424	+	+	6236	-	+	17
429	+	421	+	+	6241	-	died	
306	+	430		+	6242	-	+	15
293	+	454			6250		+	12
391	-	426	+	+	6238	-	+	died
460	-	415	+	+	6248		+	12

* + = BLV antibodies by AGID test
  - = no BLV antibodies by AGID test

** 16 = age in months at last test

DISCUSSION

From the preliminary data presented here it is evident that infectious bovine leukosis virus is not present in washed embryos from BLV infected cows which have been inseminated with sperm prepared for artificial insemination from a BLV infected bull. If BLV were present in such embryos it should have been propagated in the cells of the foetus and manifest as BLV antibodies when the calves were born. An opportunity exists to extend this study to about 100 embryo transplantations to BLV negative heifers using both reactor and non-reactor embryo donors and bulls.

Since it is recognised that BLV can be demonstrated as a persisting infection in cattle with antibodies to the virus, repeated negative AGID tests for such antibodies are a reliable indicator of no BLV infection (Olson and Baumgartener, 1976).

In this series of 6 BLV infected heifers the infection was not passed to the foetuses in 4 instances since the pre-nursing sera of 4 calves were negative for BLV antibodies. Prenursing serum was not available from the others since the calves were born at night or in a pasture and received maternal colostral antibodies before their sera could be obtained. The maternal colostral antibodies had disappeared before 4 to 7 months in 4 calves. The 2 other calves died in their first month of life. BLV antibodies have persisted for 12 months in 2 calves not a part of this report. These calves were born as twins after surgical implantation of embryos from the same recipient BLV-infected heifer. What influence the surgical implantation may have had is not known. Colostral antibodies are usually gone by 6 months of age in calves. Calves 6240 and 6243 were from embryos from the same donor but born from different BLV negative heifer recipients. Calves 6249 and 6241 were from embryos of the same donor but born to different recipient heifers, one of which was BLV infected and the other was not infected.

The question of intrauterine infection has been raised by the observation that 18% of calves had persisting BLV antibodies prior to nursing in an experimental herd where all the cattle over 30 months of age were BLV infected (Piper et al., 1979). This is a high percentage, since in calves of most herds the maternal antibodies, if present, disappear by 6 months of age and evidence of infection does not appear until they are 1 to 3 years of age and older (Olson, 1979). The possibility of such intrauterine transmission must be considered since there could be breaks in the placental blood barrier which could allow the transfer of maternal lymphocytes to the foetus, but this probably occurs only rarely. More likely is the existence of a lesion in the placenta caused by bacteria or other viruses. Such lesions could exist without being apparent but should be suspected when there is evidence of foetal infection with BLV in a herd.

SUMMARY

Although preliminary, the results in 7 calves born from BLV negative heifers to which embryos from BLV infected heifers and sired by AI from a BLV infected bull indicate that such embryo transplantation can be done without risk of BLV transmission.

REFERENCES

Baumgartener, L.E., Crowley, J., Entine, S., Olson, C., Hugoson, G., Hanson, H.J. and Dreher, W.H., 1978. Influence of sire on BLV infection in progeny. Zbl. Vet. Med. B, 25, 202-210.

Bause, I., Maas-Inderwiesen, H., Mitscherlich, E. and Schmidt, F.-W., 1978. Results of an epidemiological survey of enzootic bovine leukosis in the northern part of Lower Saxony based on serological diagnosis with agar gel immunodiffusion. Ann. Rech. Vét., 9, 756-769.

Burny, A. et al., 1980. Bovine leukemia virus: Molecular biology and epidemiology. In: G. Klein (Editor), Viral Oncology. Raven Press, New York, pp. 231-289.

Forschner, E., 1979. Erfahrungen bei der Anwendung des Immunodiffusiontestes in der Diagnostik der Rinderleukose. Fortschritte der Veterinärmedizin. Heft. 30: 13. Kongressbericht 190-193.

Lucas, M.H., Dawson, M., Chasey, D., Wiberley, G. and Roberts, D.H., 1980. Enzootic bovine leukosis virus in semen. Vet. Rec., 106, 128.

Mammerickx, M., Corman, A., Burny, A., Dekegel, D. and Portetelle, D., 1978. Eradication of enzootic bovine leukosis based on detection of the disease by the GP immunodiffusion test. Ann. Rech. Vét., 9, 885-894.

Miller, J.M. and Van der Maaten, M.J., 1979. Infectivity test of secretions and excretions from cattle infected with bovine leukosis virus. Jour. Nat. Cancer Inst., 62, 425-428.

Olson, C. and Baumgartener, L.E., 1976. Epizootiology of natural infection with bovine leukemia virus. In: J. Clemmesen and D.S. Yohn (Editors), Comparative Leukemia Research 1975. Biblio. Haemat. No. 43, pp. 255-259, Karger, Basel.

Olson, C., 1979. Progress for control of bovine leukosis. Bovine Practitioner, 14, 115-120.

Piper, C.E., Ferrer, J.F., Abt, D.A. and Marshak, R.R., 1979. Postnatal and prenatal transmission of the bovine leukemia virus under natural conditions. Jour. Nat. Cancer Inst., 62, 165-169.

Rowe, R.F., Del Campo, M.R., Critser, J.K. and Ginther, O.J., 1980a. Embryo transfer in cattle: Nonsurgical collection techniques. Am. J. Vet. Res., 41, 106-108.

Rowe, R.F., Del Campo, M.R., Critser, J.K. and Ginther, O.J.. 1980b. Embryo transfer in cattle: Nonsurgical transfer. Am. J. Vet. Res. 41, 1024-1028.

Straub, O.C., 1978. Preliminary results of a new sanitation program for the eradication of enzootic bovine leukosis. Ann. Rech. Vét., 9, 895-898.

Van der Maaten, M.J. and Miller, J.M., 1978. Susceptibility of cattle to bovine leukemia virus infection by various routes of exposure. In: P. Bentvelzen, J. Hilgers and D.S. Yohn (Editors), Advances in Comparative Leukemia Research 1977. Elsevier North Holland, New York, pp. 29-32.

DISCUSSION

R. Hoff-Jørgensen *(Denmark)*

Don't you think that you are spoiling your very good experiment by giving the colostrum because if they are positive at 2 years you don't know whether it is from the embryo or from the colostrum.

C. Olson *(USA)*

We live dangerously!

J.F. Ferrer *(USA)*

You mentioned that in the case of the twins you got the two positives. Was the recipient cow positive?

C. Olson

Yes.

SESSION VII

Epidemiology (I)

Chairmen : M. Mussgay and D. Rutili

EPIDEMIOLOGICAL STUDY OF BOVINE LEUKAEMIA VIRUS INFECTION IN FLORIDA*

M.J. Burridge, D.M. Puhr and J.M. Hennemann

Department of Preventive Medicine, College of Veterinary Medicine, University of Florida, Gainesville, Florida 32610, USA.

ABSTRACT

A serological study was undertaken to determine the prevalence and to study the epidemiology of bovine leukaemia virus (BLV) infection in Florida. Using the agar gel immunodiffusion test with a glycoprotein antigen, 47.8% of 7 768 dairy cattle and 6.7% of 4 911 beef cattle were found to have antibodies to BLV. It was demonstrated that the prevalence of BLV antibodies increased significantly (P = 0.0001) with age. After data were adjusted for age, prevalence of BLV antibodies was significantly associated with geographical area and dairy breed (P < 0.05), but not with species (Bos taurus and B. indicus) and sex (P > 0.05).

* Supported by National Cancer Institute contract no. NO1-CP-01016 and by a grant from Pitman-Moore Inc., Washington Crossing, New Jersey, USA.

O.C. Straub (ed.), Fourth International Symposium on Bovine Leukosis

INTRODUCTION

Bovine leukaemia virus (BLV) infection is an important constraint to the export of cattle and semen from the United States (Mix, 1979; Miller, 1980). Despite this, only a few superficial surveys have been conducted in the United States to estimate the regional prevalence of BLV infection (Olson et al., 1973; Baumgartener et al., 1975; House et al., 1977; Evermann et al., 1980). This paper describes a detailed investigation designed both to determine the prevalence and to study the epidemiology of BLV infection in Florida.

MATERIALS AND METHODS

Cattle

Forty-six herds (18 dairy and 28 beef) in Florida were selected for detailed study using stratified random sampling procedures. The strata considered were geographical area (Figure 1), production type (dairy and beef), herd size, and breed. This herd-sampling method was used to provide data representative of all cattle in Florida. All cattle over 18 months of age in each herd were studied, giving a total sample of 12 679 cattle (7 768 dairy and 4 911 beef). Each animal was bled for serum collection and, when available, its breed, sex and age were recorded.

Serology

Each of the 12 679 serum samples was tested for BLV antibodies using the agar gel immunodiffusion test with a glycoprotein antigen (Leukassay-B, Pitman-Moore Inc., Washington Crossing, New Jersey), according to the method of Burridge et al. (1979). Each positive reaction was interpreted to indicate past infection with BLV. This test was chosen for the present study because of its simplicity, because of its high relative sensitivity and relative specificity when compared with established tests for the serodiagnosis of BLV infection (Miller and Van der Maaten, 1976, 1977; Olson et al., 1976), and because it

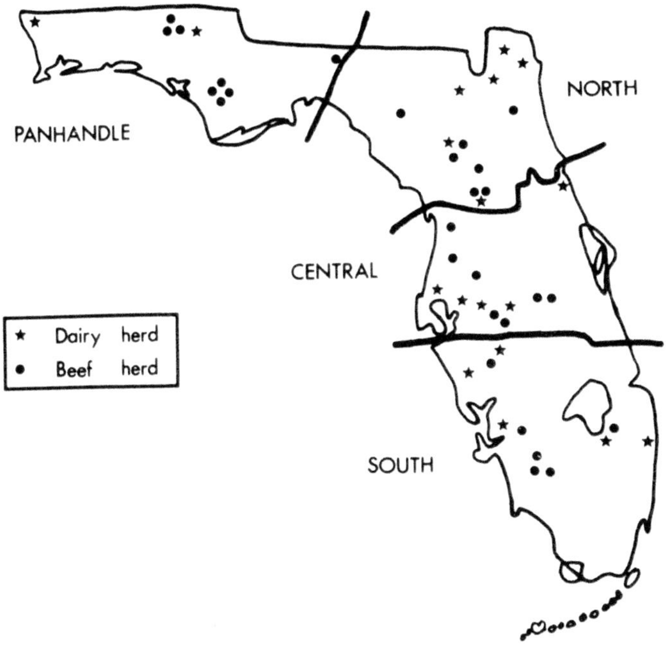

Fig. 1. Four geographical areas of Florida (Panhandle, North, Central and South) studied, showing location of each cattle herd examined.

has been recommended for field use by the member countries of the European Community (Kaaden and Stephenson, 1978).

Data analysis

The relationships between 5 variables (geographical area, species, breed, age and sex) and BLV prevalence were examined statistically using the Statistical Analysis System (SAS) programmes (SAS User's Guide, 1979). The relationship between age and BLV prevalence was investigated using the chi-square test. However, relationships between each of the other variables and BLV prevalence were analysed individually using the SAS FUNCAT procedure which models functions of categorical responses as the linear model R = A B where R is BLV prevalence, A is age in years, and B is the variable under study. Age was included in all models because of the well-documented relationship between BLV-antibody prevalence and age (Burridge et al., 1979). For analyses involving sex, only those 9 herds (all beef) containing at least 5% of each sex were examined.

RESULTS

By production type

The prevalence of BLV antibodies was 47.8% in dairy cattle and 6.7% in beef cattle.

By age

The prevalence of BLV antibodies increased significantly (P = 0.0001) with age, especially in dairy cattle (Figure 2).

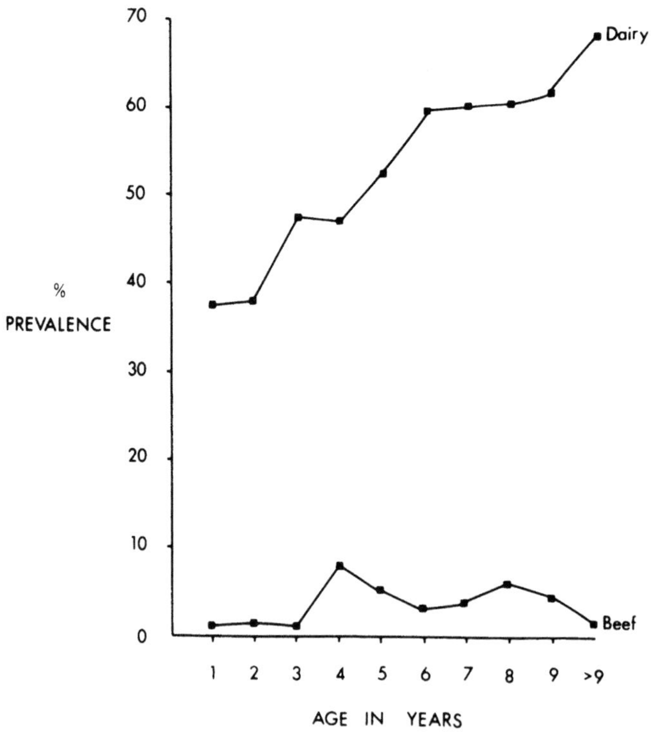

Fig. 2. Relationship between age and prevalence of antibodies to bovine leukaemia virus in cattle in Florida.

By geographical area

The prevalence of BLV antibodies in both dairy and beef cattle was significantly higher ($P < 0.0351$) in South Florida. The prevalences by area (Panhandle, North, Central and South, respectively) were 37.5%, 47.9%, 46.5% and 52.9% for dairy cattle, and 4.1%, 5.4%, 3.9% and 11.2% for beef cattle.

By bovine species

There was no significant difference ($P = 0.0700$) in prevalence of BLV antibodies between purebred *Bos taurus* and purebred *B. indicus* (Brahman) cattle. Twenty-six of 1 160 (2.2%) *B. taurus* and 5 of 548 (0.9%) *B. indicus* cattle were positive for BLV antibodies.

By breed

The prevalence of BLV antibodies in dairy cattle was significantly higher ($P = 0.0001$) in Jersey cattle than in the other breeds (Holstein, Guernsey and Brown Swiss) (Table 1). The prevalence of BLV antibodies in beef cattle is shown by breed in Table 2; the data could not be analysed using the SAS FUNCAT procedure because of an excessive number of empty cells in the cross-tabulated data. The high prevalence of 20.0% in Charbray cattle was primarily due to the influence of the 2 most southerly herds examined which were purebred Charbray herds with BLV-antibody prevalences of 42.5% (82 of 193 positive) and 14.0% (75 of 535 positive).

TABLE 1

PREVALENCE OF ANTIBODIES TO BOVINE LEUKAEMIA VIRUS IN DAIRY CATTLE IN FLORIDA BY BREED

Breed	% prevalence (no. positive/no. tested)
Jersey	63.1(159/252)
Holstein	47.4(3/234/6/826)
Guernsey	46.1(178/386)
Brown Swiss	42.8(92/215)

TABLE 2

PREVALENCE OF ANTIBODIES TO BOVINE LEUKAEMIA VIRUS IN BEEF CATTLE IN FLORIDA BY BREED

Breed	% prevalence (no. positive/no. tested)
Charbray	20.0(163/814)
Brown Swiss	10.9(7/64)
Braford	6.8(19/278)
Angus	5.0(37/743)
Charolais	4.1(6/148)
Santa Gertrudis	4.0(4/101)
Brangus	1.5(3/196)
Brahman	1.3(9/687)
Hereford	0.8(4/487)

By sex

In the 9 beef herds containing at least 5% of each sex, BLV antibodies were found in 4 of the 154 bulls (2.6%) and in 84 of the 2 335 cows (3.6%). There was no significant difference ($P = 0.3507$) in prevalence of BLV antibodies between male and female cattle when the data were adjusted for age.

CONCLUSIONS

There was serological evidence of BLV infection in virtually half (47.8%) of adult dairy cattle in Florida. The prevalence in beef cattle was considerably lower (6.7%). There was a well-defined relationship between prevalence of BLV antibodies and age, particularly in dairy cattle. Because of this association, all data must be adjusted for age before they are examined for the effects of other variables on BLV prevalence. Consequently, in this study the relationships between 4 variables (geographical area, species, breed and sex) and BLV prevalence were investigated using a statistical method that minimised the confounding effects of age.

There was no significant difference in prevalence of BLV antibodies between *B. taurus* and *B. indicus* cattle. However, apparent differences in prevalence by breed were noted. The prevalence of BLV antibodies was significantly higher in Jersey cattle than in other dairy breeds, a difference not detected in a previous one-herd study (Burridge et al., 1979). Atypically high prevalences for beef cattle were found in 2 Charbray herds from southern Florida. With the data available, it is impossible to determine if this finding reflected an influence of either breed or geographical area on BLV prevalence. Finally, no relationship between sex and prevalence of BLV antibodies was found.

REFERENCES

Baumgartener, L.E., Olson, C., Miller, J.M. and Van der Maaten, M.J., 1975. Survey for antibodies to leukemia (C-type) virus in cattle. J. Amer. Vet. Med. Ass. 166, 249-251.

Burridge, M.J., Wilcox, C.J. and Hennemann, J.M., 1979. Influence of genetic factors on the susceptibility of cattle to bovine leukemia virus infection. Europ. J. Cancer, 15, 1395-1400.

Evermann, J.F., DiGiacomo, R.F. and Huber, N.L., 1980. Prevalence of bovine leukemia virus antibody in seven herds of Holstein-Friesian cattle. J. Amer. Vet. Med. Ass. 177, 549-550.

House, C., House, J.A. and Glover, F.L., 1977. Antibodies to the glycoprotein antigen of bovine leukemia virus in the cattle population of five states. Cornell Vet. 67, 510-522.

Kaaden, O. and Stephenson, J.R., 1978. Report of the second session (Detection of BLV infection: serological methods). Ann. Rech. Vét. 9, 604-605.

Miller, J.M. and Van der Maaten, M.J., 1976. Serologic detection of bovine leukemia virus infection. Vet. Microbiol. 1, 195-202; Straub, O.C. (ed.) Elsevier Publishing Company, Amsterdam and CEC, Luxembourg.

Miller, J.M. and Van der Maaten, M.J., 1977. Use of glycoprotein antigen in the immunodiffusion test for bovine leukemia virus antibodies. Europ. J. Cancer, 13, 1369-1375.

Miller, L.D., 1980. Export testing for enzootic bovine leukosis. J. Amer. Vet. Med. Ass. 177, 620-622.

Mix, M.E., 1979. Export significance - industry observations. In: Proceedings of Bovine Leukosis Symposium. United States Department of Agriculture, Washington, pp. 183-186.

Olson, C., Hoss, H.E., Miller, J.M. and Baumgartener, L.E., 1973. Evidence of bovine C-type (leukemia) virus in dairy cattle. J. Amer. Vet. Med. Ass. 163, 355-357.

Olson, C., Baumgartener, L.E., Miller, J.M. and Van der Maaten, M.J., 1976. A comparison of tests on reference serums for BLV antibody. Vet. Microbiol. 1, 275-278; Straub, O.C. (ed.) Elsevier Publishing Company, Amsterdam and CEC, Luxembourg.

SAS User's Guide, 1979. SAS Institute Inc., Raleigh, North Carolina.

DISCUSSION

J.F. Ferrer *(USA)*

I was very interested in your comment that the Jerseys are more susceptible than other breeds. Can you speculate why this is so?

M.J. Burridge *(USA)*

I can only say that in the Florida situation the Jerseys had a higher prevalence. Whether this is due to genetic susceptibility, or different management factors, we do not know. Has anyone else any comments on this?

G.H. Theilen *(USA)*

Some years ago we studied a random sample of cattle from the island of Jersey. This was in the days when we used just the lymphocytosis test and out of 200+ animals we found one lymphocytotic animal which was normal on lymphocytosis retest. Some years later, Carl Olson's laboratory tested sera from the island for BLV p24 antibody and, as I recall it, you didn't find any infected. Is that correct?

C. Olson *(USA)*

Yes.

G.H. Theilen

So, my feeling is that the source of the Jersey cattle is probably free of BLV infection. That does not mean that they are not genetically susceptible; they become infected after they leave the island. Cattle from that island have been an isolated population for several hundred years. The authorities have forbidden the importation of cattle. During the German occupation in World War II there were some beef cattle brought on from France but they were kept apart from the general island cattle.

V. Caporale *(Italy)*

Do you find, within the herds of the same breed, an average prevalence which is more or less homogeneous? In doing a very large survey in our region, I have found a very high prevalence within certain herds. If you find situations such as this, then you could have a bias in terms of breed.

M.J. Burridge

There are very few herds where you have a large enough number of both breeds. One of those herds is our dairy research unit herd reported on this morning. There we do not have a statistically significant difference. It would be nice to find herds where you have a high prevalence area with a lot of both Holstein and Jersey. This would immediately minimise the effect of management factors, etc. We do not have that situation so I cannot give the answer. But it is a very important point to look at. If anybody is in that sort of situation it would certainly be worth investigating, and it would be very quick and easy to do.

F. Bürki *(Austria)*

We do have mixed herds in Austria and obviously they have been infected by rather recent introductions of Holstein-Friesian into the native cattle breeds of Austria. In these mixed herds the average prevalence of infection is very much higher in the Holstein-Friesian than in the native breeds.

M.J. Burridge

What we are saying, in fact, is that from the available evidence the indications are that this is probably not a true breed difference. But it certainly needs to be verified.

D.H. Roberts *(UK)*

What is the tumour incidence in Florida compared to the rest of the United States?

M.J. Burridge

Carl Olson will be able to answer this much better than I. One of the problems in Florida is that we burn our dairy cattle out rather fast - three lactations is the average - so the average age is rather low. In the dairy research unit herd, until about three years ago, we had well under 1% of animals showing tumours at one time or another. Now, it is virtually zero because the older animals have been culled. I don't know of any figures for beef cattle in Florida. But Carl Olson will be able to give a better impression of the United States generally.

C. Olson

Insofar as abattoir statistics are known, it is not a very high rate in that area. But I think you could get this from the local abattoirs and it would be very interesting.

EXTENT, DIAGNOSIS AND ERADICATION OF ENZOOTIC BOVINE LEUKOSIS IN SOCIALIST REPUBLIC OF SLOVENIA (YUGOSLAVIA)

I. Jazbec, V. Gregorović and F. Skušek

Faculty of Veterinary Science, University of E. Kardelj, Yu-61000 Ljubljana, Yugoslavia.

ABSTRACT

The development and application of diagnostic methods for establishing enzootic bovine leukosis in Slovenia are shown.

We have followed the spread of enzootic bovine leukosis on state and private farms in Slovenia by means of the successful application of the immunodiffusion test. We examined 74 large state-owned herds (85.06%). Of these, 24 were infected (32.43%). The intensity of the infection was 0.28% to 33.33%. We carried out an eradication programme by making serologic tests on all the animals in the herd, and then slaughtering or isolating all the animals which showed a positive reaction. The herd was considered to have been cleaned when the results were negative twice in a row. When a solution to the problem of financing eradication has been found, these criteria will be strengthened by the addition of a further examination.

Consistent eradication programmes for herds have been shown to be successful, whilst the disease persists in those herds which are not part of an eradication programme.

We have established that the disease is transmitted from infected herds into private co-operative farms.

O.C. Straub (ed.), Fourth International Symposium on Bovine Leukosis

INTRODUCTION

Until 1977, enzootic bovine leukosis was detected only by using the haematologic method (Jazbec et al., 1975; Jazbec, 1977a; Jazbec et al., 1979a). In 1978 we established the serological method definitively with the introduction of the immunodiffusion test (ID-test) (Jazbec et al., 1979a, 1979b; Miller and Olson, 1972; Mitscherlich et al., 1976). Before the introduction of the ID-test we managed to test 14 711 cattle on 77 state farms (Jazbec et al., 1978) and 1 004 cattle on private farms (Jazbec et al., 1977b) haematologically with the use of the electronic 'Coulter Counter ZF_6' (Jazbec, 1977a). We discovered haematologically a total of 106 (1.02%) leukosis positive reaction on 5 state farms; all the cattle on private estates were negative. The haematological diagnosis was at that time supported by pathohistological examinations.

Due to the great danger of bovine leukosis spreading in the big cattle herds, the disease was entered in the federal law 'The Law for the protection of animals against infectious diseases' (Official Gazette of SFRJ No. 43/76).

As this is a viral, infectious disease with a varying incubation period and unreliable clinical symptoms, we started an intensive effort to improve the diagnostic methods.

As the haematologic method discovers the disease only in the leukaemic stage, we have, over the last few years, been introducing serological diagnosis using the immunodiffusion test.

We have been following the extent of leukosis with the diagnostic method mentioned above, chiefly on state farms, whilst at the same time we have been introducing preventive sanitary measures. We are now extending our research to include co-operatively and privately owned herds of cattle. The results confirm that the disease is spreading from infected breeding cattle on the larger farms to the smaller private, but mainly co-operative, herds.

MATERIALS AND METHODS

Before the introduction of the serological diagnostic method, we performed haematological examinations for leukosis on 14 711 cattle older than 2 years from 77 state farms (88.5%). These farms own approximately 200 adult cattle each, with some owning more than 500. In 1978 we started planning a serological examination (ID-test) of all pedigree cattle above 6 months of age.

Up to the present, we have serologically tested cattle on 74 (85.06%) state farms, and by the end of 1980 we plan to have tested all state owned herds of cattle (approximately 17 400 pedigree cattle). Among the animals tested are pedigree bulls from the insemination centres, which are checked every year. We also carry out serologic tests on all imported animals, on animals destined for shows and animals of those private breeders who send calves to insemination centres.

Before 1973 we detected leukosis by use of the common haematological method (counting chambers) and between 1974 and 1977 we used the electronic counter (Coulter Counter ZF_6). Since 1978 we have used the serological method, i.e. the immunodiffusion test. At first we used the antigen obtained from Pitman-Moore (Leukassay-B, Pitman-Moore, Inc., Washington Crossing, N.J.) but now we use antigen obtained from the Behringwerke (Rinder-leukose-Antigen, Behringwerke A.G. Marburg, FRG).

On the basis of three years experience with the serological diagnosis (ID-test) of a large number of animals, we are convinced that this method is very sensitive and therefore suitable for routine diagnosis.

RESULTS AND DISCUSSION

Extent

Up to the present we have ID-tested 74 (85.06%) state farm herds (11 970 animals). Of these, 50 (67.57%) were seronegative and 24 (32.43%)-positive. By the end of 1980 we plan to have examined the remaining 13 herds on state farms. Among the positive herds there were 13 with up to 5% and 11 with more than 5% positive reactors. In the herd worst affected, one third of the animals reacted positively (Table 1).

We have so far found 7 private breeders with positive reactors in co-operative schemes which receive pedigree calves from large infected state owned farms.

TABLE 1

DEGREE OF INFECTION OF HERDS ON STATE FARMS IN SLOVENIA AT THE TIME OF THE FIRST TESTING

Percentage of infection		Up to 1	1.01-5.00	5.01-10.00	10.01-33.00	Total
Number of herds	n %	5 20.83	8 33.33	5 20.83	6 25.00	24
Number of reactors	n %	10 2.87	53 15.23	58 16.67	227 65.23	348

In individual herds we have to date discovered 1 to, at most, 102 (0.28% - 29.11%) positive animals during the first serological tests. In subsequent control examinations of herds which had not undergone an eradication programme, we discovered a maximum of 124 reactors and 33.33% infection. In 25% of the herds with over 10% positive animals there were more than 65% of all reactors (Table 1).

Farms AA and AB (Table 5) have a common rearing place for pedigree heifers, from which animals in an advanced state of pregnancy return to the base herd. Among the 335 heifers we have already discovered 21 (6.3%) positive animals.

Eradication

Due to the unexpectedly large extent of bovine leukosis the question of eradication and prevention of the disease has become very acute for the professional bodies as well as for the veterinary specialists.

In 1976, when with the help of the haematological method we discovered enzootic bovine leukosis in the first large herd (8.15% reactors), the breeders and veterinary inspectors co-operated on the common principle of combating an infectious disease. Only on 8th October 1976 did the new federal 'Law for the Protection of Animals Against Infectious Diseases' come into force. Bovine leukosis is enumerated in Article 1 of this law.

Since 1979, the 'Regulation of preventive inoculation and diagnostics and other examinations' in Slovenia requires that all herds with imported breeding cattle and all breeding bulls for insemination centres be serologically tested. The examination of all herds on state farms and all herds in private ownership which have more than 20 breeding cattle over the age of six months has to be completed in 1980.

A 'Regulation for the eradication of bovine leukosis' is being prepared in Yugoslavia. The regulation defines in detail diagnostic procedures and criteria for sick, suspect and non-suspect animals and herds as well as the control of traffic of animals and their waste materials.

On the basis of accumulated epizootiological data we can divide herds in Slovenia into a) negative, b) moderately infected (<5% reactors), c) highly infected (>5% reactors) and d) serologically unchecked herds.

Breeding animals can be sold only from herds which have been proven to be negative. A programme of eradication is being carried out which invloves the systematic elimination of positive reactors by slaughter or into special strictly separated isolation.

All imported breeding cattle, as well as those purchased at home, must come from herds which have been proven to be healthy. During quarantine a serological examination for enzootic bovine leukosis is compulsory.

TABLE 2

EPIZOOTIOLOGICAL SITUATION IN RELATION TO ENZOOTIC BOVINE LEUKOSIS IN STATE OWNED HERDS IN SLOVENIA IN OCTOBER 1980

Negative herds		No. %	50 57.47
Unchecked herds		No. %	13 14.94
Infected herds	< 5%	No. %	13 14.94
	> 5%	No. %	11 12.64
Total of herds			87

When all the cattle with a positive reaction have been eliminated the herd is serologically examined at intervals of 3 - 4 months until the results are negative in two consecutive tests. It is not possible to impose a third test because of the difficulties of financing the work.

TABLE 3

SURVEY OF ERADICATION OF ENZOOTIC BOVINE LEUKOSIS IN INFECTED HERDS (OCTOBER 1980)

	No.	%
Farms with eradication programme	8	33.33
Farms with partial eradication programme	4	16.67
Farms with no eradication programme	10	41.67
Leukotic herds in isolation	2	8.33
Total herds	24	

Radical and fast eradication programmes are still not possible, as the mechanism of state financing at the moment only allows for the first examination. Elimination of the cattle with a positive reaction and repeated testing until two consecutive negative results are obtained for the whole herd are in principle paid for by the owner.

The result of this is that at the moment we have 8 (33.33%) infected herds undergoing an eradication process, and 4 (16.67%) undergoing a partial eradication process. This group includes herds with a low percentage of animals with positive results, which have been separated, but where a repeated examination of the herd was not carried out.

Within the framework of the existing programme, sero-positive animals were eliminated by slaughter. In a few cases, the breeders decided to isolate the infected animals in special, well-separated breeding stations (isolation units). These animals are not used for breeding: after being used for economic reasons they are slaughtered.

The success of the eradication programme based on serological tests of herds and the elimination of sero-positive cattle, is shown in Table 4. Among 8 herds undergoing an eradication programme we found that 0.3% - 18.5% of animals were positive during the first series of tests. After isolating the positive animals, 0.9% - 5.6% of animals in 5 herds were still sero-positive in the second test. In 2 herds which had previously had a very low prevalence, all animals reacted as sero-negative. After the third and fourth tests, 5 herds were completely negative. These herds were declared to be free of BLV infection.

In Table 5 the epizootiological state from 1976 to 1980 in 5 herds with rather high percentages of sero-positive animals without the conduct of an eradication programme, is shown. In the first column the results achieved by the haematologic method, and in the others the results of the ID tests, are presented. The highly infected farm, AA, had 39 (7.22%) haematologically positive reactors in 1976. In 1977, i.e. the year of the first serological test, we found 99 (17.77%) positive reactors. During the following year, separation of positive and negative cattle was carried out by isolating infected animals. At the end of the year the animals were once again put together because of technological problems. The

TABLE 4

SUCCESS OF EBL ERADICATION IN HERDS UNDERGOING AN ERADICATION PROGRAMME

Farm	Examination				Method of eradication	Supposed source of infection - imported from:
	1	2	3	4		
A	17/18.5%/ 11.1.79, n=92	4/5.0%/ 10.12.79, n=80	0 16.5.80, n=80	0 27.10.80, n=85	Isolation	I
B	16/13.6%/ 25.11.78, n=118	7/5.6%/ 22.11.79, n=125	0 27.3.80, n=240	0 23.7.80, n=125	Slaughter	A
C	9/4.0%/ 4.4.79, n=224	7/3.0%/ 3.10.79, n=231	0 25.2.80, n=240	0 21.5.80, n=228	Isolation	G
D	18/4.2%/ 29.3.79, n=374	18/5.0%/ 16.10.79, n=358	0 3.4.80, n=285	0 16.9.80, n=295	Isolation	G
E	3/1.3%/ 5.4.79, n=238	2/0.9%/ 24.10.79, n=212	0 3.4.80, n=235	0 10.9.80, n=213	Isolation	G
F	1/0.7%/ 8.4.80, n=138	1/1.41%/ 18.9.80, n=71			Isolation	G
G	1/0.3%/ 15.2.79, n=353	0 6.6.79, n=353			Slaughter	A
H	1/2.8%/ 12.9.79, n=34	0 6.11.79, n=31	0 4.2.80, n=32		Isolation	G

TABLE 5

DEGREE OF EBL INFECTION IN HERDS WITH NO ERADICATION PROGRAMME

Method	Haematologic test	Serologic test				Supposed source of infection - imported from:
Herds	1	1	2	3	4	
AA	39/7.22%/ 8.4.76, n=540	99/17.77%/ 31.3.77, n=557	79/15.94%/ 28.3.78, n=502	102/21.52%/ 4.6.79, n=474	124/26.27%/ 4.6.80, n=472	D + G
AB	17/3.66%/ 25.5.78, n=465	50/11.57%/ 30.5.79, n=432	60/13.42%/ 26.5.80, n=447			D + G
AC	0 27.11.75, n=50	23/29.11%/ 15.2.79, n=79	12/15.79%/ 17.10.79, n=76	40/33.33%/ 17.3.80, n=120		I
AD	5/2.43%/ 20.11.76, n=206	26/10.97%/ 7.2.79, n=237	24/12.24%/ 18.3.80, n=196			A
AE	3/2.07%/ 5.6.78, n=145	7/5.12%/ 11.6.79, n=137	12/7.79%/ 14.4.80, n=154			C

number of positive animals increased in 1979 to 102 (21.52%) and in 1980 to 124 (26.27%) positives.

Farms AC and AD also started to separate cattle after the first serological test, but this procedure was not carried out consistently because of financial and technological problems. Therefore, we discovered later a higher number of positive animals than in previous years. On farm AC, we had an additional 17 new cases in addition to the 23 old cases. A marked increase in the number of positive reactors was found in herd AE as well.

This shows that a successful treatment of infected herds is only possible with systematic serological diagnosis of leukosis and consistent isolation of sero-positive animals.

CONCLUSIONS

The development and application of diagnostic methods for the determination of the presence or absence of enzootic bovine leukosis in Slovenia, are shown.

We followed the spread of enzootic bovine leukosis in state and private farms in Slovenia by means of the immuno-diffusion test and examined 74 large state-owned herds (85.06%). Of these, 24 were infected (32.43%). The prevalence of the infection was 0.28% to 33.33%. In part, we carried out an eradication programme by conducting serologic tests on all animals of a herd and then slaughtering or isolating the sero-positive animals. A herd was considered free of leukosis when the test results had been twice in a row negative. When a definitive solution to the problem of financing eradication programmes has been found, the criteria will be strengthened by a further examination.

Consistent eradication programmes for herds have been shown to be successful, whilst the disease persists in those herds which do not participate in an eradication programme.

We could also prove that the disease is transmitted from infected herds to private co-operative farms.

REFERENCES

Jazbec, I., Gregorović, V., Skušek, F. and Smrekar, D. 1975. Ugotovitve o pojavljanju goveje levkoze v Sloveniji. Zb. biotehn. fak. UL. Vet. 12/2, 273-280.

Jazbec, I. 1977a. Primjena eletronskog aparata "Counter ZF_6" u veterinarskoj laboratorijskoj diagnostici. Vet. glasn. 31/1, 49-53.

Jazbec, I., Gregorović, V. and Skušek, F. 1977b. Vpliv starosti, pasme in letnega časa na levkogram govedi v Sloveniji. Zb. biotehn. fak. UL, Vet. 14, supl. 4, 89-101.

Jazbec, I., Gregorović, V., Skušek, F. and Smrekar, D. 1977c. Študij diagnostičnih metod, razširjenosti in preventive enzootske goveje levkose na družbenem sektorju v Sloveniji. Poročilo SBK 1977/78, 1-10.

Jazbec, I., Greogorović, V., Skušek, F., Šenk, L. and Smrekar, D. 1978. Študij diagnostičnih metod, razširjenosti in preventive enzootske goveje levkose. Poročilo RSS, 1-23.

Jazbec, I., Gregorović, V. and Skušek, F. 1979a. Rezultati komparativnih istraživanja hematološke i serološke dijagnostike/ID test/enzootske govedje leukose. Vet. glasn. 23/1, 45-51.

Jazbec, I., Gregorović, V., Skušek, F. and Šenk, L. 1979b. Die enzootische Rinderleukose in SR Slowenien-Vorkomen, Diagnostik und Tilgung. XXI. Welt-Tierärztekongress, Moscow, 21-22.

Miller, J.M. and Olson, C. 1972. Precipitating antibody to an internal antigen of the C-type virus associated with bovine lymphosarcoma. J. Nat. Cancer. Inst., 49, 1459-1462.

Mitscherlich, E., Plünnecke, A., Schmidt, F.-W. and Albrecht, A. 1976. Techniques and results of immunodiffusion test in field trials. Vet. Microbiol. 1, 219-230, Straub, O.C. (ed.) Elsevier Publishing Company and CEC, Luxembourg.

DISCUSSION

A.A. Ressang *(Netherlands)*

In how many instances did you find animals positive in the third test after being negative in the first and second tests?

I. Jazbec *(Yugoslavia)*

I am afraid I do not have that data with me.

G. de Vries *(Netherlands)*

How many herds do you have in total?

I. Jazbec

There are 90 herds altogether in Slovenia.

D. Rutili *(Italy)*

You said that the rate of infection ranged from about 1% up to 33%; that is a very high variation. However, at the beginning you said that you were concerned with two kinds of herds, the large co-operative herds and the smaller private ones. Maybe there is some difference also in the type of housing of the animals, and differences in management?

I. Jazbec

It may possibly be due to the different kinds of management. The private herds have a maximum of 30 animals and the state herds have a minimum of 200.

SEROEPIDEMIOLOGICAL SURVEY OF BOVINE LEUKAEMIA VIRUS INFECTION IN CANADIAN CATTLE

B.S. Samagh[1] and J.A. Kellar[2]

[1] Agriculture Canada, Animal Diseases Research Institute NEPEAN, PO Box 11300, Station H, Nepean, Ontario, Canada K2H 8P9

[2] Agriculture Canada, Animal Health Division, 580 Booth Street, Ottawa, Ontario, Canada K1A 0Y9

ABSTRACT

In order to formulate future control programmes concerning enzootic bovine leukosis, and to study the economic impact of the disease, it was important to know the prevalence of bovine leukaemia virus (BLV) infection and the clinical disease in our cattle population. To determine, on a statistically sound basis, the prevalence of BLV infection in Canada, 38 297 serum samples from 990 herds have been examined using a glycoprotein antigen-antibody system and employing an agar gel immunodiffusion test. The overall herd infection rate is 19.7% while animal infection rate is 3.6%. However, it varies significantly in different regions. Herds in the four Atlantic (eastern) and the three western provinces have significantly lower infection rates than those in Central Canada, while animals in beef herds have lower rates than those found in dairy herds. The results of BLV infection rates in beef and dairy herds in different regions of the country are discussed.

O.C. Straub (ed.), Fourth International Symposium on Bovine Leukosis

INTRODUCTION

Enzootic bovine leukosis (EBL) is considered to be the most common malignant disease of cattle (Sørensen, 1979). Since the isolation of bovine leukaemia virus (BLV) from the leukocytes of EBL cattle (Miller et al., 1969), the virus has been confirmed as the causative agent of this disease (Abt et al., 1976; Chander et al., 1978; Devare et al., 1977). Various serological tests have been developed for the detection of antibodies to BLV and have been reviewed by Mussgay and Kaaden (1978). The agar gel immunodiffusion (AGID) test using BLV glycoprotein antigen being a specific, sensitive and simple test to conduct, was recommended as one of the methods of detecting BLV antibodies in bovine serum (Ressang (ed), 1978). In recent years various countries have completed seroepidemiological surveys for BLV antibodies in their cattle population using serological tests. In the United States, a study of 33 beef and 41 dairy herds from five states using glycoprotein AGID test (House et al., 1977), has shown that 28.2% of dairy and 2.6% of beef cattle were seropositive for BLV. Devare and Stephenson (1978), using a radioimmunoassay for p24 and glycoprotein antigen, tested serum from more than 6 000 cattle in 22 states and found that 13.5% of the cattle, including both beef and dairy breeds, were seropositive. Similar surveys have been conducted in France and Venezuela (Crespeau et al., 1978; Marin et al., 1978; Nougayerde et al., 1978).

Generally the incidence of tumour cases has been much lower than that of BLV infected animals. In Germany, for example, there were 100 - 500 cases/100 000 cattle/year in heavily infected areas (Bendixen, 1965) and this disease was considered to cause serious death losses. In Denmark, the overall incidence has been lower. In 1960, near the beginning of the Danish control programme, the incidence/100 000 was 6.0 on a national basis; 28.7 in heavily infected areas and 1.5 in lightly infected areas (Flensburg and Stryffert, 1977). In the United States condemnation records for lymphosarcoma at federally inspected slaughter establishments show less than 25 cases/100 000 animals slaughtered. On the contrary, taking into account the age of the animals and number of EBL cases which do not reach slaughter-houses, Sørensen and Beal (1979) estimated 170 cases of EBL/ 100 000 adult cattle in the USA.

A pilot study conducted in Canada had suggested that the clinical disease and BLV infection is present in almost all regions of Canada. In order to formulate rational programmes concerning EBL, it was necessary to map the true relative regional prevalence of BLV infection and the clinical syndrome. With these objectives, statistically reliable surveys were designed and the results of serological findings of BLV infection are described in this communication.

MATERIAL AND METHODS

Selection of herds for BLV serological survey

The population at risk comprised 206 900 herds[1]. A 967 herd sample size was chosen at random to provide a 95% confidence level, with a tolerated error of 0.03 between the real and estimated values of 'P' (*a priori* decision had assumed herd infection level approximately up to 35%). The sampling frame was structured to assure that it was representative of the herd sizes and dairy/beef distribution of each of seven geographic regions of Canada, namely:

1. Atlantic (Eastern) Provinces, i.e. Newfoundland, Prince Edward Island, New Brunswick and Nova Scotia.
2. Quebec,
3. Ontario,
4. Manitoba,
5. Saskatchewan,
6. Alberta, and
7. British Columbia.

[1] Statistics Canada, Agriculture Livestock Census, 1976

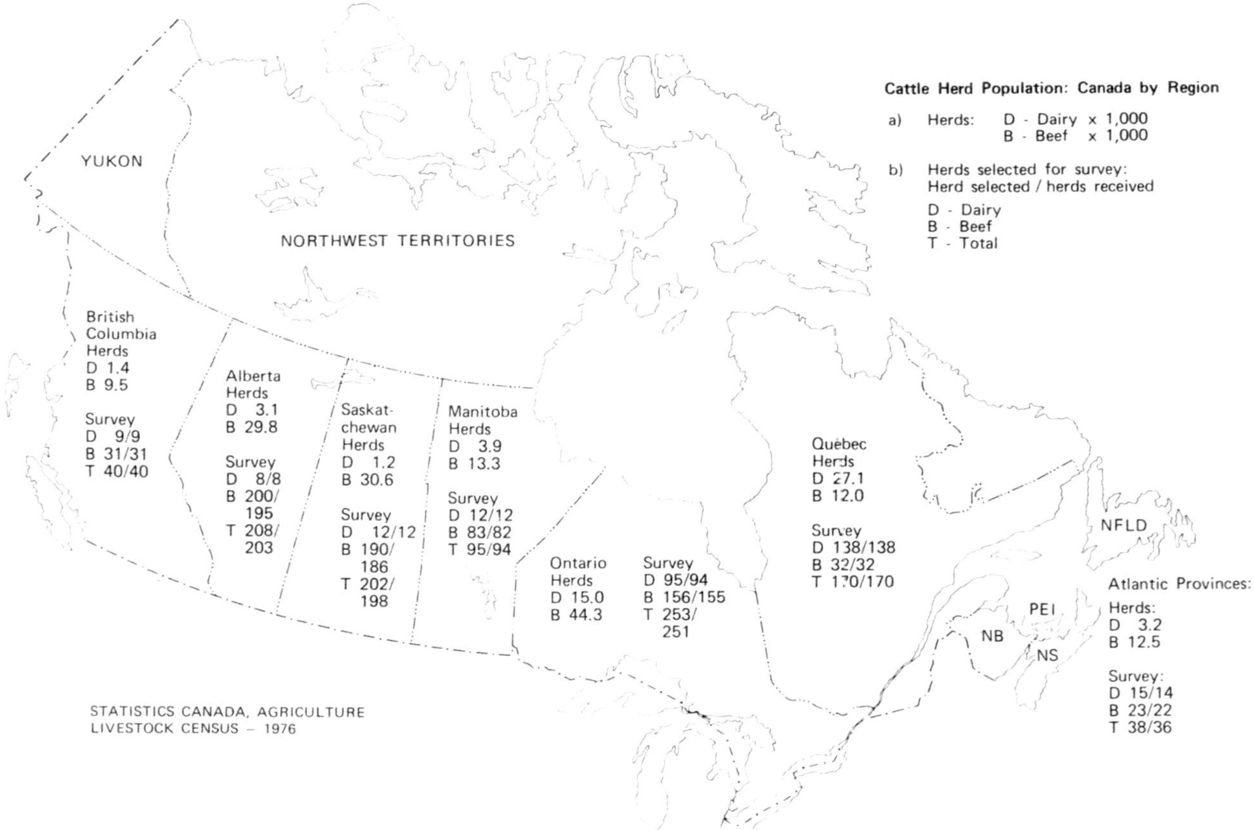

Fig. 1. Herd population and number of herds selected from different regions of Canada for bovine leukaemia virus infection survey.

The herd basis of selection was designed to depict accurately BLV infection on both a herd and an animal basis and to reflect the intra-herd distribution of infection. Allowing for potential sample losses the sample size was incremented to 1 004 herds, of which 990 herds (comprising a total of 38 297 animals) had been bled from April 1979 - March 1980 and tested for BLV antibodies. Following guidelines established for standard brucellosis testing, animals bled were 6 months of age or older. Details of the total number of herds in each of the above regions, as well as number of herds selected and received for testing, are illustrated in Figure 1.

Agar Gel Immunodiffusion (AGID) test

The antigen used for the AGID test was 30% ammonium sulphate precipitate of the BLV infected cell culture fluid of foetal lamb kidney. The AGID test system was balanced to detect glycoprotein antibodies in the cattle sera. The preparation of the antigen, reference serum and AGID test were the same as previously described (Samagh et al., 1978).

RESULTS

Prevalence of BLV infection in Canadian herds

The prevalence of BLV infection in Canadian herds was studied by determining the presence of BLV antibodies using the AGID test. The presence of one or more sero-positive animals in a herd constituted herd infection. In a total of 990 herds, 287 dairy and 703 beef herds were tested; 195 herds (116 dairy and 79 beef herds) were found to be infected, giving an overall BLV prevalence rate of 19.7 ± 2.5%[1] (dairy 40.5 ± beef 11.2 ± 2.3%). The national and regional distribution of herd infection on a dairy, beef and composite[2] basis is outlined in Figure 2.

[1] 95% confidence intervals as employed throughout this paper

[2] An overall or weighted average of all dairy and beef incidence rates

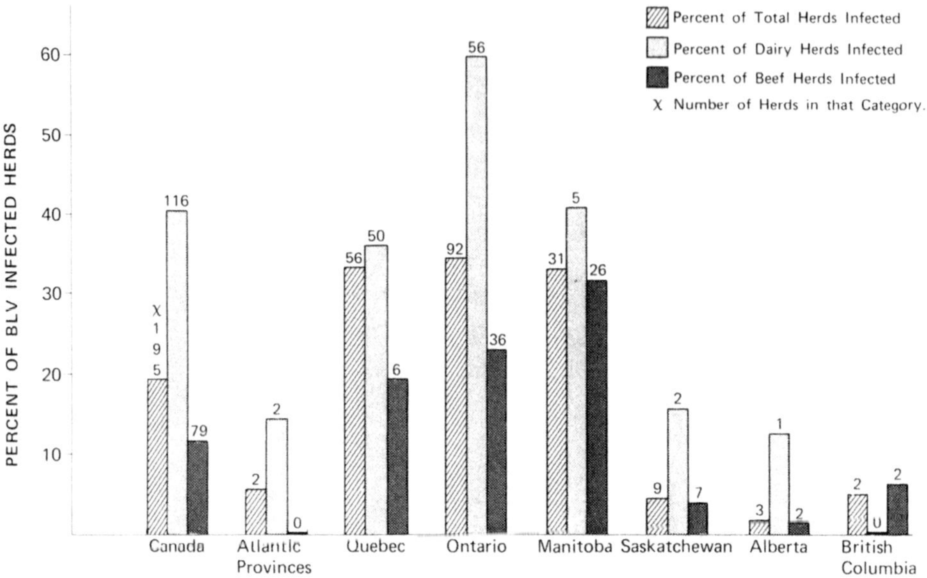

Fig. 2. Distribution of bovine leukaemia virus infected herds in different regions of Canada

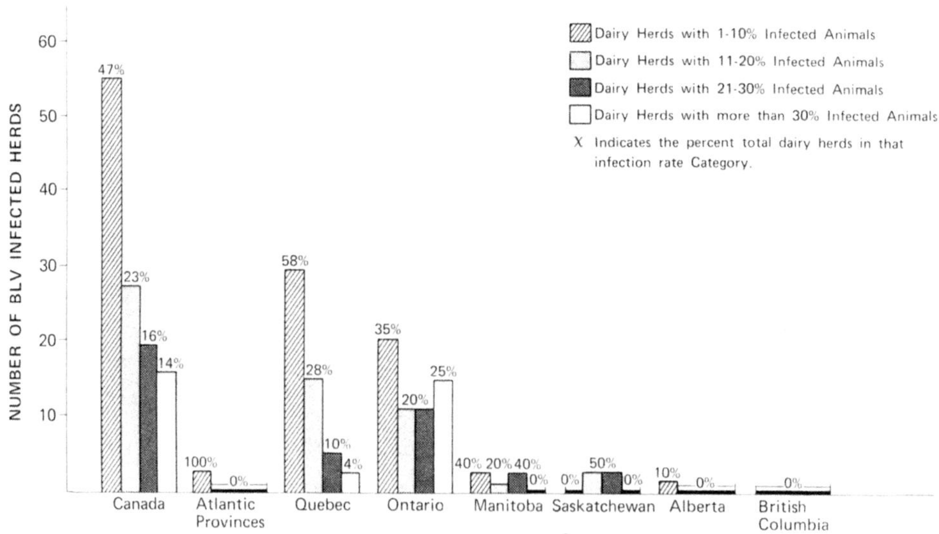

Fig. 3. Degree of bovine leukaemia virus infection in dairy herds in different regions of Canada

The apparent regional prevalence of BLV infection varied greatly. The degree of herd infection was comparatively much higher in the three central provinces as compared to the four Atlantic and three Western provinces. The prevalence rate in the Atlantic provinces was 5.5 ± 7.5%, 2 of 14 dairy herds (14.3 ± 18.3%) tested were found to be infected, whereas all 23 beef herds tested were negative. In Saskatchewan, Alberta and British Columbia the composite prevalence rates were 4.5 ± 2.9%, 1.5 ± 1.7% and 5.0 ± 6.8%; the dairy herd rates 16.7 ± 21.1%, 12.5 ± 22.9% and 0%, and the beef herd rates 3.8 ± 2.7%, 1.0 ± 1.4% and 6.5 ± 8.6% respectively. The smaller sample size in some provinces is reflected in the wider confidence intervals.

The three central provinces, Quebec, Ontario and Manitoba have 55.8% of the total herd population of Canada (83.8% dairy; 45.8% beef). They contain, however, 90.2% of the infected herds in the country (95.7% dairy; 86.1% beef). The overall prevalence rate for BLV infected herds in Quebec, Ontario and Manitoba is 32.9 ± 7.5%, 36.9 ± 6.0% and 32.6 ± 9.5%, respectively; with respective prevalence rates in dairy herds of 36.2 ± 8.0%, 59.6 ± 9.9% and 42.0 ± 27.9% and in beef herds of 19.0 ± 13.5%, 23.2 ± 6.6% and 32.0 ± 10.1%.

Degree of BLV infection in Canadian dairy and beef herds

In order to study the distribution of infection rates within the dairy and beef herds across the seven Canadian regions, the herds were grouped according to their individual BLV infection rates. Four arbitrary ranges indicating 1 - 10%, 11 - 20%, 21 - 30% and >30% seropositive animals were selected. Of the survey's 116 infected dairy herds, 54 herds (47%) had 1 - 10%, 27 herds (23%) had 11 - 20%, 19 herds (16%) had 21 - 30% and 16 herds (14%) had >30% seropositive animals (Figure 3). Of the survey's 79 infected beef herds, 52 herds (66%) had 1 - 10%, 12 (15%) had 10 - 20%, 8 (10%) had 21 - 30% and 7 herds (9%) had >30% seropositive animals (Figure 4).

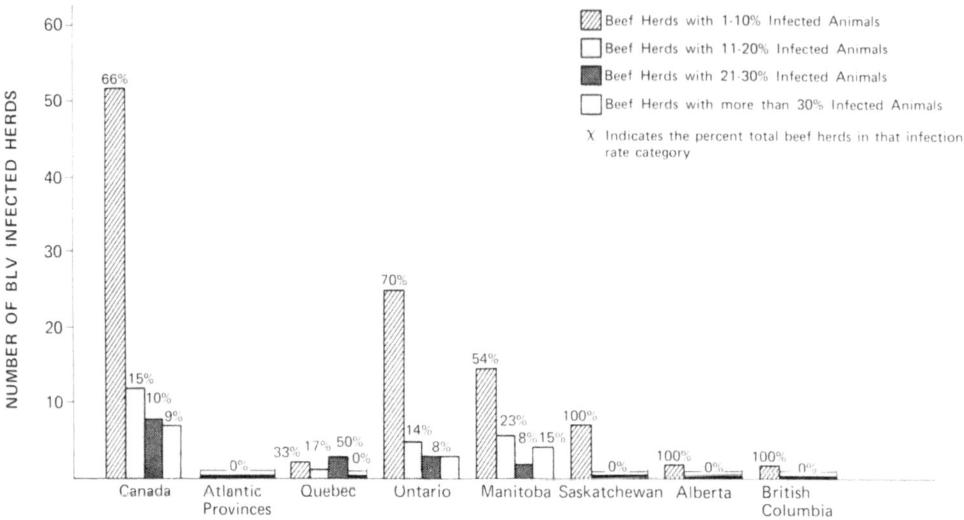

Fig. 4. Degree of bovine leukaemia virus infection in beef herds in different regions of Canada.

The degree of rate of BLV infection in individual dairy and beef herds of the seven regions follows a similar pattern of prevalence to the BLV infected herds. In British Columbia all the dairy herds tested were seronegative, in Alberta 1 out of 1 infected herd and in Atlantic provinces 2 out of 2 infected herds had 1 - 10% seropositive animals. In Saskatchewan out of 2 infected dairy herds, one had 11 - 20% and the other had 21 - 30% seropositive animals. All the beef herds tested in Atlantic provinces were completely negative and none of the beef herds tested in three western provinces had >10% seropositive animals. In Saskatchewan 7 out of 7, in Alberta 2 out of 2 and in British Columbia 2 out of 2 infected beef herds had 1 - 10% seropositive animals.

Among the three central provinces, Manitoba and Ontario had higher infection rates in beef herds, whilst Quebec and Ontario showed a higher infection rate in dairy herds. Out of 26 infected beef herds in Manitoba 14 herds (53.8%) had 1 - 10%, 6 herds (23.1%) had 11 - 20%, 2 (7.7%) had 21 - 30% and 4 herds (15.4%) had >30% infected animals. In Ontario, the beef herds had almost the same distribution of infection rates as in

Manitoba, out of 36 infected beef herds, 25 herds (69.5%) had 1 - 10% infected animals, 5 herds (13.9%) had 11 - 20% and 3 herds (8.3%) in both the 21 - 30% and >30% infection rate categories. In Quebec none of 6 infected beef herds had >30% infection rate: 2 herds (33%) had 1 - 10%, 1 herd (17%) had 11 - 20% and 3 herds (50%) had 21 - 30% seropositive animals.

Out of 5 infected dairy herds in Manitoba 2 herds (40%) each fell into 1 - 10% and 21 - 30% infection rate categories and 1 herd (20%) had 11 - 20% seropositive animals. In Ontario, out of the 56 infected dairy herds, 20 herds (35.7%) had 1 - 10% infected animals, 11 (19.6%) herds each had 11 - 20% and 21 - 30% seropositive animals and 14 (25%) herds had >30% infection rate. In Quebec out of 50 infected dairy herds, 29 herds (50%) had 1 - 10%, 14 herds (28%) 11 - 20%, 5 herds (10%) had 21 - 30% and 2 herds (4%) had a >30% infection rate category.

It may be concluded that in the survey Ontario and Manitoba had 7 out of 7 beef herds, Ontario and Quebec had 16 out of 16 dairy herds showing >30% BLV seropositive animals in the country.

DISCUSSION

The BLV infection prevalence study demonstrates the relative predominance of infection in Canada's three central provinces and its markedly diminished levels in the Atlantic (eastern) and western areas of the country. These three central provinces, Quebec, Ontario and Manitoba, have an estimated 90.2% of the national infected herds (95.7% dairy; 86.1% beef). Such regional variations in BLV infection within countries have been previously noted. Devare et al. (1977) with a limited number of samples showed that the rate of BLV infection varied from a low of 2% to a high of 41% in 22 states of the USA. Crespeau et al. (1978) tested 295 herds serologically in the south-west of France and found 64% of herds infected, whereas Nougayerde et al. (1978) serologically examined 763 herds in the west of

France and found only 1.44% of herds infected with BLV. Such regional divergence of BLV infection may be related to the regional difference in management practices, production methods and herd contact (Piper et al., 1975). The high survey rate of infected herds demonstrated in the three central provinces of Canada suggests that the focus of BLV infection is in these provinces and that the spread of infection to the east and west is currently limited.

These studies reveal that 19.7% of the total herds, 40.4% of the dairy and 11.2% of the beef herds are infected with BLV, which reflects approximately four times more infected dairy than beef herds.

Baumgartener et al. (1975) found 66% of the dairy and 14% of the beef herds infected in a survey of 150 herds in Iowa, Michigan, Minnesota, Nebraska, South Dakota and Wisconsin. Since BLV is transmitted horizontally mainly by contact (Samagh et al., 1978), the high degree of herd to herd movement of animals which occurs in dairy husbandry, plus the facts that dairy herds have older animals and the animals spend more time indoors in close contact, could be responsible for the significantly higher numbers of infected dairy herds. Burridge et al. (1979) have suggested the genetic influence on the susceptibility of animals to BLV infection but further investigations of herds from a wider geographical area are required to confirm this hypothesis.

House et al. (1977) tested 1 295 beef and dairy cattle from 33 beef and 41 dairy herds in Georgia, Pennsylvania, New York, Texas and Wisconsin and found that 2.6% of animals in beef and 28.2% of animals in dairy herds were infected with BLV. Marin et al. (1978) tested 6 081 dairy and 8 948 beef animals in Venezuela for BLV antibodies and showed 49.1% of dairy and 20.9% of beef animals were seropositive. In this study a total of 38 297 animals were tested for BLV antibodies and an overall rate of infection was found to be 3.6 $\pm$ 0.2% (9.3 $\pm$ 0.4% in dairy and 0.5 $\pm$ 0.1% in beef animals).[1]

[1] The influence of BLV infection on breed, age and sex will be presented in another communication.

Many investigators have shown that herds experiencing clinical cases of EBL have significantly higher rates of BLV infection than those with no clinical evidence of disease. Abt et al. (1976) have shown that 12 herds having multiple cases of EBL had on average 48% of the animals infected with BLV compared to 20% BLV infection rate in 7 contact herds with no clinical disease. House et al. (1977) have found a BLV seropositive rate of 51.8% in herds experiencing clinical EBL compared to 13.7% infection rate in animals from 29 herds known to be free of clinical disease. In this study only 16 dairy and 7 beef herds had infection rates of >30%; and, out of these, only dairy and 6 beef herds experienced an infection rate of $\geq$41%. This suggests that 1.7% of the dairy (5/287) and 0.8% (6/703) of the beef herds in this country are at increased risk of experiencing one or more clinical cases of EBL at some time throughout the herd's history.

In order to find the incidence of clinical EBL, surveys have been designed and information is being collected from bovine practitioners, veterinary colleges, provincial and federal animal pathology laboratories and abattoirs in the country. The preliminary results[1] indicate that death losses due to clinical diseases are not of sufficient economic importance to warrant a nationwide control programme, although the BLV infection rate being high in a low percentage of herds may lead to death losses numerous enough to suggest a preventive programme in these herds. The ever-increasing requirement of importing countries for BLV negative breeding animals will restrict the movement of BLV infected cattle in international trade. The epidemiological study of BLV infection and clinical disease will be used to study the economic impact of EBL in Canada. The results of this study will be used to assess the justification for control programmes in the country.

[1] Interim results from a random survey of bovine practitioners estimate the 1979-80 losses from clinical EBL as 670 animals in a population of 14 million, giving 4.8 cases/100 000 animals (dairy 22.5; beef 1.1).

ACKNOWLEDGMENTS

The authors thankfully acknowledge the technical assistance of Mrs. Rita Groulx and Mr. M.K. Krishnamurthi for conducting serological tests. The authors also thank the numerous practising veterinarians of the Food Production and Inspection Branch, Agriculture Canada without whose wholehearted co-operation this study could not have been completed.

REFERENCES

Abt, D.A., Marshak, R.R., Ferrer, J.F., Piper, C.E. and Bhatt, D.M., 1976. Studies on the development of persistent lymphocytosis and infection with bovine C-type leukemia virus (BLV) in cattle. Vet. Microbiol., 1: 287-300; Straub, O.C. (ed.), Elsevier Publishing Company Amsterdam and CEC, Luxembourg.

Baumgartener, L.E., Olson, C., Miller, J.M. and Van der Maaten, M.J., 1975. Survey for antibodies to leukemia (C-type) virus in cattle. J. Amer. Vet. Med. Assoc., 166: 249-251.

Bendixen, H.J., 1965. Bovine enzootic leukosis. Adv. Vet. Sci., 10: 129-204.

Burridge, M.J., Wilcox, C.J. and Henneman, J.M., 1979. Influence of genetic factors on the susceptibility of cattle to bovine leukemia virus infection. Eurp. J. Cancer, 15: 1395-1400.

Chander, S., Samagh, B.S. and Greig, A.S., 1978. BLV-antibodies in serial sampling over five years in a bovine leukosis herd. Ann. Rech. Vet., 9: 797-802.

Crespeau, J.P.S., Vuillaume, A., Levy, D., Parodi, A.L., 1978. A two year seroepidemiological survey of bovine leukemia virus (BLV) infection in high incidence area of the South-West of France. Ann. Rech. Vet., 9: 747-754.

Devare, S.G., Chander, S., Samagh, B.S. and Stephenson, J.R., 1977. Evaluation of radioimmunoassay precipitation for the detection of bovine leukemia virus infection in domestic cattle. J. Immunol., 119: 277-282.

Devare, S.G. and Stephenson, J.R., 1978. Radioimmunoassay for the major internal antigen (p24) and envelope glycoprotein (gp51) of bovine leukemia virus. Ressang, A.A. (Ed.): The serological diagnosis of bovine leukosis. Commission of the European Communities. Luxembourg. pp. 43-55.

Flensburg, J.C. and Stryffert, B., 1977. The control of bovine leukosis in Denmark. Epidemiological and diagnostic aspects. Nord. Vet. Med., 29: 49-67.

House, C., House, J.A. and Glover, F.L., 1977. Antibodies to the glycoprotein antigen bovine leukemia virus in the cattle population of five states. Cornell Vet., 67: 510-522.

Marin, C., De Lopez, N.M., Alvarez, L., Lozano, O., Espana, W., Castanos, H. and Leon, A., 1978. Epidemiology of bovine leukemia in Venezuela. Ann. Rech. Vet., 9: 743-746.

Miller, J.M., Miller, D.L., Olson, C. and Gillette, K.G., 1969. Virus-like particles in phytohemagglutinin-stimulated lymphocyte culture with reference to bovine lymphosarcoma. J. Natl. Cancer Inst., 43: 1297-1305.

Mussgay, M. and Kaaden, O-R., 1978. Progress in studies on the etiology and serologic diagnosis of enzootic bovine leukosis. Current topics in Microbiol. and Immunol., 79: 43-72.

Nougayerde, P., Quentel, C. and Gayot, G., 1978. Enzootic bovine leukosis: An epidemiological survey among cattle in the west of France by precipitating antibody detection. Ann. Rech. Vet., 9: 755-760.

Piper, C.E., Abt, D.A., Ferrer, J.F. and Marshak, R.R., 1975. Seroepidemiological evidence of horizontal transmission of bovine C-type virus. Cancer Res., 35: 2714-2716.

Ressang, A.A. (Ed.), 1978. The serological diagnosis of enzootic bovine leukosis. Commission of the European Communities. Luxembourg. p 208.

Samagh, B.S., Chander, S., Greig, A.S. and Boulanger, P., 1978. Serological diagnosis of bovine leukemia virus infection using dual (glycoprotein and p24) viral antigen. Ressang, A.A. (Ed.): The serological diagnosis of enzootic bovine leukosis. Commission of the European Communities. Luxembourg. pp 69-79.

Sørensen, D.K., 1979. Clinical manifestations of bovine leukosis. In: Proc. Bovine Leukosis Symposium, College Park, Maryland. May 22-23, 1979. Published by United States Department of Agriculture, Hyattville, Maryland. pp 5-17.

Sørensen, D.K. and Beal, Jr., V.C., 1979. Prevalence and economics of bovine leukosis in the United States. In: Proc. Bovine Leukosis Symposium, College Park, Maryland. May 22-23, 1979. Published by United States Department of Agriculture, Hyattsville, Maryland. pp 33-50.

DISCUSSION

G. de Vries *(Netherlands)*

I would like to know the total number of herds. I estimate that out of 40 million there must be about 300 000, so the thousand herds are less than half a percent of the total. Is that statistically sound?

B.S. Samagh *(Canada)*

From the survey we did we had a 35% infection rate. We sent that to a statistician and he told us that this was the number of herds we should check. But I can see that where the infection rate is low we might have to test more herds.

A.A. Ressang *(Netherlands)*

Is EBL native in Canada, or is it due to importation? If you look in the literature, every country claims that EBL has been imported, no country admits to it being a native disease.

B.S. Samagh

I think we imported it from Europe, and now we are sending it back!

O.-R. Kaaden *(FRG)*

Did you say that all herds carrying more than one positive animal were considered to be positive?

B.S. Samagh

One or more animals in the herd means an infected herd.

O.C. Straub *(FRG)*

There are a few countries that do not claim to have imported EBL. One of them is East Prussia. If you read the old papers by Knuth and Volkmann (1916) they state this. In my paper I mentioned that some countries recognised that they had the disease; Estonia is another example. So, not all of them deny it.

OBSERVATIONS ON SEROLOGICALLY WEAK-POSITIVE REACTIONS WITH THE IMMUNODIFFUSION TEST (IDT) IN THE DIAGNOSIS OF ENZOOTIC BOVINE LEUKOSIS (EBL) INFECTIONS

R.J. Lorenz[1], U. Wernery[2], T. Zimmermann[2] and O.C. Straub[1]

[1] Bundesforschungsanstalt für Viruskrankheiten der Tiere, D-7400 Tübingen,

[2] Veterinäruntersuchungsamt des Landes Schleswig-Holstein, D-2350 Neumünster, Federal Republic of Germany.

ABSTRACT

Eight hundred and sixty one cattle herds in Schleswig-Holstein, where at least one weak-positive reactor was observed, were selected for the study. The mean age of strong - and weak-positive reactors significantly exceeded the mean age of <u>*all cattle*</u>*. In addition, weak-positive reactors had a larger mean age than strong-positive reactors. In herds which had formerly been unsuspected, weak-positive reactors were on average younger than in those herds where the EBL-infection had already been diagnosed (on the basis of haematological testing).*

O.C. Straub (ed.), Fourth International Symposium on Bovine Leukosis

INTRODUCTION

According to the official diagnostic rules for EBL in the European Community (EC) a blood sample is assessed serologically as either 'positive', 'questionable' or 'negative' for the presence of antibodies against the EBL virus.

A series of comparative tests revealed that a blood sample found as questionable in one laboratory may be found positive or negative in other laboratories. The reason for this lack of reproducibility between laboratories is attributed to a variation in the sensitivity of the IDT. In general, however, questionable results are obtained from samples with a low antibody titre called weak-positive reactors - as distinct from positive and negative reactors.

Veterinary officers in the Federal Republic of Germany dealing with the control of EBL reported:

1) Questionable IDT results as isolated events in a herd occur very rarely. If a questionable result is observed in a herd, then in almost all cases positive results are also found.

2) Questionable results are found predominantly among older cattle.

It is noticeable that a number of veterinarians had the impression that the proportion of questionable test results seems to increase with time.

These observations - provided they can be confirmed - are not in full agreement with the intuitive concept of the role and the genesis of weak-positive reactors in the frame of epizootiology.

According to this concept the antibody titre of a newly infected animal is at first low and remains for a period of time below the sensitivity threshold of the testing system. Animals in this stage of infection will therefore not be detected as reactors. The concentration of antibodies increases with time, however, and eventually passes the threshold. The animal is then recognised as a weak-positive or positive reactor. As the degree of increase of the antibody titre is assumed to vary from animal to animal, the time interval between infection and crossing the threshold may also differ.

Furthermore, it is very likely that the increase of the titre is not a steady movement from low to high values. There is evidence that it is in many cases a fluctuating up-and-down-movement with a general tendency to an increase. This can be concluded from observations on cattle which are diagnosed seropositive in a first, negative in a second test some months later and again positive and/or negative in later tests. If this picture of the development of seropositivity is correct, the age structure of serologically weak-positive cattle should - on the whole - be the same as that of positive reactors. It was therefore interesting to investigate this matter by means of a controlled study.

MATERIALS AND METHODS

The basis of the study was a sample of 861 herds in Schleswig-Holstein, where serologically 'questionable' test results had been obtained. These herds were tested between September 1978 and September 1979 as part of a series of the first IDTs performed which means that earlier herd tests were based on haematology.

From 47 361 cattle tested, 5 627 were strong-positive and 1 440 weak-positive.

The age distribution of all cattle in Schleswig-Holstein was obtained from the results of the animal census of December 1979. This distribution was used as a general control. Unfortunately, it was not possible to obtain the ages of all those cattle under study.

The age distribution of strong-positive reactors was determined by an independent survey using 1 303 positive cattle in Schleswig-Holstein.

Cattle in the animal census are divided into 3 groups of age: 0 - 1 year, 1 - 2 years and above.

RESULTS

Figure 1 gives the age distributions

- of the total cattle population in Schleswig-Holstein,
- of 1 303 strong-positive reactors,
- of the 1 440 weak-positive reactors.

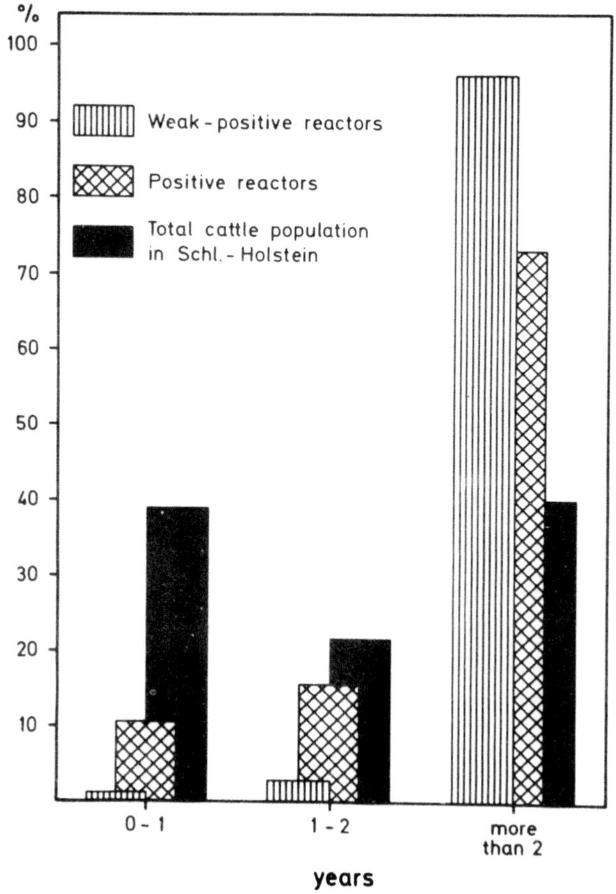

Fig. 1. Age distributions of weak-positive and positive reactors and of the total cattle population.

It is obvious that the mean age of reactors is significantly greater than that of the total population.

Between the strong-positives and weak-positives (Figure 2) a more differentiated comparison was possible. The ages of these animals were classified according to a 7-stage scale. The mean age of weak-positive reactors is significantly greater than that of the positive reactors. In other words: the proportion of old animals is greater in the population of weak-positive reactors than in the population of positive reactors.

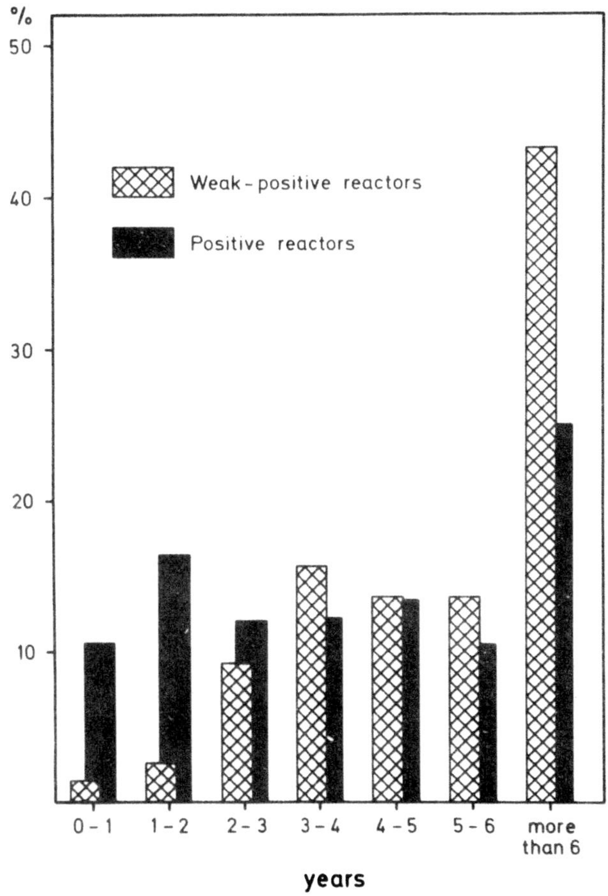

Fig. 2. Age distributions of weak-positive and positive reactors on a 7-stage scale of years of age.

Next we investigated the question of whether or not questionable test results are always associated with positive results in the same herd. Twenty per cent (172) of the herds contained only questionable but no positive results. The mean number of questionable results/herd was 1.10. This indicates that a herd with only questionable results is not exceptional. But it is also true that in almost all such herds not more than a single questionable result is found. In the remaining 80% of the herds, questionable results were associated with positive results. The mean number of questionable results/herd was 1.82. This means that in this group of herds the weak-positives have a higher frequency of occurrence (per herd) than in the other group.

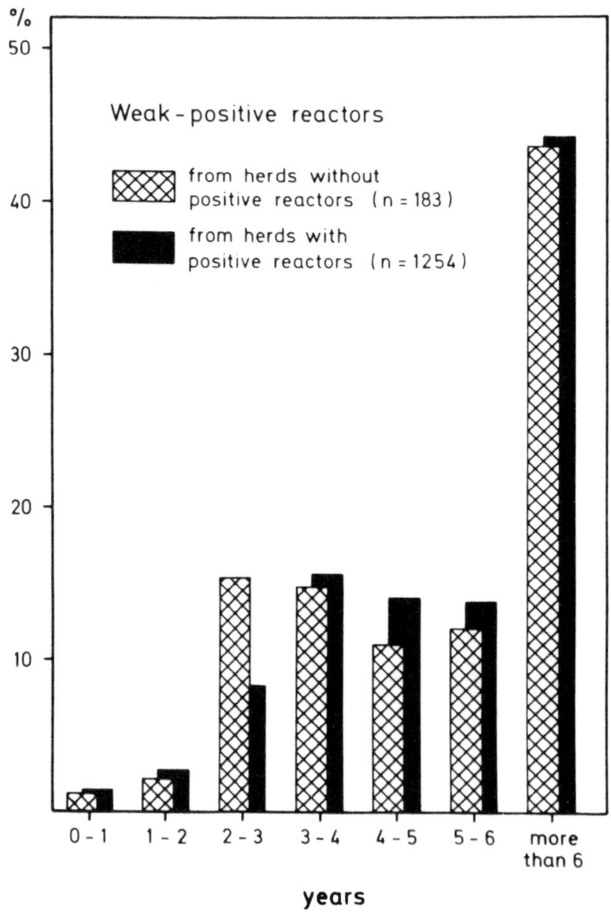

Fig. 3. Age distributions of weak-positive and positive reactors
a) from herds without positive reactors b) from herds with positive reactors

We compared the age distributions of weak-positives in both groups of herds and did not find a remarkable difference (Figure 3).

We then subdivided the herds with regard to another criterion

- into those herds which were known to be infected,
- and into those herds which had formerly been unsuspected.

This was possible only with 83 herds which had this information available at the time of the survey. Figure 4 shows the age distributions of weak-positive reactors in both groups of herds. In the group of infected herds the proportion of old animals is greater than in the group of formerly unsuspected herds.

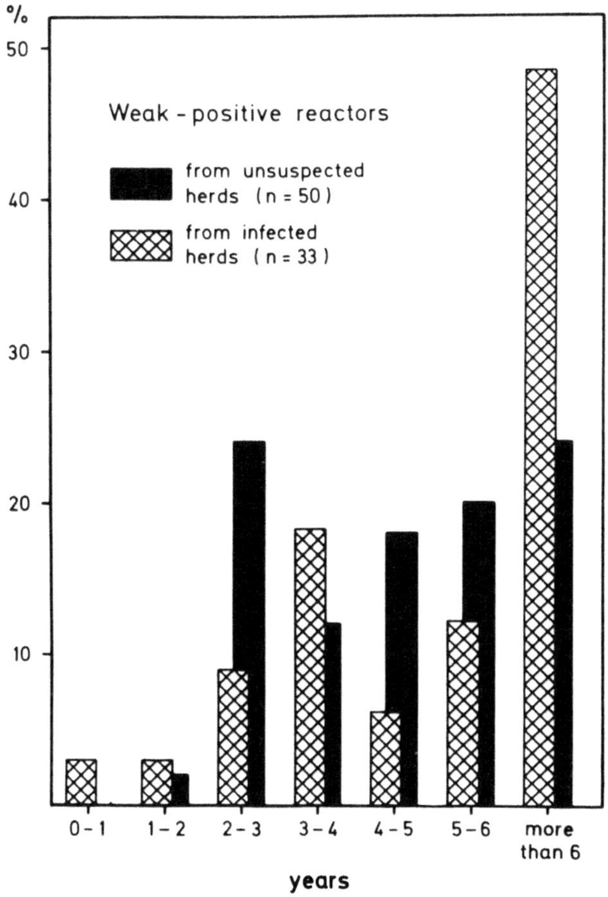

Fig. 4. Age distributions of weak-positive reactors
a) from formerly unsuspected herds b) from infected herds

The findings can be summarised as follows:

1) The mean age of strong-positive reactors exceeds that of the total cattle population.

2) The mean age of weak-positive reactors exceeds that of strong-positive reactors.

3) In 20% of the herds investigated weak-positive reactors occurred as isolated events; 80% of the herds contained weak-positives and strong-positives. There was no difference in the age distributions.

4) Weak positive reactors in herds known to be infected have a greater mean age than weak-positive reactors in formerly unsuspected herds.

The question then is whether an explanation for these observations can be given.

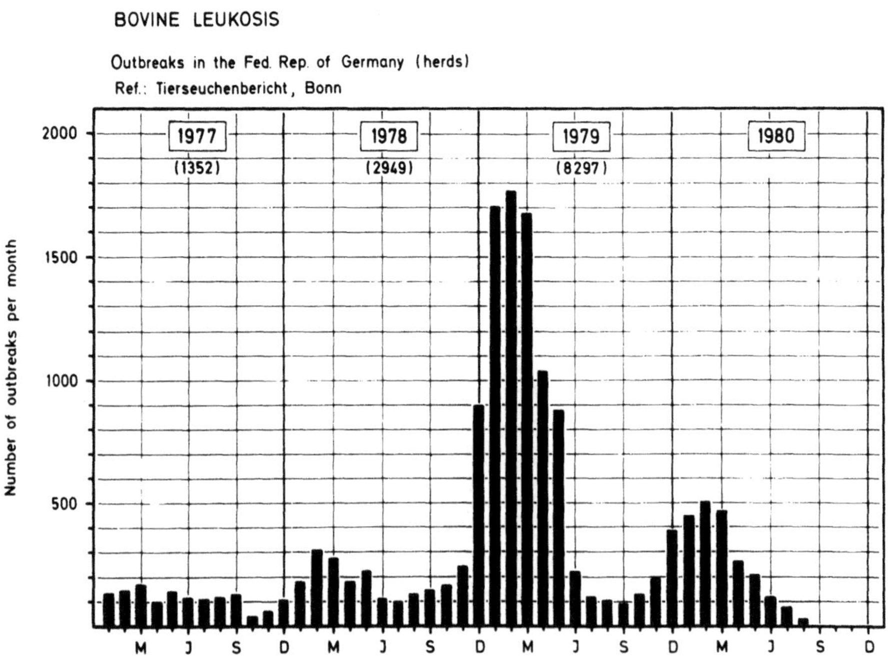

Fig. 5. Number of outbreaks of EBL (per month) in the Federal Republic of Germany since 1977.

CONCLUSIONS

First of all, we tried to check the possibility that we were fooled by some artificial effects, the presence of which can never be safely excluded from a survey of this kind. We realised, for example, that the various samplings had been taken from different populations (or from different strata of the basic population of all cattle in Schleswig-Holstein). But so far we have been unable to detect any source of bias inherent in the data. We may assume therefore that the variations observed in the age structures reflect relevant effects.

The high proportion of old animals among the weak-positive reactors is supposed to be the result of an accumulating process. Cattle detected as seropositive in the first test may have contracted the infection many years ago but remained undetected under the haematological test programme. This is strongly confirmed by the data presented in Figure 5, which gives the number of outbreaks (i.e. infected herds) per month in the Federal Republic. By the first serological test (winter season 1978/79) about four times as many reactors were detected than in the preceding winter season.

Can an explanation then be offered for the statement that the mean age of weak-positive exceeds the mean age of strong-positive reactors?

We suppose that the population of weak-positive reactors is composed of two or more subpopulations. The first one consists of newly horizontally infected cattle showing a 'normal development' of antibodies with increasing but still low antibody titres. The age structure of this subpopulation is assumed to be more or less identical with the age structure of the positive reactors.

The other subpopulation consists of cattle with another history of BLV infection. Calves infected either prenatally or immediately after birth may not be fully immunocompetent and carry the virus during the whole life. These animals may produce antibodies of a very low level. Some of these cattle have a dam which was BLV-infected. So far, there has been no case where the dam was non-infected.

A further group of permanent weak-positivity consists of cattle which had weak-positive dams which transmitted insufficient amounts of colostral antibodies to their calves which were then infected at a rather young age.

DISCUSSION

A.A. Ressang *(Netherlands)*

Would you define what you mean by a 'weak' reaction.

R.J. Lorenz *(FRG)*

A reaction which shows a very low antibody titre.

A.A. Ressang

By 'weak' reaction, do you mean that the line of precipitation is close to the well containing the serum?

O.C. Straub *(FRG)*

Yes, but there are still some loose ones and if you concentrate them they are nicely positive, just as we described it a few months ago. You concentrate them one or two fold, and then they are strongly positive.

A.A. Ressang

So this also includes the curving of the reference line?

O.C. Straub

Yes, of course.

A.A. Ressang

I wonder what happens if you introduce viral tests routinely in your system. These weakly positive animals may be virologically positive in 90% of cases. If they are virologically positive they are potentially viral shedders. So would it not be better to divide your animals into virologically positive or negative rather than weakly and strongly positive ones? Virological testing is no problem.

O.C. Straub

Well, this survey actually was done in Schleswig-Holstein with thousands and thousands of animals. Under those circumstances, you could not do any virological work. The laboratory where the testing was done is a State diagnostic laboratory.

A.A. Ressang

You are presuming that it is a complicated test.

O.C. Straub

No, I am just stating that in a State diagnostic laboratory it is impossible to engage in this type of virological work.

D.H. Roberts *(UK)*

Have you examined the negative herds with questionable results?

R.J. Lorenz

A negative herd is a herd where neither positive nor questionable results have been observed.

D.H. Roberts

I thought you referred to 1.1% of 'questionable herds', herds that did not have the virus, or did not have the infection.

R.J. Lorenz

Well, we don't know whether they have the virus. We only had a sample of herds where questionable test results were obtained.

D.H. Roberts

In clean herds?

R.J. Lorenz

No. There is a routine test and at least one so-called questionable result was observed. Is that a clean herd or is it not a clean herd?

D.H. Roberts

But have you examined these herds in detail, for infection?

R.J. Lorenz

It was observed that in the whole herd there was no other positive or questionable result. The history of those cases was not followed in this study.

D.H. Roberts

So we are not certain whether they are infective or positive?

R.J. Lorenz

No.

R. Hoff-Jørgensen *(Denmark)*

I hope that I am still right that when we are talking about the diffusion test, we know that it can show negative when the animal is infected but I presume it is not being suggested that it can show weak-positive reaction if the animal is not infected.

R.J. Lorenz

We are inclining more and more to the view that a questionable result should be judged as positive. The problem of this paper was not a technical one; there were so many animals that were weak-positive and will remain weak-positive over a long period. The question was whether it was a case of another aspect rather than a technical one.

A. Burny *(Belgium)*

My question has been partially answered. If these herds were to be followed now, and if these animals are really viral shedders, then the rate of spread of the infection in these herds must be expected to be high. So then, virus shedding, or not virus shedding, becomes irrelevant.

R.J. Lorenz

Of course, but this is more the practical aspect. We wanted to know why these animals differed in the age structure. We could not find a ready answer, it was a curious result.

PROBABLE HORIZONTAL SPREAD OF BOVINE LEUKOSIS VIRUS NOT FOLLOWED BY SECONDARY DISEASE OUTBREAKS

G. Hugoson and R. Brattström
National Veterinary Institute, S-750 07 Uppsala, Sweden.

ABSTRACT

The northern part of Sweden has been a low prevalence area for bovine leukosis (BL) for decades. All the northern herds which had been registered for BL cases for a twelve year period were traced and when possible investigated for the BL serological picture and the routines of management and recruitment. Serological results were compared to random abattoir sampling carried out within the area as well as within the high BL prevalence area in the south. Serological examinations were also carried out on trade animals delivered from the south and twice in 12 herds following the addition of seropositive or seronegative animals.

In spite of only one single occurrence of manifest BL, 16 out of 29 herds and 61 out of 386 animals showed seropositive findings compared to 1.1% of abattoir animals in the north and 27.1% of the animals in the south. No clear indications of horizontal virus transmission were received related to kinds of management routine or to recent addition of seropositive animals.

(The complete paper is published in Zentralblatt für Veterinärmedizin, B27, 304-312, 1980).

SESSION VIII

Epidemiology (II)

Chairmen : L. Bellani and J.C. Flensburg

LARGE SCALE SURVEY OF BOVINE LEUKOSIS VIRUS INFECTION IN CENTRAL AND SOUTHERN ITALY

D. Rutili[1], M. Severini[2], G. Bertorotta[2] and F. Titoli[1]

([1]) Istituto Zooprofilattico Sperimentale dell'Umbria e delle Marche - I-06100, Perugia, Italy.

([2]) Istituto di Ispezione degli Alimenti di Origine Animale - Facoltà di Medicina Veterinaria - I-06100, Perugia, Italy.

ABSTRACT

The results of a large scale serological survey for detection of enzootic bovine leukosis (EBL) in herds of 8 regions are reported. Using the immunodiffusion test with gp antigen, 19 139 animals were examined. Of 1 496 herds tested, 91 were positive and 771 animals showed antibodies to bovine leukosis virus (BLV). The infected herds consisted of Holstein-Friesian dairy cattle alone or included animals of other breeds. Imported cattle play an important role in the onset and spread of EBL.

O.C. Straub (ed.), Fourth International Symposium on Bovine Leukosis

INTRODUCTION

The causative agent of enzootic bovine leukosis (EBL) is a virus (BLV) that can be transmitted both horizontally and vertically. Infected animals can be identified by detection of specific BLV antibodies found in their sera.

In Italy, the disease was recognised for the first time in 1974 (Rampichini et al., 1975). Subsequently, some epidemiological studies have been carried out in central Italy (Rutili et al., 1978) which indicate that BLV infection is quite widespread in the country, contrary to previous opinions formed in the absence of data from large scale haematological investigations and based on a few cases of recognised lymphosarcoma which had been reported previously (Gentile, 1976).

It was demonstrated that infected animals were present in a high percentage of herds in which cases of lymphosarcoma had never been recognised.

It was deemed necessary, therefore, to undertake a large scale investigation aimed at discovering the extent of distribution of BLV infection in the entire national territory. This programme was financed by the Ministry of Health and our group was assigned to performing the study in central, southern and insular regions.

In the present work we report the results related to the first part of this epidemiological study, which refers to the data gathered in 1979.

MATERIALS AND METHODS

The sera of 19 139 animals of various breeds and cross-breeds from 1 496 herds in 7 regions of central, southern and insular Italy (Toscana, Lazio, Umbria, Campania, Puglia, Calabria and Sicilia) were used in the agar gel immunodiffusion test, according to the method described elsewhere (Severini et al., 1981). The antigen was obtained commercially (Pitman Moore, USA).

For a certain number of herds (see Tables) it was possible to gather precise information on the size of the herd, the breed, the origin of the first nucleus of animals, the successive introduction of other cattle, the type of stabling and the type of insemination adopted.

Methods used in the analysis of the data

Sample size estimation was made according to the following formula:

$$P = \frac{X}{T} \times \frac{X-1}{T-1} \times \frac{X-2}{T-2} \times \ldots\ldots\ldots\ldots \times \frac{X-N}{T-N}$$

where: P is the confidence level; X is the number of uninfected animals or herds; T is the number of animals or herds in the population; N + 1 is the required sample size.

In the absence of information on the frequency of BLV infection in Italy, the percentage rates assumed were those found in the sample examined either on animal or herd level.

For comparisons reported in the various Tables, the Chi-square statistic witn correction of the continuity of Yates was used. When necessary, comparison between the prevalence rates was made with Fisher's exact test (2 tailed).

RESULTS

According to the high frequency found, the sample we considered is quantitatively representative.

Out of 19 139 animals examined which were older than 1 year, 771 (4.0%) were found to be sero-positive and distributed in 91 (6.1%) of the 1 496 herds studied.

Table 1 presents the results relating to 445 herds in which it was possible to verify the breed of the animals. By examining this Table one sees that the infected herds consisting of the Holstein-Friesian breed or of Holstein-Friesian cross-breds represent 19.1% of the general total. The infected herds consisting of one or more breeds other than the Holstein-Friesian, and with eventual cross-breds, constitute only 0.9% of the total herds. The comparison between these two groups of herds showed that those herds consisting of the Holstein-Friesian breed only, or containing the Holstein-Friesian breed, are significantly ($P < 0.01$) harder hit than the others (Table 2).

TABLE 1

FREQUENCIES OF SEROLOGICALLY POSITIVE HERDS ACCORDING TO BREED

Herds by breed	Positive	Negative	No. herds examined	Percentage (*) prevalence
Holstein Friesian	79	187	266	17.75
Chianina	-	42	42	-
Other pure breeds	-	16	16	-
Holstein-Friesian cross-breds	6	90	96	1.35
Mixed breeds without Holstein-Friesian	4	21	25	0.90
Total	89	356	445	20.00

(*) Prevalence refers to total herds examined (445).

Out of 10 044 Hostein-Friesian cattle, 698 (6.9%) were found to be sero-positive.

A comparison between herds of less than 50 animals and those with more than 50 animals shows that in the latter the frequency of BLV infection is significantly ($P < 0.01$) higher (Table 2).

TABLE 2

PREVALENCE OF HERDS WITH SERO-POSITIVE ANIMALS ACCORDING TO DIFFERENT FACTORS

	Breed		Size		Type of stabling		Origin of animal nuclei	
	H-F*+others mixed with H-F	Others breeds without H-F	≤50 head	≥50 head	Animals in tied stalls	Animals raised in paddocks	Local	Foreign - out of the region - both
No. of herds with positive animals	85	4	45	40	29	40	37	25
No. of herds with negative animals	277	79	238	39	185	85	139	21
Fisher's exact test (2 tailed)	P = 0.00							
χ^2	=		39.554 (P<0.01)		15.448 (P<0.01)		18.500 (P<0.01)	

*H-F = Holstein-Friesian

A comparison of the herds in which the animals are permanently kept on pastures, or are raised in large paddocks, with those in which the animals are raised in tied stalls shows that the frequency of BLV infection is significantly ($P < 0.01$) higher in the former herds (Table 2).

Herds formed with an initial nucleus of animals from foreign countries or from other regions of Italy, showed a frequency of BLV infection significantly ($P < 0.01$) higher than those originally formed with animals of local origin (Table 2).

The subsequent introduction (sporadic or frequent) of animals into the herd did not cause a significant difference in the frequency of BLV infection, either in herds formed with a nucleus of animals originating outside the region, or in those formed with a nucleus of animals of local origin (Table 3).

Lastly, results show that the type of insemination (natural, artificial, or both) does not cause a significant difference in the frequency of BLV infection, taking into consideration both the origin of the initial nucleus of animals and the herd size (Table 3).

TABLE 3

PREVALENCE OF HERDS WITH SERO-POSITIVE ANIMALS ACCORDING TO DIFFERENT FACTORS

	Subsequent introductions (local origin of nuclei)		Subsequent introductions (foreign origin of nuclei)		Insemination (local origin of nuclei)		Insemination (foreign origin of nuclei)		Insemination (herds with ≤ 50 head)		Insemination (herds with > 50 head)	
	none	sporadic or frequent	none	sporadic or frequent	N*	A**	N	A	N	A	N	A
No. of herds with positive animals	26	8	6	17	23	13	12	12	17	16	20	13
No. of herds with negative animals	91	38	6	15	79	54	9	12	76	57	21	12
χ^2	0.220		0.024		0.088		0.032		0.150		0.000	

N* - Natural or natural and artificial insemination

A** = Artificial insemination

CONCLUSIONS

The cumulative results of our survey show that BLV infection is present in the cattle herds of central, southern and insular Italy. BLV antibody positive animals are considerably widespread among herds consisting of the Holstein-Friesian breed or of other breeds raised together with Holstein-Friesian cattle. Serologically positive animals were never found in herds comprising cattle of one or more native breeds other than Holstein-Friesian. The prevalence of infected herds is very low among those comprising one or more breeds other than Holstein-Friesian but including cross-breds. The breed of the parents of these cross-breds is not known with certainty.

BLV infection is mainly prevalent in herds which were formed initially with animals imported from abroad (USA, Canada and Holland) or from other regions of Italy, particularly the north.

Since we have observed that successive introductions of animals do not seem to have an important influence, it would seem that the presence of the BLV infection is due mainly to the animals which constituted the original nuclei of the herds.

In spite of this, it was verified that in the majority of the infected herds, which had been composed originally of nuclei of local origin, there had been successive introductions of cattle from abroad (USA, Canada or Holland) or from northern Italy. In these, therefore, the successive introductions of animals could have played a determining role in the origin of the BLV infection.

With regard to the infected herds composed exclusively of cattle of regional origin, it is necessary to point out that they are, for the most part, small in size. However, these small farms nearly always acquire animals from local medium or large size herds which are mainly composed of cattle nuclei imported from abroad or from northern Italy. The origin of BLV infection, therefore, does not seem to be truly local, but must be attributed to the preceding sequence of importations.

From our data it can be seen that the herds harder hit by BLV infection average more than 50 head and it is mainly herds of this dimension which resort to the foreign or extra regional market. This fact also explains why BLV infection is more frequent in herds where the animals are raised in large paddocks. This method of raising cattle is particularly widespread among herds of medium and large size in the country.

Lastly, it can be seen that no significant differences exist in the frequency of BLV infection among herds which use different methods of insemination (natural or artificial) leading to the assumption that semen or sire have no influence.

In conclusion, the survey has shown that BLV infection in herds of central, southern and insular Italy is correlated with the presence of cattle of the Holstein-Friesian breed from abroad, particularly from the USA, Canada, Holland, and from northern regions of Italy.

In order to prevent or minimise the spread of BLV infection, it will therefore be necessary to adopt control measures immediately, at least in the medium and large herds of cattle consisting of the Holstein-Friesian breed and to be particularly careful in the acquisition of new animals especially from abroad or from northern Italy.

It would be advisable, also, to avoid uncontrolled breeding between cattle of local breeds and cattle of the Holstein-Friesian breed in order to protect the important and valuable autochthonous livestock still essentially free of BLV infection.

ACKNOWLEDGMENTS

This study was supported by Ministry of Health, Direzione Generale Servizi Veterinari, and was conducted with the cooperation of Dr. P. Agrimi, Dr. M. Palarchi, Dr. G. Micozzi, Dr. D. Amaddeo (Ist. Zooprofilattico Lazio e Toscana), Dr. A. Capurso (Ist. Zooprof. Campania e Calabria), Dr. L. Sobrero (Ist. Zooprof. Puglia e Basilicata), Dr. S. Caracappa (Ist.Zooprof. Sicilia). The authors thank S. Buchetti and L. Ferraguzzi for technical assistance.

REFERENCES

Gentile, G., 1976. La Leucose Bovine en Italie. Bull. Off. int. Epiz. 85: 1-10.

Rampichini, L., De Castro Portugal, F.L., Severini, M. and Rutili, D., 1975. Leucosi Enzootica dei Bovini e Studio di Particelle di tipo C in una Bovine Adulta con Leucemia Linfatica Acuta e in Bovine dello stesso Allevamento con Linfocitosi Persistente. Tumori 61: 261-270.

Rutili, D., Severini, M., Rampichini, L. and Titoli, F., 1978. Epidemiologic Study on Enzootic Bovine Leukemia in Italy. Ann. Rech. Vet. 9: 761-764.

Severini, M., Rutili, D., Fruganti, G., Rampichini, L. and Cenci, G., 1981. Experimental Transmission of Enzootic Bovine Leukosis in Calves. IV International Symposium on Bovine Leukosis, Bologna, Nov. 5-7, 1980 (this publication).

DISTRIBUTION OF BLV INFECTION IN SOME PROVINCES IN NORTHERN ITALY

C. Cavrini[1], G. Gentile[2], G. Vacirca[3], L. Giordani[3]
[1]Ministry of Health - Veterinary Services - Rome, Italy
[2]University of Bologna - Veterinary Medical Clinic
Viale Q. Filopanti n. 5 - I-40126 Bologna - Italy.
[3]University of Milan - Veterinary Medical Clinic
Via Celoria n. 10 - I-20100 Milan - Italy.

ABSTRACT

Bovine enzootic leukosis has been reported in Italy only in recent years. A serological survey has been urged by the Ministry of Health in order to evaluate the present distribution of the disease in Italian cattle herds. This paper concerns investigations made in some provinces of northern Italy which are among the most developed from the zootechnical point of view, and where the largest importation of cattle from other countries has been recorded. The serological survey was carried out using the immunodiffusion test. The results are discussed taking into account the significance of imported animals and the need for health checks with regard to BLV.

O.C. Straub (ed.), Fourth International Symposium on Bovine Leukosis

INTRODUCTION

During the last few years there has been a radical change in the diagnosis of bovine leukosis, thanks to the development of serological tests which started in 1972 with the first observations by J.M. Miller on the presence of BLV antibodies in the serum from BLV infected animals. This approach was officially recognised at the international meeting on 'The Serological Diagnosis of Enzootic Bovine Leukosis' held in Rotterdam (August 29 - 30, 1977) where it was concluded that, "for the early diagnosis of enzootic bovine leukaemia (EBL) a serological examination is indispensable". The undoubted diagnostic reliability of serological procedures (especially of the AGID, due to its easy execution) provides more precise information on the distribution of the disease along with data which will make it possible to prepare an epizootiological map needed for the control of the condition, for eradication programmes and for the measures to be enforced with regard to both national and international trade exchanges. As a contribution to the execution of such an epizootiological map, our Ministry of Health has recommended and supported this present survey, aimed at establishing the distribution of the disease in Italy where there is now cause for concern about the enzootic form of bovine leukosis following the reports by Rampichini et al. (1975) and Gentile et al. (1980) and the documented importation from abroad of bovine animals with BLV antibodies (Gentile et al., 1980).

MATERIALS AND METHODS

The serological survey involved a total number of 51 685 animals above 1 year of age in 7 provinces of northern Italy. Provinces were chosen which were most likely to represent as exactly as possible the zootechnical trends of the respective regions, which are among the most advanced from the zootechnical standpoint; in particular, the investigations were performed in the provinces of Milan, Piacenza, Turin, Vicenza, Modena, Bologna and Bolzano. According to prevailing local animal production practice, the various provinces were investigated either by checking a few large herds (Milan and Piacenza) or many small herds (Vicenza, Modena, Bologna and Bolzano). In particular, in the provinces of Modena and Bologna, the farms were located in different areas and a random selection was made among large and small farms; whenever possible the randomisation was made among both hill and plain areas, with or without reports of recent importations. None of the herds had any history of clinical enzootic leukosis. In some provinces in particular, the prevalence of recently imported cows was high; the number of animals bred from cattle which had been imported from Canada was even higher because of the importance of Canadian blood in the genetic improvement of Italian dairy herds in recent years. With the exception of the provinces of Turin and Bolzano, all the control cows were Friesian. The animals investigated in the Turin province belonged to a total of 268 farms and included 5 961 Friesian and 1 221 Piedmontese; both breeds were often housed on the same farm. In the district of Bolzano there were Simmental cattle and a minor quantity of local breeds as well as Friesians. In this province where small family herds are typical, 8 953 animals from 1 033 farms averaging 8.66 head/farm were controlled. The serological test used for the studies was the agar gel immunodiffusion test with BLV glycoprotein antigen (Leukassay B test of Pitman-Moore). The research was carried out during 1979.

RESULTS AND CONCLUSIONS

The initial data show that at present investigations are at different stages and need to be completed. It is, however, possible to make a first tentative evaluation of the presence of enzootic bovine leukosis in some provinves of northern Italy. The results and considerations may be summarised as follows:

1. All the areas investigated, without exception, show the presence of animals with BLV antibodies.

2. The different sizes of the herds checked in the individual areas make significant comparisons impossible; in general, in most of the provinces studied, the prevalence of the infection appears to vary from 0.76 to 2.65% of animals examined. In the same areas, stables with animals seropositive to BLV vary from 2.61 in Bolzano to 9.70 in Turin, with an average of 6.05 (Table 1). In this evaluation, the inquiries which have been made in the province of Milan and Piacenza have been deliberately excluded, because they have particularly high numbers of positive animals. The infection rate calculated in these provinces (19.28% of the animals tested) might be altered by further more detailed research involving not only a large number of animals, but also - and chiefly - a larger number of farms. In fact, it is reasonable to believe that the above figure may be due to the high infection rates in the individual herds investigated rather than expressing the real distribution of EBL in the province; the individual farms examined were in fact low in number (Table 1) and all of them consisted of high numbers of animals, a large proportion of which have been imported from abroad.

TABLE 1

SEROLOGICAL INVESTIGATION FOR EBL IN NORTHERN ITALY

Province	Farms			Animals		
	Tested	Seropositive		Tested	Seropositive	
	No.	No.	%	No.	No.	%
Turin	268	26	9.70	7 182	182	2.53
Vicenza	574	40	6.96	10 241	81	0.79
Modena	612	56	9.15	9.986	265	2.65
Bologna	963	60	6.23	11 434	125	1.09
Bolzano	1 033	27	2.61	8 953	68	0.76
	3 450	209	6.05	47 796	721	1.51
Milan Piacenza	45	25	55.55	3 889	750	19.28
				51 685	1 471	2.84

3. The highest seropositive rates were recorded in farms where animals were more concentrated. Apparently, these farming conditions are more favourable for the spread of the infection (mass interventions, vaccinations, etc.). In mountain and hill areas, serological positivity was lower than in lowland areas solely because in the former zones herds generally contained a smaller number of animals.

4. The data for the province of Turin, though scarce, seem to indicate, at least as far as the two breeds considered are concerned, that there are no relevant differences in their susceptibility to BLV; once present in a herd, under favourable conditions the infection may equally affect both Friesian and Pièdmontese animals.

5. In those provinces where serological testing was performed on a larger number of farms, it appears that the infection is already present at varying levels, on farms throughout the whole provincial area. This observation is substantiated by the high ratios of infected herds/examined herds and even more by the fact that infected farms, although having different serological positivity rates and different numbers of animals, were territorially distributed among 28 communes from 46 in the province of Modena and among 38 communes from 60 in the province of Bologna.

6. In the animals examined in the provinces of Bologna and Modena, we tried to establish some relationship between the rate of infection and the age of the animals (Table 2). The results appear to be hardly significant in the province of Bologna due to the comparatively low number of animals and to the small size of the farms checked, where sporadic seropositive cases were recorded. In the province of Modena, where 3 030 animals of various age groups (265 of them were seropositive for BLV) belonging to fairly large herds were examined, the infection rate was directly proportional to the age of the animals with values increasing progressively from 1.20% in infected animals aged 1 to 2 years up to 16.29% in animals

TABLE 2

DISTRIBUTION BY AGE GROUPS OF THE CATTLE TESTED AND INFECTED IN FARMS OF THE PROVINCE OF MODENA

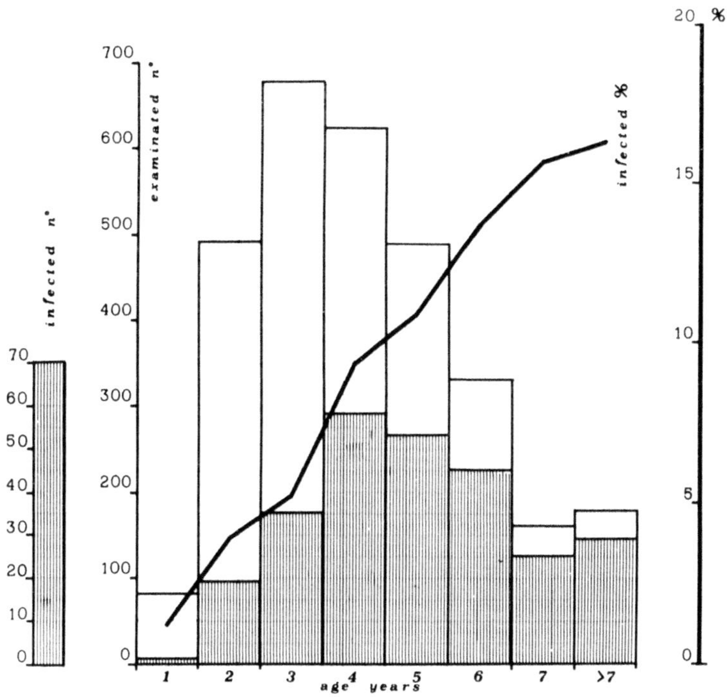

number examined	83	491	677	623	487	331	160	178
number infected	1	19	35	58	53	45	25	29
% infected	1.20	3.86	5.16	9.30	10.88	13.59	15.62	16.29

above 7 years of age. Although some differences were noticed in age groups with the highest numbers of infected animals, the above observations agree with those by previous authors (Crespeau et al., 1978; Valikhov, 1978) who consider them significant in supporting the concept of the horizontal transmission of the disease in the herd.

ACKNOWLEDGEMENTS

Serological tests for the provinces of Turin, Bolzano and Vicenza respectively, were performed at:

- Istituto Zooprofilattico Sperimentale del Piemonte, Liguria e Vallé d'Aosta;
- Istituto Zooprofilattico Sperimentale delle Tre Venezie;
- Sezione Zooprofilatticà di Bolzano.

We would like to thank our colleagues working at these laboratories.

REFERENCES

Crespeau, F., Sarsat, J.P., Vuillaume, A., Levy, D. and Parodi, A.L., 1978. A two years seroepidemiological survey of bovine leukemia virus (BLV) infection in a high incidence area of the south-west of France. Ann. Rech. Vét. 9, 747-754.

Gentile, G. and Schiavio, A., 1976. Sporadic enzootic leukosis in Italy. Vet. Microbiol. 1, 337-345. Straub, O.C. (ed.), Elsevier Publishing Company Amsterdam and CEC, Luxembourg.

Gentile, G. and Testi, F., 1978. Ulteriori osservazioni su un focolaio di leucosi enzootica e trasmissione sperimentale. Atti Soc. Ital. Buiatria, vol. X, 291-301.

Gentile, G., Rutili, D. and Ferrari, G., 1980a. Preliminari indagini sierologiche sulla presenza della leucosi bovine in allevamenti dell' Emilia. Clinica vet., 103, 128-131.

Gentile, G., Cinotti, S., Giordani, L. and Stefanon, G., 1980b. Indagini sierologiche per BLV (Bovine Leukemia Virus) in bovini di importazione. Clinica vet., 103, 146-147.

Marin, C., De Lopez, N.M., Alvarez, L., Lozano, O., España, W., Costanos, H. and Leon, A., 1978. Epidemiology on bovine leukemia in Venezuala. Ann. Rech. Vét., 9, 743-746.

Miller, J.M. and Van der Maaten, M.J., 1976. Serological detection of bovine leukemia virus infection. Vet. Microbiol. 1, 195-202. Straub, O.C. (ed.), Elsevier Publishing Company Amsterdam and CEC, Luxembourg.

Rampichini, L., De Castro Portugal, F., Severini, M. and Rutili, D., 1975. Leucosi enzootica dei bovini e studio di particelle in una bovina adulta con leucemia linfatica acuta e in bovine dello stesso allevamento con linfocitosi persistente. Tumori, 61, 261-270.

Rutili, D., Severini, M., Rampichini, L. and Titoli, F., 1978. Epidemiologic study on enzootic bovine leukemia in Italy. Ann. Rech. Vét., 9, 761-764.

Valikhov, A.F., 1978. Studies on the morphology and on some immunological properties of bovine leukemia virus. In: The serological diagnosis of enzootic bovine leukosis. (A.A. Ressang Ed.) Commission of the European Communities, 172-187.

DISCUSSION

G. de Vries *(Netherlands)*

Does Italy officially demand for animals imported from the United States and Canada to be free of leukosis, to be serologically examined before shipment?

G. Poli *(Italy)*

This will be the subject of the next paper.

F. Bürki *(Austria)*

Do you do anything beyond detecting BLV? Do you do anything to control it?

D. Rutili *(Italy)*

All this is preliminary work done to draw some conclusions whether we should introduce some control measures or an eradication programme. The interest in this disease is so high that something will surely be done.

J.C. Flensburg *(Denmark)*

You were talking about BLV infection, have you any tumour statistics?

D. Rutili

There are only a few results concerning investigations in this respect. There is a paper by Professor Gentile that reports a very low prevalence of lymphosarcoma, about 0.02 per 100 000 animals.

SEROLOGICAL INVESTIGATIONS FOR BLV INFECTION ON IMPORTED CATTLE IN ITALY

L. Bellani[1], G. Gentile[2], G. Vacirca[3] and G. Poli[4].

[1]Direzione Generale dei Servizi Veterinari, Ministero della Sanità, Roma

[2]Istituto di Patologia Speciale e Clinica Medica Veterinaria, Università di Bologna, I-40126 Bologna

[3]Istituto di Patologia Speciale e Clinica Medica Veterinaria, Università di Milano, I-20100 Milan.

[4]Istituto di Microbiologia e Immunologia Veterinaria, Università di Milano, I-20100 Milan
Italy

ABSTRACT

During the period July 1979 - October 1980 all cattle imported for reproduction were examined for the detection of bovine leukaemia virus (BLV) antibodies. All the sera from 23 601 animals were tested by the agar gel immunodiffusion test. The animals were divided according to the country of origin.

O.C. Straub (ed.), Fourth International Symposium on Bovine Leukosis

INTRODUCTION

As Cinotti et al. (1980) rightly claim, Italy ranks among the countries 'with a high importation index' of cattle partly destined to breeding farms, partly to beef production. Beef cattle, which by their nature are confined to special feeding centres and slaughtered shortly after their arrival, do not represent a real danger for the diffusion of BLV infection. The grave and impending danger is when breeding cattle, imported from infected areas or herds, or BLV carriers, are introduced without previous control onto national breeding farms.

This is the reason why the General Direction of Veterinary Services promoted the systematic control for enzootic leukosis of breeding cattle imported from other countries.

During the period July 1979 - October 1980 a total of 23 601 imported cattle were tested, of which 21 068 were from Switzerland and Austria and 2 533 from Canada and the United States.

The research was conducted with the agar gel immunodiffusion test, according to EC regulations, on blood samples collected by State Veterinary Officers upon arrival of the cattle, using antigens of different makes (Pitman Moore, USA, and Behring, FRG). In a number of cases the tests were also performed with an antigen prepared by the exporting country, with identical results.

RESULTS

The results obtained during the first period (July 1979 - March 1980) are reported in Table 1. The high percentage of BLV reacting cattle imported from Canada and the USA induced the National Veterinary Service officers to take the matter up with the competent authorities in the exporting countries. It was decided that a health certificate must be issued for animals exported to Italy, confirming that:

1. The animals come from a herd where no clinical cases of leukosis have been recorded during the past three years.
2. Sixty days at least prior to exportation the animals were tested by the agar gel immunodiffusion test for specific BLV antibody, with negative results.
3. Since the first test the animals were isolated from the other cattle on the breeding farm.
4. During the 30 days prior to exportation the animals were tested by immunodiffusion tests a second time, always with negative results.

It was also agreed with the Veterinary Services of the exporting countries that the cattle will be tested again by immunodiffusion tests upon arrival in Italy and accepted only if the results are negative (the latter point has been already effective as of January 1980).

TABLE 1

BLV SEROLOGY OF IMPORTED CATTLE (JULY 1979 - MARCH 1980)

	No. of imported animals	No. of positive tests	%
Austria	16 033	6	0.037
Switzerland	5 035	-	-
Canada	1 156	12	1.03
USA	525	31	5.90

These sanitary regulations, effective as of April 1980, have determined a consistent reduction in BLV positive imported cattle, as shown in Table 2.

This proves that the enforcement of protective measures, application of which is not exceedingly difficult, considerably reduced the risk of introducing BLV carriers from the countries mentioned in Table 2.

TABLE 2

BLV SEROLOGY OF IMPORTED CATTLE (APRIL - OCTOBER 1980)

	No. of imported animals	No. of positive tests	%
Canada	698	2	0.28
USA	154	3	1.94

With regard to cattle imported from Austria it is worth mentioning that the few animals with positive test results refer only to the first period of our investigation, and that no animal imported from Austria has since been found positive by the immunodiffusion test.

REFERENCE

Cinotti, S., Giordani, L., Stefanon, G. and Gentile G., 1980. Indagini sierologiche per BLV (bovine leukemia virus) in bovini di importazione. Clin. Vet., 103: 146.

DISCUSSION

J.F. Ferrer *(USA)*

You said that according to your regulations that animals have to be isolated after they have been proved negative in the first test. Do you mean isolated individually or as a group?

G. Poli *(Italy)*

We had discussions with the representatives of the Canadian and United States Commissions on the matter. Apparently there is a centre where all the export cattle are collected.

J.F. Ferrer

What happens if, for example, you have five cattle and one of them turns out to be positive when they arrive in Italy. Do you reject the whole group or only the infected animal?

G. Poli

Only the one positive animal. Up till now we have just sent back or slaughtered the positive animal. We are now making plans to be able to follow the imported cattle for at least six months.

L.M. Markson *(UK)*

Can you tell me why you have this system of import controls, pre-import testing, when EBL already exists in Italy and you have no control programme?

G. Poli

I take your point but it is certainly not going to help the situation if we import more infected animals.

F. Bürki *(Austria)*

With regard to Dr. Ferrer's question, perhaps I could explain what we do since Austria is probably the largest exporter of breeding cattle in Europe. Commissions send representatives to buy these cattle; they visit the herds of origin of the cattle. There they select and check the health status of those herds. The selected animals are then sent to a centre where they stay for three weeks. During this period they are tested for at least six, and sometimes eight, infectious diseases of cattle. In addition, they are vaccinated against foot and mouth disease and only then are they shipped.

M.J. Burridge *(USA)*

Dr. Poli, I see that the 5 000 cattle you imported from Switzerland were all negative. Does anybody have any data on the situation of BLV infection in Switzerland?

G. Poli

Generally speaking, they say that Switzerland is leukaemia free. I should stress that the animals to which you refer were a different breed, Brown Swiss. From Canada and the States we import Holstein-Friesian.

O.C. Straub *(FRG)*

Results have been published in Switzerland which show that having tested sera from animals all over the country, they are completely negative.

F. Bürki

Five Aberdeen Angus bulls were imported into Switzerland from England; they were all seropositive and subsequently killed.

W.A. Watson *(UK)*

Has the speaker any information on the part of the United States from which the cattle have been coming this year?

G. Poli

We are awaiting that information ourselves from the States.

V. Caporale *(Italy)*

We have carried out a small survey on about 5 000 animals in our region where we have quite a few Brown Swiss cattle, mostly imported from Switzerland. We have found seropositive animals. Now, I certainly cannot say that the cattle had been already infected when they were imported.

EPIDEMIOLOGY OF BOVINE LEUKOSIS VIRUS INFECTION IN SOME SELECTED HERDS

D. Rutili[1], M. Severini[2], F. Titoli[1], L. Rampichini[2] and G. Bertorotta[2]

[1]Istituto Zooprofilattico Sperimentale dell'Umbria e delle Marche, I-06100 Perugia, Italy.

[2]Istituto di Ispezione degli Alimenti di Origine Animale, Facoltà di Medicina Veterinaria - I-06100 Perugia, Italy.

ABSTRACT

The results of serological investigations in 8 herds examined at one year intervals are reported. The animals of one herd were examined for five years in order to gain some experience in the control of enzootic bovine leukosis taking into account economic factors which apply to the herd.

O.C. Straub (ed.), Fourth International Symposium on Bovine Leukosis

INTRODUCTION

In recent years a large amount of information regarding the epidemiological aspects of enzootic bovine leukosis (EBL) has been collected. The identification and characterisation of bovine leukosis virus (BLV), regarded as the causative agent of EBL, have led to the development of sensitive and specific serologic methods for the identification of BLV infected cattle. The serological test that is widely used for the diagnosis of BLV infection is the agar gel immunodiffusion (AGID) test. The AGID test, utilising BLV glycoprotein antigen, represents a valid and practical tool for the routine diagnosis and control or eradication of EBL (House et al., 1977; Rutili et al., 1977; Maas-Inderwiesen et al., 1978; Frenzel et al., 1978; Mammerickx et al., 1978; Van der Maaten and Miller, 1979).

Seroepidemiological surveys have shown that BLV infections are prevalent in the cattle population of many countries and that their frequency is higher in dairy cattle than in beef cattle. The results of these investigations and the evaluation of incidence rates of BLV infection have allowed the development of control or eradication programmes in some European countries (Mammerickx et al., 1978; Straub, 1978).

In Italy a nationwide serological investigation has recently been undertaken in order to ascertain the prevalence of BLV infection in cattle herds. Our group was involved in the examination of the herds of central and southern Italy and the results of this survey show that the prevalence of BLV infected animals is 6.1% (Rutili et al., 1980).

In order to gather more detailed information regarding EBL, which at present has a relatively low frequency in Italy, and before taking into consideration eventual plans for prophylaxis, it appears to be of primary interest to study extensively the characteristics of distribution of BLV infection within the herds. This report presents the results of an investigation carried out on 8 dairy herds with BLV infected animals and on 1 infected dairy herd where some control measures were practised and which had been under our surveillance for the last 4 years.

MATERIALS AND METHODS

Herds

Nine dairy herds containing Holstein-Friesian cattle were tested. In one herd there were also several Brown Swiss cows. The total size of these herds ranged from 50 to 300 cattle. These herds were self-contained, without introduction of new animals. Artificial insemination or natural insemination with own bulls was used. In two herds the cattle were kept in tied stalls. In the others separated groups of 30 - 40 animals were raised in paddocks. The separation of the various groups was done with wooden or metal fences. The cows calved in a separate building. The newborn calves received colostrum from their own dams and were then fed with powdered milk. Up to the age of one year the calves were housed separately from the adult cattle.

All herds examined were controlled every year for brucellosis and tuberculosis. The animals were vaccinated yearly against foot-and-mouth disease.

In the above herds there was no history of lymphosarcoma.

Serological tests

All animals over one year of age belonging to herds 1 - 8 were sampled twice at a twelve month interval. In herd 9 all cattle above one year of age were bled at twelve monthly intervals for two years and for the next two years at six monthly intervals.

The sera collected were stored at -30°C until used in the AGID test for the detection of BLV antibodies. The test was carried out as described elsewhere (Severini et al., 1980). The

BLV-glycoprotein antigen was obtained commercially (Pitman-Moore, USA).

Estimation of infection rates

The prevalence and incidence of BLV infection according to the age and the type of stabling was determined in herds 1 - 8. In herd 9 the prevalence and the incidence of the BLV infected animals were determined with regard to some control measured applied to minimise the spread of BLV infection.

This control programme was based on the gradual removal of serologically positive animals as soon as possible after their detection and taking into account economic factors relevant to the particular farm. Moreover, for the blood sampling and for any other similar operation one needle was used for each animal. The calves born from BLV infected cows were immediately removed from their dams and received colostrum from negative cows.

Analysis of the data

For the herds tested the percentage incidence of new serologically positive animals/year was calculated (Schwabe et al., 1977; Wilesmith et al., 1980). The animals at risk were determined in the following manner:

Animals at risk = Number of negative animals present at beginning of the period ± ½ x number of animals not present during the whole period.

The percentage incidence rate/year was calculated as follows:

Percentage incidence rate/year =

$$\frac{\text{Number of animals becoming serologically positive}}{\text{Animal days at risk}} \times 365 \times 100$$

where: Animal days at risk = Animals at risk x length of inter-test time in days

The Chi-square statistic was calculated with the continuity correction of Yates when one among the expected frequencies was lower than 50. When necessary Fisher's exact test (2 tailed), using the tables of logarithms of natural number factorials, was employed.

For the analysis of the evolution of prevalence and incidence rates the coefficient of linear regression with the control of statistic significance was calculated.

RESULTS

In Table 1 the results of investigations performed in herds 1 - 8 serologically examined in autumn 1978 and autumn 1979 are reported. The cumulative prevalence of serologically positive animals (Table 2) found at the first survey was 11.0% and in the second 10.5%. The prevalence according to the type of stabling was 9.4% (autumn 1978) and 9.5% (autumn 1979) for animals in tied stalls, while for animals raised in paddocks the prevalence was 11.2% (autumn 1978) and 10.6% (autumn 1979). With regard to age, the highest prevalence observed was 6.2% in the first age class, 12.6% in the second and 21.1% in the third. The cumulative incidence/year of new serologically positive animals found in herds 1 - 8 was 3.9% (Table 3).

In herds with animals in tied stalls the incidence rate was 2.5% and in herds in which the animals were raised in paddocks the incidnce was 4.1%. The incidence rates according to age, were 3.2%, 3.8% and 6.2% for the three age groups (Table 3). Comparing these incidence rates statistically, there is no significant difference between either the two different types of stabling or among the three age groups (Tables 4 and 5). Table 6 shows the general situation of BLV infection in herd 9 after 7 controls. The prevalence of serologically positive animals in this herd reached its highest rate (15.0%) in the second test and then showed a progressive reduction in successive tests, achieving a rate of 1.8% in the last test.

TABLE 1

GENERAL SITUATION OF ENZOOTIC BOVINE LEUKOSIS IN HERDS 1 - 8 AFTER TWO SUCCESSIVE CONTROLS

Type of stabling	No. animals examined				Reactors			Reactors eliminated			New reactors		
	Total	1-3*	3-6*	>6*	1-3	3-6	>6	1-3	3-6	>6	1-3	3-6	>6
Autumn 1978													
Animals in tied stalls	128	22	85	21	-	9	3	-	1	1			
Animals raised in paddocks	1013	462	404	147	30	52	31	9	11	14			
Total	1141	484	489	168	30	61	34	9	12	15			
Autumn 1979													
Animals in tied stalls	137	28	53	56	-	1	12				-	-	3
Animals raised in paddocks	1119	532	401	186	24	56	39				16	16	8
Total	1256	560	454	242	24	57	51				16	16	11

* Age in years

TABLE 2

POINT PREVALENCE (%) OF SEROLOGICALLY POSITIVE ANIMALS BY AGE AND STABLING TYPE IN HERDS 1 - 8 TWICE TESTED

		Age in years			Cumulative prevalence by stabling
		1 - 3	3 - 6	>6	
Animals in tied stalls	Autumn 1978	-	10.6	14.3	9.4
	Autumn 1979	-	1.9	21.4	9.5
Animals raised in paddocks	Autumn 1978	6.5	12.9	21.1	11.2
	Autumn 1979	4.5	4.7	1.0	10.6
Cumulative prevalence by age	Autumn 1978	6.2	12.5	20.2	11.0
	Autumn 1979	4.3	12.6	21.1	10.5

TABLE 3

PERCENTAGE INCIDENCES/YEAR OF SEROLOGICALLY POSITIVE ANIMALS BY AGE AND STABLING TYPE IN HERDS 1 - 8

	Age in years			Cumulative incidence by stabling
	1 - 3	3 - 6	>6	
Animals in tied stalls	-	-	8.3	2.5
Animals raised in paddocks	3.4	4.5	5.6	4.1
Cumulative incidence by age	3.2	3.8	6.2	3.9

TABLE 4

COMPARISON OF INCIDENCE RATES BETWEEN DIFFERENT TYPES OF STABLING IN HERDS 1 - 8

Stabling type		Frequencies of serologically positive animals +	-
Animals in tied stalls		3	118*
Animals raised in paddocks		40	930
Fisher's exact test (2 tailed)	P = 0.56		

* The frequencies refer to the animals at risk

TABLE 5

COMPARISON OF INCIDENCE RATES ACCORDING TO THE AGE OF THE ANIMALS IN HERDS 1 - 8

Groups of age		Frequencies of serologically positive animals +	-
a) 1 - 3		16	480*
b) 3 - 6		16	400
c) > 6		11	167
χ^2 test of differences between:			
	(a) and (b) = 0.107		
	(a) and (c) = 2.254		
	(b) and (c) = 1.073		

* The frequencies refer to the animals at risk

TABLE 6

PREVALENCE AND INCIDENCE RATES OF SEROLOGICALLY POSITIVE ANIMALS IN HERD 9

Date of herd test	8/76	8/77	8/78	2/79	8/79	2/80	8/80
No. of animals tested	257	234	286	274	287	278	282
No. of reactors	30	35	34	32	15	8	5
Prevalence rate (%)	11.7	15.0	11.9	11.7	5.2	2.9	1.8
No. of reactors eliminated	9	5	9	18	9	7	-
No. of new positives	-	14	4	7	1	2	4
Animal days at risk	-	80 300	83 037	45 716	46 994	49 640	50 279
One year percentage incidence rate	-	6.4	1.8	5.6	0.8	1.5	2.9

This decrease of prevalence occurred at an annual rate of 3.1%, which is statistically significant (Figure 1). The percentage incidence rates/year of new serologically positive animals in the six inter-test periods in herd 9 are reported in Table 6. Comparing these rates statistically, no significant difference can be noted. Table 7 shows the comparison of incidence rates in four inter-test seasonal periods. There is no statistically significant difference between the incidence rates found in the spring/summer periods and those which occurred in the autumn/ winter periods.

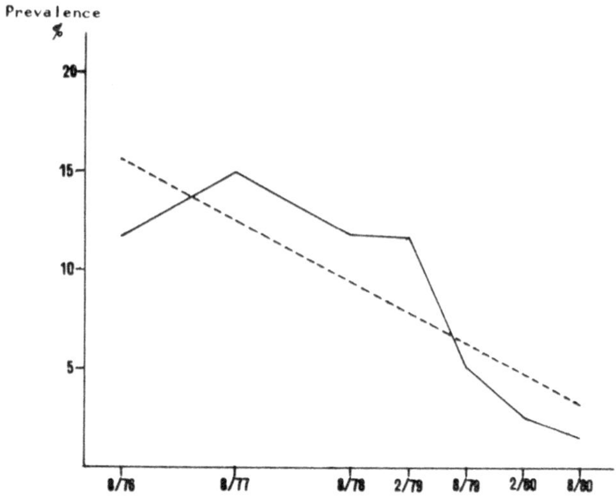

Fig. 1. Sequential point prevalences (%) of antibody positive animals in herd 9 (continuous line) and linear regression of prevalence rates (dotted line).

b = -3.1% t = 3.417 ($P < 0.05$)

TABLE 7

COMPARISON OF INCIDENCE RATES IN FOUR INTER-TEST PERIODS IN HERD 9

Inter-test period	Frequencies of serologically positive animals +	-
a) 8/78 to 2/79	7	243*
b) 2/79 to 8/79	1	256
c) 8/79 to 2/80	2	270
d) 2/80 to 8/80	4	271
Fisher's exact test (2 tailed) of differences between:		
Periods (a) and (b) P = 0.06		
Periods (a) and (d) P = 0.44		
Periods (b) and (c) P = 1.00		
Periods (c) and (d) P = 0.70		

* The frequencies refer to the animals at risk

CONCLUSIONS

The prevalence rates of serologically positive animals for BLV antibodies found in the 9 herds (11.0% - 11.7%) are moderately higher than those reported for the Holstein-Friesian breed (6.9%) in central and southern Italy (Rutili et al., 1980).

There was no substantial change in the prevalence rates in herds 1 - 8 in the two tests performed at an interval of one year. Similarly, significant differences were not observed for the prevalence rates regarding either the type of stabling or the age of the animals.

The cumulative percentage incidence/year of BLV antibody positive animals in herds 1 - 8 (3.9%) has to be considered in relation to the husbandry methods of the herds examined. In fact, it relates to closed herds in which, during the year, a certain number of animals is eliminated (sold or culled) as required by standard herd management.

The differences in the prevalence rates regarding the type of stabling and the age of the animals were not statistically significant. Nevertheless, it appears evident that there exists a higher incidence in adult animals as compared to the young. This leads us to believe that horizontal transmission may assume a predominant role in the spread of BLV infection.

Though the small size of the sample and the limited number of tests carried out do not enable us to attribute significance to the incidence rates found, these preliminary data seem to be interesting nevertheless in that they refer to herds in which a case of lymphosarcoma has never been reported and in which the introduction of new animals is practically non-existent. In such conditions, therefore, the incidence of BLV infection represents an important indication of the natural transmission of BLV among animals in a herd.

On the basis of these considerations it is clear that the normal management of a closed herd in itself leads to a rather low frequency of serologically positive animals for BLV.

This fact seems important because it demonstrates that the control of BLV infection in these types of herds may be carried out by resorting to control measures that are not excessively burdensome from an economic point of view. The results obtained in the investigation conducted in herd 9, in which no case of lymphosarcoma was reported, indicate that the initial prevalence rate found is comparable to that observed in the 8 preceding herds, that being roughly 11%.

This prevalence decreased at a yearly rate of 3.1% during the overall period of time we considered. This statistically significant decrease appears important, because the control measures applied against the spread of BLV infection were not drastic and were economically bearable, and because it must be considered in relation to the time that was necessary to reach very low prevalence rates. In fact, a prevalence of 1.8% was obtained after 4 years.

The incidence rates found in herd 9 in six inter-test periods are variable and there are no statistically significant differences among them. However, it is clear that from the beginning of the control programme until the last test, a noticeable decrease of the incidence rates occurred. We believe, therefore, that by limiting the possibility of the spread of BLV infection within the herd, with practical and relatively inexpensive control measures, positive results can be obtained in a long-term eradication programme.

Regarding the influence of seasonal factors on the spread of BLV infection, it was not possible to find any significant difference in the incidence rates observed in the various seasonal periods.

In all the seven tests carried out in herd 9, a total of 11 animals of 1 year of age were found to be BLV antibody positive. Bearing in mind that the calves born to infected dams had received colostrum from negative cows and that all the calves were housed separately from the adults until 1 year of age, this leads us to suppose that these positive animals either acquired the virus before birth or became infected by contact with other calves that were born infected. It can be noted, therefore, that - even if with a very low frequency - a prenatal transmission of BLV from infected cows to their foetuses occurred in herd 9. In fact, it has been demonstrated that this type of transmission can occur even if only in a limited percentage of cases (Ferrer, 1979). The role of vertical transmission (*in utero* or via milk) was also pointed out during our research on an experimental herd (Severini et al., 1980). We believe, therefore, that calves born to infected dams, besides taking colostrum from negative cows, should be tested in the first days of life and eventually eliminated if found positive.

On the basis of the data reported, although in a preliminary way, we can conclude that for the type of herds considered in our investigation, which constitute a standard representative sample of the Holstein-Friesian herds of our regions, it is more suitable to apply control measures for EBL rather than drastic eradication programmes.

ACKNOWLEDGEMENTS

The authors thank S. Buchetti and O. Cortona for their technical assistance.

REFERENCES

Ferrer, J.F., 1979. Bovine Leukosis: Natural Transmission and Principles of Control. J. Amer. Vet. Med. Ass. 175: 1281-1286.

Frenzel, B., Kaaden, O.R. and Mussgay, M., 1978. Untersuchung über die Häufigkeit und Verteilung von Antikörpen gegen ein Glykoproteinantigen des Rinderleukosevirus in leukoseverseuchten Bestanden. Dtsch. Tierärztliche Wschr. 85: 45-47.

House, C., House, J.A. and Glover, F.L., 1977. Antibodies to the Glycoprotein Antigen Bovine Leukemia Virus in the Cattle Population of five states. Cornell Vet. 67: 510-522.

Maas-Inderwiesen, F., Albrecht, A., Bause, I., Osmers, M. and Schmidt, F.W., 1978. Zum Einfluss der Leukosebekämpfung auf die Entwicklung der enzootischen Rinderleukose in Niedersachsen. Dtsch. Tierärztl. Wschr. 85: 309-313.

Mammerickx, M., Cormann, A., Burny, A., Dekegel, D. and Portetelle, D., 1978. Eradication of Enzootic Bovine Leukosis based on the detection of the disease by the gp immunodiffusion test. Ann. Rech. Vét. 9, 885-894.

Rutili, D., Severini, M., Rampichini, L. and Titoli, F., 1977. Haematological, Serological and Electron Microscopical Diagnosis of Bovine Leukemia. I - Preliminary Investigation on Some Herds of Umbria. Bovine Leucosis: Various Methods of Molecular Virology. Burny, Brussels, EUR 5685e, 171-176.

Rutili, D., Severini, M., Bertorotta, G. and Titoli, F., 1981. Large Scale Survey of Bovine Leukosis Virus Infection in Central and Southern Italy. Proceedings of the Fourth International Symposium on Bovine Leukosis, CEC, Bologna - Italy, 1980 (this publication).

Schwabe, C.W., Riemann, H.P. and Franti, C.E., 1977. Epidemiology in Veterinary Practice. Lea and Febiger, Philadelphia.

Severini, M., Rutili, D., Fruganti, G., Rampichini, L. and Cenci, G., 1981. Experimental Transmission of Enzootic Bovine Leukosis in Calves. Proceedings of the Fourth International Symposium on Bovine Leukosis, CEC, Bologna - Italy, 1980 (this publication).

Severini, M., Rutili, D., Titoli, F., Rampichini, L. and Vizzani, A., 1981. Development of Bovine Leukosis Virus Infection in Cattle of an Experimental Station. Proceedings of the Fourth International Symposium on Bovine Leukosis, CEC, Bologna - Italy, 1980. (this publication).

Straub, O.C., 1978. Preliminary Results of a New Sanitation Program for the Eradication of Enzootic Bovine Leukosis. Ann. Rech. Vét. 9, 895-898.

Van der Maaten, M.J. and Miller, J.M., 1979. Appraisal of Control Measures for Bovine Leukosis. J. Amer. Vet. Med. Ass. 175, 1287-1290.

Wilesmith, J.W., Straub, O.C. and Lorenz, R.J., 1980. Some Observations on the Epidemiology of Bovine Leukosis Virus Infection in a Large Dairy Herd. Res. Vet. Sci. 28, 10-16.

DISCUSSION

M.J. Van der Maaten *(USA)*

If I understood you correctly, in the first test you had 30 positive animals and you removed 9. On what basis did you choose these 9?

D. Rutili *(Italy)*

There was no real basis for it. We had to take account of the economic interests of the farmer in a voluntary situation.

J.C. Flensburg *(Denmark)*

And you think in this way you can keep the prevalence to a low level?

D. Rutili

Yes, I think so, on the basis of the herds we have examined. At the present time the economic factor is the primary one.

THE DEVELOPMENT OF ANTIBODIES TO BLV IN A LEUKOSIS CATTLE HERD

B. Hofírek
University of Veterinary Medicine, Department of Diagnostics, Therapy and Prophylaxis, Brno, Czechoslovakia

ABSTRACT

The development of antibodies to BLV in a leukotic herd containing 207 animals using the immunodiffusion test has been studied. The active antibodies, as a consequence of the infection, were demonstrated at the earliest age of 9 - 12 months. The transmission of passive colostral antibodies from infected mothers to calves, appearing in the calf serum shortly after colostrum intake but not lasting longer than 6 months, has also been demonstrated. The detection of precipitating antibodies in new-born calves, prior to colostrum intake, was infrequent (10%). Under defined conditions the decisive role of infected dams on leukosis incidence in their progeny has not been established. The experiments have shown that, under natural conditions, enzootic bovine leukosis is most often transmitted horizontally; the vertical (prenatal) transmission being also possible.

The results of the experiments show that the time course for antibody appearance and the development of persistent lymphocytosis in infected animals is influenced by genetic factors.

O.C. Straub (ed.), Fourth International Symposium on Bovine Leukosis

INTRODUCTION

Numerous epizootological studies have shown that enzootic bovine leukosis, once being brought into a herd, spreads and gradually afflicts growing numbers of animals. The introduction of serological methods into the diagnosis of enzootic leukosis in cattle has provided facilities for the investigation of leukosis development in herds of cattle. We have, therefore, focused our attention on antibody incidence in a leukotic herd, the goal being the elucidation of its dynamics under natural conditions. At the same time, we have attempted to contribute to the clarification of the vertical and horizontal transmissions of this serious disease.

MATERIALS AND METHODS

A herd of Danish Red cattle, with a long record of enzootic leukosis (22 years) during which the disease was not suppressed for experimental reasons, has been followed. The infestation of the original herd of dams was found to be 53.1% (detected by the immunodiffusion test) at the time of our experiment.

The following animal breeding and rearing method was used in the fore-mentioned herd: calves born from both positive and negative dams were left with their mothers for 10 - 14 days and fed naturally. They were then transferred to a calf-house and received milk substitutes. Having changed to herbivorous nutrition the calves were kept separately from their dams in a young cattle-rearing house. Heifers, selected for breeding, returned to a maternal herd and the remaining cattle were left for fattening. The stable layout is illustrated in Figure 1.

Antibodies were detected by the method of double radial diffusion using the commercial Pitman-Moore glycoprotein antigen. The detection was carried out repeatedly during 2 years on all cattle categories.

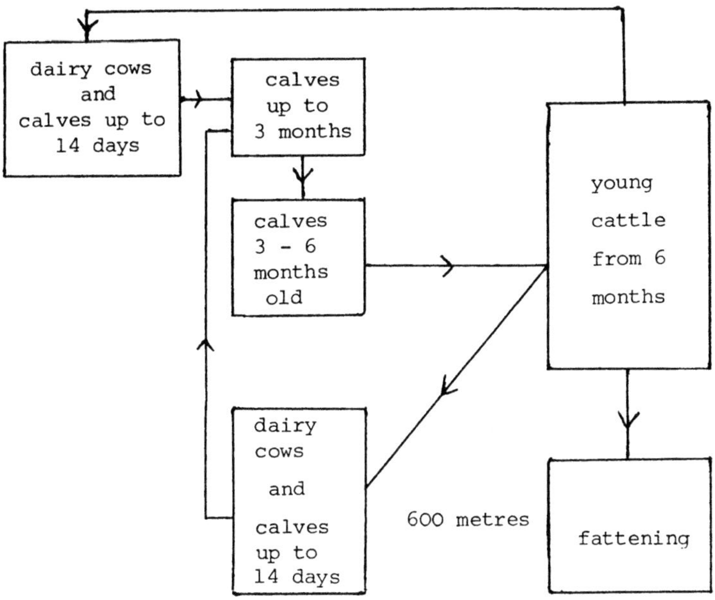

Fig. 1. The layout of the leukosis herd, showing the methods of animal transport during rearing.

In this experiment antibodies were also studied in a group of 14 cows (12 Bohemian Spotted and 2 Black Pied Lowland). These animals came from herds where enzootic leukosis did not appear, they were serologically negative and were placed in our leukosis herd in two separate experiments so that they only came into contact with calves and young cattle of this herd. The duration of contact was one year.

The scope of the examination has enabled us to follow not only the antibody incidence in dams but also in their progeny (daughters) of F_1 generation. The evaluation of the progeny of 51 dams with demonstrable antibodies, and of 38 dairy cows, in which precipitating antibodies were not detected, was possible. The influence of three bulls in the herd could also be evaluated from the material obtained, namely the antibody distribution in the progeny of F_1 generation of 3 Danish Red bulls (Dai 2, Dev 2 and Dom 3) serving both positive and negative mothers. The antibodies were detected and evaluated in progeny 2 - 3 years old.

The precipitating antibodies, detected by immunodiffusion as an expression of BLV infection, were followed in 207 cattle (calves prior to and post colostrum intake, young cattle and dairy cows).

RESULTS

Four variants of the course of antibodies to BLV were detected in calves (Figure 2).

The antibody distribution in young cattle and the maternal herd of dairy cows (Table 1) was followed in a later stage of our experiment. The relatively low antibody frequency in animals of younger age categories (0.5 - 3 years) was found. The percentage of animals with antibodies gradually increased with age, reaching 100% in cattle older than 7 years.

TABLE 1

DISTRIBUTION OF PRECIPITATING ANTIBODIES TO BLV GLYCOPROTEIN ANTIGEN IN ANIMALS FROM THE LEUKOSIS HERD IN RELATION TO THEIR AGE

Age, in years	Number of all animals	Animals with antibodies		Animals without antibodies	
		Number	%	Number	%
0.5 - 1	39	7	17.9	32	82.1
1 - 2	28	7	25.0	21	75.0
2 - 3	25	9	36.0	16	64.0
3 - 4	25	17	68.0	8	32.0
4 - 5	16	15	93.7	1	6.3
5 - 6	19	16	84.2	3	15.8
6 - 7	15	14	93.3	1	6.7
7 and more	8	8	100.0	0	0.0
Total	175	93	53.1	82	46.9

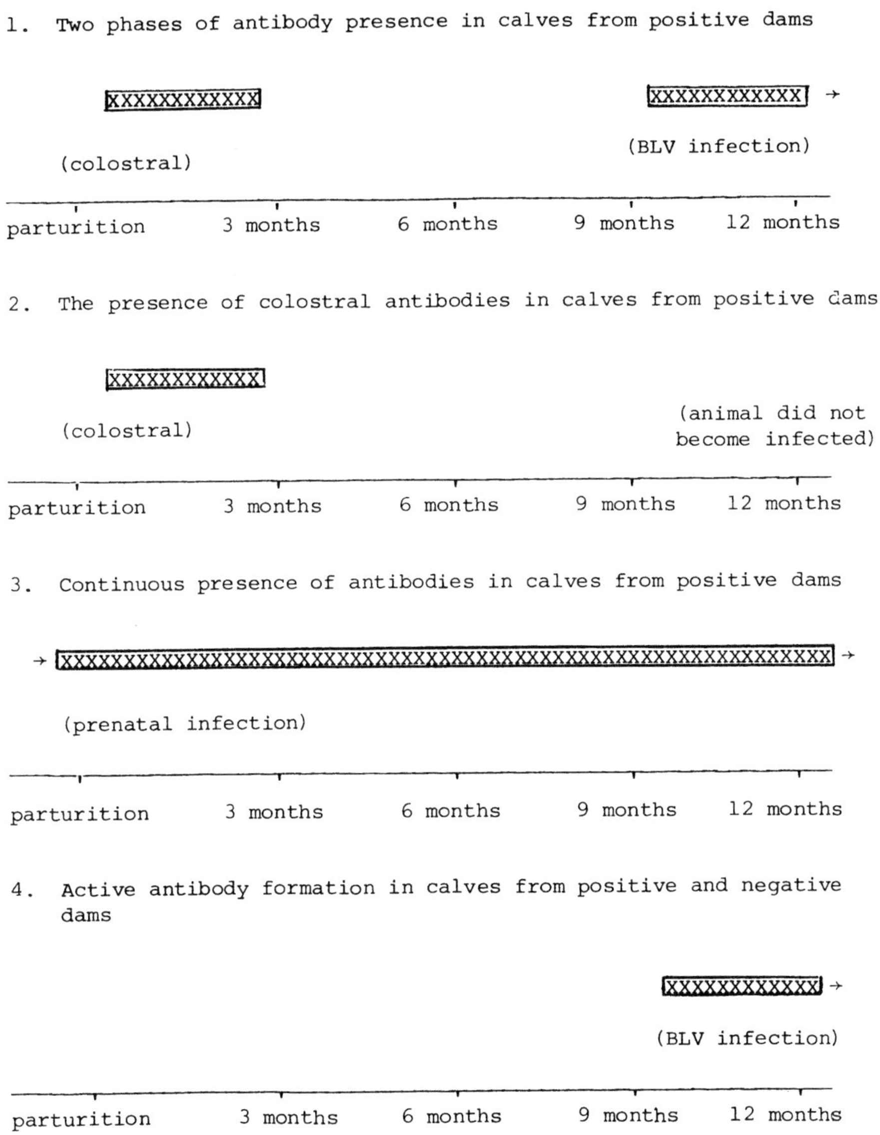

Fig. 2. Four variants of the course of antibodies to BLV in calves

XXXXXXXXX = seropositive phases

The distribution of precipitating antibodies to BLV-gp_{70} glycoprotein antigen in animals from the leukosis herd, in dependence on their age, is shown in Table 1.

When studying the enzootic bovine leukosis transmission from Danish Red breeds to healthy Bohemian Spotted and Black Pied Lowland breeds, the precipitating antibodies to BLV were demonstrated in two cases after contact for 12 months. The condition after one year's contact and the layout of the animals' locations are presented in Figure 3a and 3b, respectively

From the experiment conducted we have also evaluated the antibody incidence in progeny of F_1 generation from positive and negative dams. The findings are presented in Table 2 where the result of haematological examination (persistent lymphocytosis) is included for comparison.

TABLE 2

INCIDENCE OF PRECIPITATING ANTIBODIES TO BLV GLYCOPROTEIN ANTIGEN AND THE RESULT OF HAEMATOLOGICAL EXAMINATION IN THE PROGENY OF F_1 GENERATION OF POSITIVE AND NEGATIVE DAMS

Dams (n - 89)	Positive dams (n - 51)		Negative dams (n - 38)	
Progeny	Positive	Negative	Positive	Negative
F_1 generation (serologically)	35 (68%)	16 (32%)	25 (66%)	13 (34%)
F_1 generation (haematologically)	19 (38%)	32 (62%)	10 (26%)	28 (74%)

The performance of 3 bulls and the incidence of precipitating antibodies and of persistent lymphocytosis in their progeny of F_1 generation was similarly evaluated. The results are shown in Table 3.

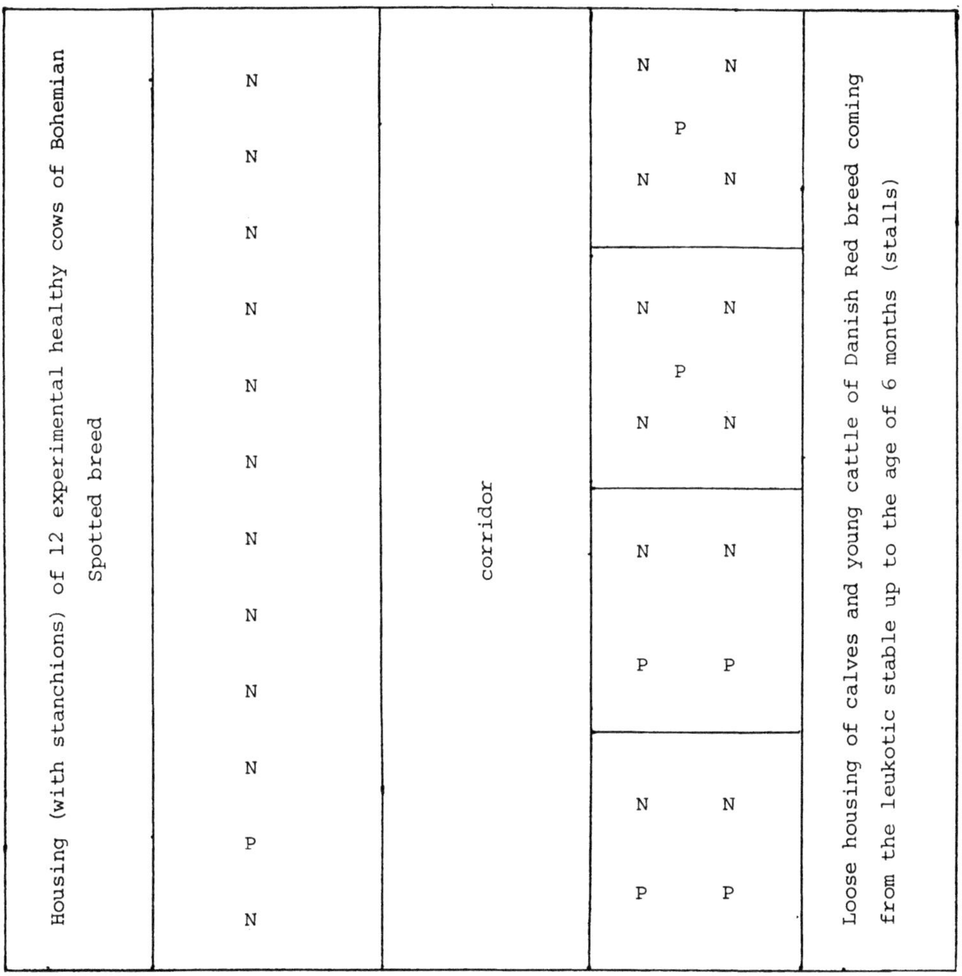

P - animals in which precipitating antibodies to BLV glycoprotein antigens were detected during one year of the experiment

N - animals in which precipitating antibodies were not detected

Fig. 3a. The study of horizontal transmission of enzootic bovine leukosis. Stable layout plan with the location of animals in which antibodies were detected when studies on leukosis transmission under natural conditions from young cattle of the Danish Red breed to dairy cows of Bohemian Spotted breed were carried out.

Housing (with stanchions) of 20 young cattle at the age of 6 - 18 months of Danish Red breeds from leukotic stable		corridor		Housing (with stanchions) of 18 young cattle at the age of 6 - 18 months of the Danish Red breed from a leukotic stable, and the lay-out plan of the lacation of two experimental healthy Black Pied Lowland cows
	N		N	
	N		N	
	N		N	
	N		N	
	N		N	
	N		N	
	N		N	
	N		N	
	N		N	
	N		N	
	P		N - exper.	
	P		P - exper.	
	P		N	
	N		N	
	N		N	
	N		N	
	N		N	
	N		P	
	P		N	
	N		N	

P - animals in which precipitating antibodies to glycoprotein antigen were detected during one year of the experiment

N - animals in which precipitating antibodies were not detected

Fig. 3b. The study of horizontal transmission of enzootic bovine leukosis. Stable layout plan with the location of animals in which antibodies were detected when studies on leukosis transmission in natural conditions from young cattle of the Danish Red breed to dairy cattle of the Black Pied Lowland breed were carried out.

TABLE 3

INCIDENCE OF PRECIPITATING ANTIBODIES TO BLV GLYCOPROTEIN ANTIGEN AND OF PERSISTENT LYMPHOCYTOSIS IN THE PROGENY OF F_1 GENERATION OF 3 BULLS

Bull Dev 2	Dams (n - 27)	Positive (n - 13)		Negative (n - 14)	
	Daughters	Positive	Negative	Positive	Negative
	F_1 generation (serologically)	9 (69%)	4 (31%)	10 (71%)	4 (29%)
	F_1 generation (haematologically)	3 (23%)	10 (77%)	2 (14%)	12 (86%)
Bull Dai 2	Dams (n - 37)	Positive (n - 27)		Negative (n - 10)	
	Daughters	Positive	Negative	Positive	Negative
	F_1 generation (serologically)	16 (59%)	11 (41%)	2 (20%)	8 (80%)
	F_1 generation (haematologically)	0 (0%)	27 (100%)	1 (10%)	9 (90%)
Bull Dom 3	Dams (n - 25)	Positive (n - 11)		Negative (n - 14)	
	Daughters	Positive	Negative	Positive	Negative
	F_1 generation (serologically)	10 (91%)	1 (9%)	13 (93%)	1 (7%)
	F_1 generation (haematologically)	4 (36%)	7 (64%)	3 (22%)	11 (78%)

DISCUSSION

Serological methods yield more objective results when compared with the haematological method, which dominated for several decades in the diagnosis of bovine enzootic leukosis and which did not facilitate an entirely objective study of the spread of infection in infected herds (Hoffrek and Hojovcová, 1976). The data we obtained from immunodiffusion studies prove this opinion.

When analysing the antibody incidence in the youngest age category of cattle in the infected herd (calves) by the previously defined method of calf rearing (Figure 1), 4 principal variants of antibody incidence were observed (Figure 2 - 1, 2, 3 and 4). Variant 1, and occasionally variant 2, is most frequently found in calves from positive dams. The cases where antibodies were detected immediately after calf birth prior to colostrum intake were rare (10%, variant 3). Prenatal infection was considered in these cases. Variant 4 was found to be most frequent in calves from negative dams. Virtually identical results can be found in works of other authors (Chander et al., 1978; Ferrer and Piper, 1978; Ferrer et al., 1976; Baumgartener and Olson, 1978; Straub, 1978), the differences in the antibody incidence in relation to calf age being caused by the character of the experiments and observations.

Later results have shown that the separation of young cattle from the infected maternal herd, or a very short stay (10 - 14 days) of calves with their dams, plus colostrum and milk intake, decreases the risk of infection. This is evident from data presented in Table 1 where, in the age categories from 0.5 to 2 years, when calves and young cattle were isolated from the maternal herd, the leukosis incidence remains relatively low (17.9 and 25%). However, it increases rapidly in the maternal herd of dairy cows, reaching 100% after 7 years of age. All these finding demonstrate the significance of horizontal transmission of enzootic bovine leukosis, the range of this transmission being dependent on the possibilities of contact infection, i.e. on the percentage of positive animals (possible infection transmitters) present in a stable. We must, therefore, consider the horizontal transmission as the primary source of enzootic bovine leukosis, this fact also being demonstrated by our further experiment with transmission from the Danish Red breed to Bohemian Spotted and Black Pied Lowland cattle (Figure 3).

We suppose, as does Bech-Nielsen et al. (1978), that blood sucking insects play a major role in the transmission of this infection. The influence of colostrum or milk intake can be considered as one of the pathways of enzootic bovine leukosis horizontal transmission but, as found by Ferrer and Piper (1978), the infection does not occur frequently. Passively acquired colostral antibodies seem to induce a remarkable resistance to BLV infection. This observation is supported by our results presented in Table 2. When comparing animals receiving colostrum or milk from leukotic dams with those receiving colostrum or milk from healthy dams under comparable conditions to our leukotic herd, the larger number of animals with antibodies was not detected. It is necessary, however, to point out that calves remained with their infected dams for only a short period (10 - 14 days), the intake of colostrum or milk being limited to this period only.

In agreement with Ferrer and Piper (1978), we conclude that calves are endangered by infection first of all through contact with infected dams or other infected dairy cows. Pre-natal infection, however, cannot be excluded, this fact being evidenced by the demonstration of antibodies in 10% of calves prior to colostrum intake in our experiment. This mode of transmission is, however, less frequent, which is in accordance with observations of other authors (Chander et al., 1978; Ferrer et al., 1976). Both possible modes of transmission have to be taken into consideration in sanitation programmes.

The role of genetic factors in the pathogenesis of enzootic bovine leukosis appears to be a very interesting and serious question. Ferrer et al. (1978) reported the significant role of these factors in the development of persistent lymphocytosis and possibly of lymphosarcoma. Our studies on this problem have shown that persistent lymphocytosis tends to occur more frequently in progeny whose mothers also suffered from persistent lymphocytosis (Table 2). These facts have been known for a long time (Verter and Gehrke, 1965) but were ascribed a different meaning.

It has been shown by our observations that in the development of persistent lymphocytosis even the genetic background of fathers can play a significant role (Table 3), possibly significantly influencing the percent of persistent lymphocytosis incidence. Our results have shown that no persistent lymphocytosis was observed in serologically positive daughters of the bull Dai 2, whereas in progeny of the bull Dom 3 the incidence of persistent lymphocytosis was relatively high (36%) when compared with the mean of the herd (15.3%). If we compare the bull Dai 2, in whose progeny no persistent lymphocytosis was found, with the remaining 2 bulls of the herd a new fact appears. This bull also had the lowest number of serologically positive daughters at the age of 2 - 3 years both from positive and negative dams. These facts lead to the conclusion that genetic factors can either facilitate or aggravate the incorporation of viral DNA into cell, or possibly its replication.

Taking into account the fact that a long period of contact with animals from a leukotic herd leads almost always to infection and to a serological response (demonstration of antibodies) then the influence of genetic factors is only temporarily effective. In practice this means that genetically predisposed animals in a leukotic herd develop persistent lymphocytosis sooner when compared with animals possessing genetically coded resistance. Nevertheless, we believe that genetic selection could also have a practical significance.

CONCLUSIONS

The development of antibodies to BLV in a leukotic herd containing 207 animals using the immunodiffusion method has been studied. The active antibodies, as a consequence of the infection, were demonstrated at the earliest age of 9 - 12 months. The transmission of passive colostral antibodies from infected mothers to calves, appearing in the calf serum shortly after colostrum intake, but not lasting longer than six months, has also been demonstrated. The detection of precipitating antibodies in newborn calves prior to colostrum intake was infrequent (10%). Under defined conditions the decisive role of infected dams on leukosis incidence in their progeny has not been established. The experiments have shown that under natural conditions, enzootic bovine leukosis is most often transmitted horizontally, the vertical (prenatal) transmission being also possible.

The results of the experiments show that the time course for antibody appearance and the development of persistent lymphocytosis in infected animals is influenced by genetic factors.

From the practical point of view of sanitation programmes concerning enzootic bovine leukosis, the results of our studies have shown the significance of individual serological diagnosis. The sanitation programme and the isolated rearing of calves and young cattle apart from the infected maternal herd can create preconditions for the successful eradication of this dangerous enzootic disease.

REFERENCES

Baumgartener, L.E. and Olson, C., 1978. Immunodiffusion antibodies to P_{24} and gp antigens in cattle. The serological diagnosis of enzootic bovine leukosis. (A.A. Ressang, ed.) Commission of the European Communities, Brussels-Luxembourg, 148-155.

Bech-Nielsen, S., Piper, C.E. and Ferrer, J.F., 1978. Natural mode of transmission of bovine leukemia virus: role of blood-sucking insects. Am. J. Vet. Res., 39: 1089-1092.

Chander, S., Samagh, B.S. and Greig, A.S., 1978. BLV-antibodies in serial sampling over five years in a bovine leukosis herd. Ann. Rech. Vét., 9: 797-802.

Ferrer, J.F., Piper, C.E., Abt, D.A., Marshak, R.R. and Bhatt, D.M., 1976. Natural mode of transmission of the bovine c-type virus (BLV). Bibliotheca Haemat., 43: 235-237.

Ferrer, J.F. and Piper, C.E., 1978. An evaluation of the role of milk in the natural transmission of BLV. Ann. Rech. Vét., 9: 803-807.

Ferrer, J.F., Marshak, R.R., Abt, D.A. and Kenyon, S.J., 1978. Persistent lymphocytosis in cattle: its cause, nature and relation to lymphosarcoma. Ann. Rech. Vét., 9: 851-857.

Hofírek, B. and Hojovcová, M., 1976. Diagnostics of enzootic bovine leukosis in South Moravian District. Brno. (not published)

Straub, O.C., 1978. Horizontal transmission studies on enzootic bovine leukosis. Ann. Rech. Vét., 9: 809-813.

Verter, W. and Gehrke, E., 1965. Die Ausbreitung der Leukose in Kuhfamilien. Mh. Vet. Med., 20: 533-537.

SESSION IX

Control and Eradication

Chairmen : M.J. Burridge and J.F. Ferrer

RESULTS AND OBSERVATIONS OF AN EBL ERADICATION PROGRAMME BASED ON AGIDT DIAGNOSIS AND CULLING OF REACTORS

F.-W. Schmidt
Tierärztliches Institut der Universität Göttingen,
Geiststr. 7, D-3400 Göttingen,
Federal Republic of Germany

ABSTRACT

Two hundred and nine EBL infected herds have been under observation for three and a half years. An eradication programme has been carried out within these herds by performing AGID tests on all animals more than six months of age, in half year sequences, and by the slaughter of reactors. Epidemiological data are presented, which show that eradication of EBL by this programme was successful in most of the infected herds.

O.C. Straub (ed.), Fourth International Symposium on Bovine Leukosis

INTRODUCTION

To combat Enzootic Bovine Leukosis (EBL) a programme has been introduced in the Federal Republic of Germany which is based on the methods given in the following scheme:

<u>Total cattle population</u>

serological test (AGIDT) of all animals above two years of age

Negative results: 'unsuspicious herd'
↓
serological tests (AGIDT) of all cattle more than 2 years of age every year

Positive results in one or more animals: 'Leukosis-infected herd'. Herd is closed etc.
↓
immediate slaughter of reactors
↓
retest of all animals more than 6 months of age
↓
immediate slaughter of reactors
↓
after 3 negative tests carried out at intervals of at least 4 months: herd sanitised

To evaluate the efficiency of this programme, 209 EBL infected herds have been under observation for three and a half years. Results are presented in Table 1, Figures 1 - 4, and described below.

RESULTS

In the first test, using AGIDT-p24, 8 467 cattle were tested in the 209 herds. In all herds reactors were found, giving a total of 7% positive and 3% 'doubtful' antibody carriers. After slaughter of these reactors, in the second test the reactor incidence was reduced to 2% positive and 2% 'doubtful', which were present only in 47% of the 209 herds. Fifty-three per cent showed no reactors.

Despite the slaughter of these reactors, the introduction of gp-antigen during the third AGID test again brought the number of reactors to 12% positive and 2% 'doubtful', which were present in again 89% of the 209 originally infected herds. This demonstrates again, that AGIDT-gp detects more BLV antibody carriers than AGIDT-p24.

TABLE 1

RESULTS OF ERADICATION PROGRAMME IN 209 EBL INFECTED HERDS

Test, at 6 month intervals	Antigen	% Herds with	without reactors	No. of cattle in % -	±	+	total
1	p 24	100		90	3	7	8 467
2	p 24	47	53	96	2	2	9 062
3		89	11	86	2	12	10 388
4		56	44	95	1	4	10 651
5	gp	37	63	97	0.5	2.5	10 157
6		20	80	99		1	10 716
7		7	93	99.7		0.3	11 217

Immediate slaughter of reactors found during the following herd tests led to a steady reduction, leaving 0.3% reactors in 7% of the 209 herds after the seventh test.

Figure 1 shows once again the decrease in the number of herds with reactors during the course of the combating programme.

Although the total decrease of incidence of infected herds is remarkable and demonstrates the effectivity of the combating programme, the question remains whether, once sanitised, herds can stay free or whether and how frequently 'reinfections' occur.

Taking 89% of the 209 herds (186 herds), which in the third herd test (the first gp test) again showed positive reactors, we followed the history of infection through the fourth to seventh test in respect of reinfections. The results are given in Figures 2 - 4.

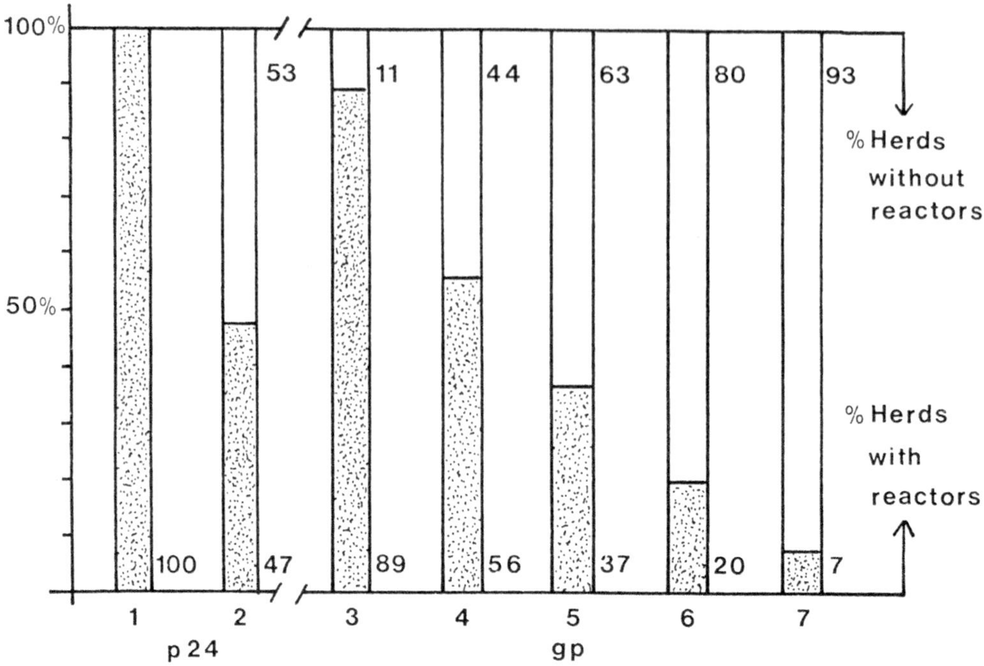

Fig. 1. Results of eradication programme in 209 herds

Dotted field: herds with new reactors
Free field: herds without new reactors

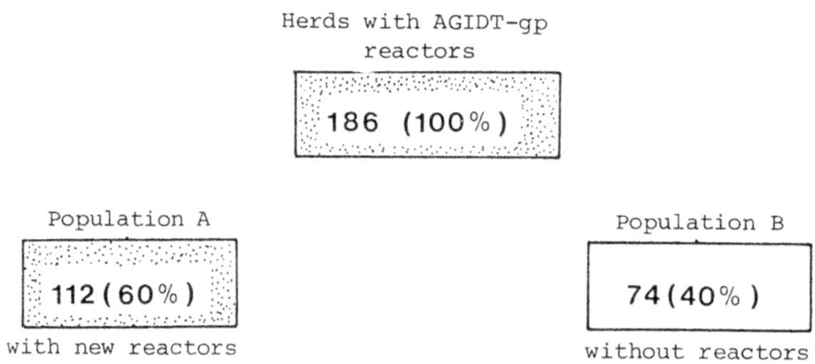

Fig. 2. History of EBL infection in 186 herds

Six AGIDT-gp in half-year sequences, slaughter of reactors

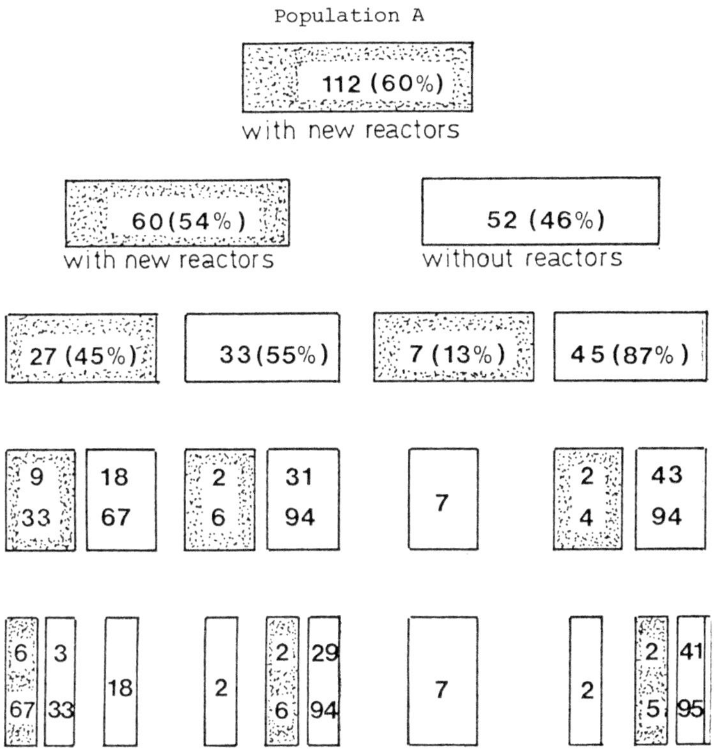

Fig. 3. Dotted field = herd with new reactors
Free field = herd without reactors

After AGIDT-gp reactors in the 186 herds were slaughtered, the following test 6 months later showed 112 (60%) herds once again with new reactors. These herds will be referred to as 'Population A'. On the other hand, 74 (40%) of the 186 herds remained free, and these will be referred to as 'Population B'.

When comparing the herds in 'Population A' with those in 'Population B', there were two marked differences. The average herd size of the reinfected herds in 'Population A' was 53 animals, whereas those herds in 'Population B' had an average of only 37 animals. Besides this, the average number of reactors at the first AGID-gp test was higher in herds of 'Population A' (7 reactors) than in 'Population B' (4 reactors).

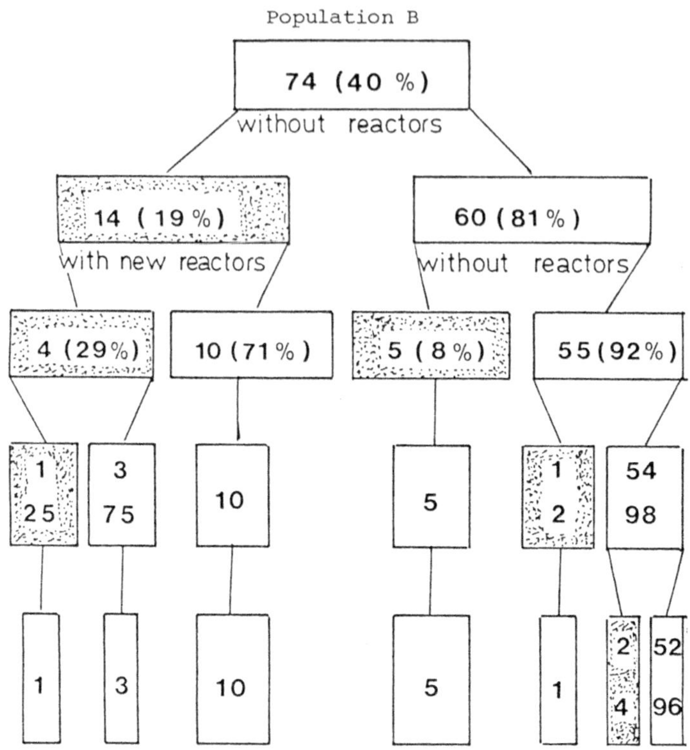

Fig. 4. Dotted field = herds with new reactors
Free field = herds without reactors

The development of sanitation in 'Population A' (112 herds with new reactors after the first AGID-gp test) is shown in Figure 3.

About 30 - 60% of the still positive herds showed new reactors in the following test, whereas from those herds which were once negative, about 80 - 95% stayed negative throughout.

The last test result showed 8 herds with reactors, originating from the positive herds in test 2, but only 2 herds with reactors were left originating from the sanitised herds in test 2.

Figure 4 demonstrates the development of sanitation in 'Population B' (74 herds sanitised after the first AGIDT-gp). Here reinfections occurred less seldom so that the last test showed only 2 herds left with new reactors. It is remarkable that these 2 herds originated from herds which did not show new reactors for 3 years after their first sanitation. Only one reactor was found in each of these 2 herds. The origin of the infection could not be traced.

A summary of the results reveals that after 3½ years of the combating programme as described above, 12 herds (6%) from a total of 209 EBL infected herds still showed BLV antibody carriers in AGIDT-gp. From these, 6 herds (3%) showed new reactors in each test which had been undetected in the previous test. Another 4 herds originated from those herds which showed no more reactors in the second test ('Population B').

CONCLUSIONS

It can be concluded that the combating programme, based on AGID tests and the slaughter of reactors, in combination with official veterinary regulations such as trade control etc., is effective, but takes some time (about 3 - 4 years under our conditions).

The slaughter of totally infected herds after the first serological test would perhaps have led to a faster elimination of EBL. However, since an economical comparison between the slaughter of single reactors on the one hand, and total herd slaughter on the other, showed the latter to be about 4 times as expensive (data to be published elsewhere), the combating programme described in this paper can be fully recommended for conditions found in Lower Saxony.

DISCUSSION

J.C. Flensburg *(Denmark)*

Your experiments are very important to us all and we shall look forward to seeing your results in the coming years. You were talking about reinfection in the herds where you had four clean tests and then reappearance. Have you any indication where this comes from? Is it, in fact, an old infection which has been going through the whole system, or have infective animals been introduced?

F.-W. Schmidt *(FRG)*

These herds are closed in that they cannot sell any animals for purposes other than slaughter. They can buy, but this did not happen with these particular herds. We don't know where these infections come from but it must be a case of an old infection, unless it is contact from the pastures and so on which seems unlikely. (For comparison see paper by Lorenz et al. in this issue).

J.F. Ferrer *(USA)*

How long after the animals are detected as positive are they removed from the herd?

F.-W. Schmidt

About two weeks later, as soon as possible in fact.

D.H. Roberts *(UK)*

I see that the tumour incidence has been reduced from 10 per 100 000 to 3 per 100 000. Looking at the costing side of it, it appears that the whole cost of the programme has only resulted in a saving of 5 or 6 cows per year. What other savings are there?

F.-W. Schmidt

I think this calculation is a little wrong. You cannot consider the tumour cases alone. There are other aspects of course, trading aspects. Also, I think we all agree that if you do not do anything with a heavily infected herd the tumour cases will just go on increasing.

(See introductory paper for additional explanations)

SEROLOGICAL EVIDENCE OF INFECTION WITH BOVINE LEUKAEMIA VIRUS (BLV) IN DANISH CATTLE: AN ACCOUNT OF THE ENZOOTIC BOVINE LEUKOSIS (EBL) CONTROL PROGRAMME 1979/80

J.C. Flensburg

Danish Veterinary Services,
Frederiksgade 21, DK-1265 Copenhagen K, Denmark.

ABSTRACT

A short description of the 3 Danish EBL control programmes 1959 - 68, 1969 - 78 and 1979 - 81 is given. During the 20 months from 1 January 1979 to 31 August 1980, altogether 22 herds have been found to contain serological (ID) reactors. At the routine monitoring 0.04% of the examined animals were found to be reactors and 0.45% of the examined herds contained reactors. Out of previously suspect herds 1.4% were found to contain reactors. Out of 98 herds with a leukotic tumour case one contained one reactor. In the 22 infected herds an average of 2.2% of the animals were reactors. Only 7 herds had 3 or more reactors. Nearly half of the infected herds were of the Jersey breed, while only 18% of the national herd is of that breed. A few reactors may apparently be present in a herd over a period of as much as 10 years without leukotic tumour cases and even without cases of persisting lymphocytosis occurring.

O.C. Straub (ed.), Fourth International Symposium on Bovine Leukosis

INTRODUCTION

The leukosis control programme in progress in Denmark at the moment is part of a programme begun in 1959. On 1 January 1979 the use of total lymphocyte counts as a diagnostic tool in leukosis work was abandoned completely. The purpose of this paper is to give an account of the findings since that date. It is necessary to summarise the programme from 1959 - 78 which preceded the present programme, and which was based on haematology and histology as diagnostic tools. Administratively it was based on the following assumptions:

1. Persisting lymphocytosis (lymphocytotic blood picture for more than 2 months) is an indication of leukosis.
2. More than one leukotic (persisting lymphocytosis or tumorous leukosis) animal in a herd is indicative of EBL.
3. A leukosis herd can only be made leukosis free by slaughter of the whole herd followed by the establishment of a new herd recruited from leukosis free herds.

MATERIALS AND METHODS

Programme 1959 - 68

Suspect tumours of bovines was a notifiable disease, and material from such cases, whether found at meat inspection or as clinical cases, had to be submitted for histological examination. When leukosis was established in an animal, an epidemiological examination was carried out including a haematological examination of all adult animals in the herd of origin and in-contact herds. Herd diagnosis and disease eradication was carried out according to the 3 assumptions mentioned above. Herds considered to be suffering from EBL were closed (animals could only leave the herd directly for slaughter with a movement permit) and a public subsidy, determined by the number and age group of the animals in the herd, was offered in order to induce the owner to slaughter the whole herd. Such a drastic herd slaughter policy was only possible because the overall prevalence of disease was low, and because, for other reasons, there was a rapid decline in the number of cattle herds anyway, particularly on the eastern islands where most of the disease was found. Under this programme altogether 603 herds considered to be suffering from EBL were identified.

Programme 1969 - 78

During the first period it became clear that a herd could be infected, and spread infection, for many years without a clinical case. Development of electronic cell counters made large numbers of white blood cell counts possible, and routine haematological herd tests of all herds in the country were initiated in 1969. The first countrywide haematological test was done during 1969 - 71, the second in 1972 - 74 and the third in 1975 - 78. During the third period investigations of serological methods developed during the early seventies were carried out. The main work was done with an immunodiffusion test. It became clear almost immediately that this was a very valuable diagnostic tool, the test was specific and considerably more sensitive than the haematological test, and it was hence used in connection with haematologic or histologic evidence of leukosis. Under this programme 468 EBL herds were identified. Together with the EBL herds identified during the previous programme this constitutes about 1% of the total number of herds during the period.

Programme 1978 - 81

The present programme is planned for the 3 year period 1979 - 81. As from 1 January 1979 the use of the haematological leukosis test was discontinued, and routine blood tests only carried out as an immunodiffusion test using a glycoprotein antigen. A routine herd test comprises all animals above the age of 24 months and calves up to 6 months of age (maternal antibodies). Special herd tests on suspect herds (i.e. in connection with finding an animal with leukotic tumours) comprises all animals irrespective of age. During the three year period all herds on the eastern islands (previous high incidence area) are to be examined by the routine test, and during the same time a special test will be performed on all herds in which one leukotic animal has been found since 1969. All herds delivering animals to AI stations and performance testing stations must have passed a routine test within the past 3 years.

RESULTS

The findings in connection with this programme are summarised in 3 tables:

Table 1 is a summary of the serological herd examinations during the 20 months from 1 January 1979 to 31 August 1980. 'A' is a summary of the routine herd monitoring in the former high incidence area (eastern islands). It shows that out of 2 665 herds examined (calves and adults) 12 herds were found to contain 28 reactors. Out of the examined animals 0.04% were reactors and out of the examined herds 0.45% contained reactors. 'B' shows that 6 herds containing 17 reactors were found by 'follow up' examinations of the 1978 routine haematological examinations and of herds in contact with the infected herds found in the present programme. 'C' is a summary of a special examination in the low incidence area (Jutland and Funen) of 216 herds previously under quarantine for 2 years due to the finding of one leukotic animal (haematology or histology). Three herds (1.4% of the examined) were found to contain altogether 10 reactors. 'D' shows that out of 98 herds examined because tumorous leukosis was found in them, only one herd contained 1 reactor (the tumorous animal). This summary shows that the incidence of reacting herds (0.45%) and reacting animals (0.04%) is very low even in the former high incidence areas. It also shows that the herds previously quarantined due to EBL suspicion in the low incidence area of Denmark constitute a higher risk, but even among such herds only 1.4% are found to contain reactors. Finally it shows that 97 out of 98 leukotic

TABLE 1

SUMMARY OF DANISH LEUKOSIS CONTROL PROGRAMME 1 JANUARY 1979 - 31 AUGUST 1980

	No. of herds examined	No. of reactors	No. of herds with reactors	% reactors	% herds with reactors	No. and % of reactors per reacting herd		Total no. of animals per reacting herd (range)
						No.	%	
A	2 665	28	12	0.04	0.45	2.3	1.7	140 (23 - 928)
B	-	17	6	-	-	2.8	3.1	90 (47 - 130)
C	216	10	3	-	1.4	3.3	3.3	102 (51 - 200)
D	98	1	1	-	1.0	1	16.7	6
Total		56	22			2.5	2.2	115

A Routine programme.

B Contagious contact herds.

C Special examinations of previously suspect herds outside 'routine area' (tumour or haematology).

D Examination of herds with leukotic tumours 1 January 1979 - 31 August 1980.

tumours found during the 20 month period are apparently unconnected to EBL infections. It is noticeable that nearly half of the 22 herds are Jersey herds, while only 18% of Danish cattle are of that breed.

Table 2 is a summary of the 105 leukotic tumours reported during the 20 month period. Ninety eight tumours were found in herds considered EBL free at 3 previous haematological herd examinations. On the basis of serological tests of all animals in the herd in which tumours were found, only one tumour case in an adult animal could be connected with EBL infection. Forty five tumours in animals > 24 months were apparently unconnected with EBL infection, similarly 42 tumours in animals < 24 months and 10 tumours of the skin type. Seven tumours in adult animals were found in about 40 herds under leukosis quarantine pending slaughter during the period.

TABLE 2

SUMMARY OF LEUKOTIC TUMOURS FOUND 1 JANUARY 1979 - 31 AUGUST 1980

Herd status	BLV tumours (serological herd test)	Sporadic leukotic tumours (serological herd test)		
		Juvenile leukosis	Skin leukosis	Sporadic adult form
EBL free	1	42	10	45
EBL infected	7	0	0	0

Table 3 is an account of epidemiological investigations in connection with finding 22 herds with reactors. The investigations are based on the District Veterinary Officer's routine report and on the records kept at the Veterinary Services head office. No special epidemiological investigations were carried out. Some interesting facts can be seen in this table: 8 out of the 22 herds have already been strongly suspect (2 years quarantine) during the time of haematology, and only 6 herds have no immediately recognisable epidemiological connection to EBL records. Only one case of tumorous leukosis has ever been recorded in all of the 22 herds. That is the one herd with one

TABLE 3

SUMMARY OF 22 NEW HERDS FOUND TO BE SUFFERING FROM EBL 1 JANUARY 1979 - 31 AUGUST 1980

Herds identified through	Routine programme 2 665 herds examined	Contagious contact herds	Special examination of 216 previously suspect herds outside 'routine area' (tumours or haematology)	Examination of 98 herds with leukotic tumours 1 Jan 1979 - 31 Aug 1980
No. of EBL herds identified	12	6	3	1
No. of herds previously suspect (haematology)	5	0	3	0
No. of herds with history of contagious contact	2	5	0	1
Tumour history (no. of herds/no. of tumours)	0	0	0	1/1
No. of herds with no previous contact	5	1	0	0

reactor (the tumorous animal) out of the 98 'tumour herds' (Tables 1 and 2).

CONCLUSIONS

Summarising the findings two striking facts stand out:

1. The very low number of reactors per reacting herd, on average 2.2% of the entire herd. Out of the 22 herds found, only 7 have 3 or more reactors (3 x 3, 1 x 5, 1 x 6, 2 x 8).
2. Outside the known leukosis herds it is very rare to find leukotic tumours connected with EBL.

These facts are, of course, due to the control programme carried out over the past 20 years, and including the 3 haematological tests of all herds. The result of that programme is the virtual eradication of EBL as a clinical disease and very near eradication of EBL infection as determined by the immunodiffusion test.

However, it is worrying to note the extremely insidious nature of this infection in some cases. It appears, when scrutinising the available herd histories, that several of the 22 herds with reactors have been infected with BLV for 10 years or more. The virus has been able to survive during those years without giving rise to clinical cases or to more than single cases of lymphocytosis at the three haematological tests carried out from 1969 to 1978. In most cases the serological herd test now reveals only one or very few reactors.

REFERENCES

Bendixen, H.J., Gaede, T., Geersbro, K., Gørtz. and Holmen, T., 1972. Den systematiske bekaempelse af kvaegets leukose i Danmark 1959-71. (The systematic control efforts in connection with bovine leukosis in Denmark 1959-71). Danske Dyrlaegeforen. Medlemsbl. 55, 900-911.

Broberg, B., Flensburg, J., Friis, N., Holmen, Ths., Hoff-Jørgensen, R. and Nørgaard, J., 1979. Bovin Enzootisk Leukose. En Oversigt over Kontrol- og Bekaempelsesforanstaltninger 1959-78. (Enzootic Bovine Leukosis. A Summary of Control and Eradication Measures 1959-78). Dansk Vet. Tidsskr., 62, 24, 1137-1142.

Flensburg, J.C. and Streyffert, B., 1977. The Control of Bovine Leukosis in Denmark. Epidemiologic and Diagnostic Aspects. Nord. Vet.-Med. 29, 49-67.

Hoff-Jørgensen, R., 1980. Determination of antibodies for Bovine Leukosis Virus by the ELISA technique. In: L.M. Markson (ed.) CEC Scientific Workshop on Bovine Leukosis. CEC Brussels-Luxembourg, EUR 6897 EN, 55-65.

DISCUSSION

G. Hugoson *(Sweden)*

I think we have a problem of definitions again here. In general, we have in our country only one case per herd. If we have one clinical case over a long period of time and we define it as sporadic leukosis, then most of the problem would disappear.

J.C. Flensburg *(Denmark)*

But nowadays you cannot define it as sporadic leukosis before you have tested each animal in the herd by serology and found that it is negative.

PROGRESS AND PROBLEMS IN THE ERADICATION OF EBL IN THE NETHERLANDS

G. de Vries
Veterinary Surgeon, National Animal Health Committee,
Bachmanstraat 48, The Hague, Netherlands.

ABSTRACT

At the beginning of the official eradication programme of Enzootic Bovine Leukosis (EBL) in May 1977 there were serological positive animals on about 50 farms. All these infected animals and their offspring were slaughtered immediately. Most of them had been imported but on several farms autochthonous cattle had also been infected by the horizontal route.

By 1979 the majority of the so-called 'infected' farms had already passed a two year period of herd examinations with negative results, and at that time only 17 farms were still under control.

In 1980 three large farms are still under control, since the risk of infection spreading on large farms is greater. Nevertheless, it is expected that these farms may also be considered free again by the beginning of 1981.

Due to a decision of the CEC in April 1980, the Netherlands were no longer authorised to demand a guarantee against EBL on all imported cattle. In consequence there is a possibility that very young animals have once more brought new infections into the country. Therefore, a constant screening system on the incidence of EBL is desirable for the future. From the beginning of 1981 every herd of cattle intended for slaughter will have to be identified individually. The examination of blood samples of slaughtered animals will be a good guard against the outbreak of new infections of EBL.

O.C. Straub (ed.), Fourth International Symposium on Bovine Leukosis

We can establish that EBL has never been a real problem in the Netherlands. When in 1970 the first cases were found in imported cattle, a period began in which every year three new cases were diagnosed. In May 1977, when we started the official eradication programme there were 17 herds considered to be infected from a total of about 130 000 farms. Most of the infected herds had only one or two seropositive animals and after these had been removed, it was possible for the most part to have a sequence of five negative examinations during a period of two years and then the herd could once again be declared free. Only in six herds did the infection expand and the herd have to be slaughtered. Some big herds with over 400 head of cattle gave a few problems but now, after three years of control, even these herds can be considered to be free of EBL.

In the beginning of 1980 only 6 herds were still under control but we expect that in the beginning of 1981 the periodical examinations for these herds can also be stopped.

Looking over the period from 1970 to 1980 it may be concluded that the EBL problem, as far as it existed, has been solved in our country. However, we still have to be careful. Due to our control system we obtained approval from the CEC to ask for a guarantee when cattle were imported from member countries. In 1979, about 3 200 head of cattle were imported. Although they had a certificate of examination and originated from a herd in which no case of leukosis had ever been diagnosed, 6 animals were found positive when examined on arrival.

It was very disappointing that in April of 1980 the CEC did not renew its approval for the EBL certificate. We may expect that, in the near future, more positive cases of EBL may be discovered in imported cattle, and since we know more about the real character of the disease, we shall not stop our efforts to keep our country free of new cases. However, all the tumour cases that are found in the slaughterhouses are traced back to the herd of origin. Fortunately in 1979 only 17 leukotic tumours were found in adult cows, on which the same number of herds was also examined, but no new EBL cases resulted.

In spite of its favourable situation, the Netherlands, as a cattle exporting country, cannot take risks and so we have made plans for a more intensive screening programme.

During the last few years a screening programme has already been carried out with the help of the blood samples taken for brucellosis control. Last year 75 000 samples were examined. However, these samples are mainly from herds that do not produce milk and, therefore, are not representative of the total cattle population of the country.

Since hardly any cases of tuberculosis are found during the yearly examinations, there are plans to stop the tuberculinations and to intensify the *post mortem* examinations of slaughtered cattle. From 1st January 1981 the control on the identification of every animal that is sent to the slaughterhouse will be intensified. As may already be known, every cow in the Netherlands is individually identified using a form on which the pattern of the hide is drawn and this also contains complete information about the herds to which the animal has belonged. The intensification programme will mean that the animal must be accompanied by the correct form before slaughter, otherwise it cannot be slaughterd, except under restricting conditions. The manpower required for this programme will facilitate collection of blood samples from slaughtered animals.

Since 30% of cattle from dairy farms are culled yearly, it is possible to get a good representative sample of the total cattle population. With the help of a computerised administration system it is also possible to centralise brucellosis and leukosis control in cattle. The centralisation of these routine examinations is necessary because the infection rates of the diseases are too low for it to be worthwile examining all the animals in every herd. By bringing in modern methods of automation we hope to build up a less expensive and more efficient and reliable system for the control of cattle diseases including EBL.

Nevertheless the final solution for the eradication of EBL can only be reached if all the EC countries will co-operate and begin an overall national programme. In my opinion it is not necessary, and not always even desirable, that a complete harmonisation be carried out, so long as every country uses the serological tests that have already proved effective in a manner that suits their own EBL situation.

DISCUSSION

A. Burny *(Belgium)*

How many times did you have to check large herds before you considered them to be free, was it more than twice?

G. de Vries *(Netherlands)*

Yes, after we find the first positive animal we repeat the examination every six weeks until we have a negative result for the whole herd. Then you need a sequence of five negative examinations. These herds needed more so far. The first year we tested the large herds nearly every six weeks, until we had negative herds. And now, for the last two years, these large herds have remained free during a sequence of five examinations.

A. Burny

And you used the immunodiffusion test?

G. de Vries

Yes, We do the normal routine tests in the laboratories of our animal health service but as soon as we discover a reaction that is not really negative, we send it over to Dr. Ressang and he does all the tests possible which are available.

F. Bürki *(Austria)*

How are the five negative tests spaced in time?

G. de Vries

At six monthly intervals, so it takes two years. Such programmes may not be right for every country but in the Netherlands we are anxious to export cattle and we hope that the costs of the programme will be offset by our exports.

J.C. Flensburg *(Denmark)*

You were talking about slaughterhouse monitoring by taking blood samples from your slaughter cattle. Have you any idea what percentage of the slaughtered animals you are going to take samples from?

G. de Vries

We will build it up gradually. We will start on 1st January 1981. Of course you cannot start with the whole system. I would be satisfied if in the first three months we control that we have the right form with the right animal. That will be enough trouble in the beginning. The controller will have plenty of time to take samples. Obviously, we have to be able to identify the animals from which we have taken samples, so we leave the left ear on the slaughtered animal and it has a tag on it. The number on the tag corresponds with the number on the form on which the details are recorded. The first thing we have to check for is tuberculosis but I would like to build in more checks because obviously we do not find more than the odd one or two cases of Tb in a year. So at the beginning of next year maybe we will take samples from 10 or 20%; it depends on how much time the controller has, and the more he gets into a routine, the more samples he will be able to collect. We also have a computer into which we feed the information.

EXPERIENCES GAINED AND PROGRESS ACHIEVED WITH BLV ELIMINATION FROM AUSTRIAN LIVESTOCK

F. Bürki
Institut für Virologie, Veterinärmedizinische Universität,
A-1030 Vienna, Austria.

ABSTRACT

At the 1978 symposium a concept for the nationwide detection and sanitation of bovine leukosis in Austrian cattle was presented, which had gone into action a year before and was to run for 2 additional years. It largely relied on ID testing with glycoprotein antigen which, in doubtful cases, was supplemented by immunofluorescence inhibition tests. The experiments made on large numbers of cattle sera have shown that this is a highly reliable and efficient procedure to detect infected herds as well as individual animals, permitting fast sanitation of infected herds, whose owners are willing to submit to our eradication programme.

Our screening was performed on 4 135 cattle, concentrating on the 6 oldest animals per herd and performed at low cost, because these sera were residual from Austria's brucellosis control programme done biannually. Seroreactors were detected in 7 out of 9 federal states (with Burgenland and Vienna exempted), and in all of the 5 Austrian cattle breeds, although in no place in high density. Among the 757 herds screened, 46 proved infected, harbouring 100 (2.4%) positive plus 8 (0.2%) doubtful animals.

In addition, in 37 herds all animals older than 6 months were subjected to a serotest, either because they contained (a) case(s) of lymphosarcomatosis and/or cattle with elevated leukocyte counts. Among these 522 animals screened serologically 12 (2.2%) positive and one (0.2%) doubtful reactors were detected.

As outlined in 1978, owners of BLV infected herds were invited to join our eradication programme, run on a voluntary basis under a three year project financed by the Ministry of Health and Environmental Protection. Essentially, this part of the project was adopted by the federal states of Salzburg, Lower Austria, Carinthia, and Vorarlberg.

O.C. Straub (ed.), Fourth International Symposium on Bovine Leukosis

All cattle over 6 months old from 32 co-operating herd owners have been serotested every half year, followed by the slaughtering of reactors with a small financial compensation. Of the 783 animals in this programme, with the 81 (10.3%) positive plus 11 (1.4%) doubtful animals in the first test, the percentage of infected animals has gradually receded to 3.6% in the second test and 2.5% in the third test. Eleven herds have achieved official freedom from BLV. The federal states of Salzburg and Lower Austria have achieved the best progress in our sanitation programme.

The herd owners who were unwilling to join our eradication programme may be divided in two groups. Those with 40 to 60% seroreactors, for whom the financial compensation available per capita was too weak an incentive to sanitise their herds. On the other hand, there were those with a very low incidence of BLV, who therefore judged BLV not important enough to eradicate it.

Having learnt through our screening that BLV did occur in some of their herds, the important cattle exporters among the federal states, later followed by the others, extended ID screening in 1979 to a total of 174 463 animals over 2 years old, among which 304 (0.17%) seroreactors were found. Some federal states have raised budgets to pay higher compensation for slaughtered seroreactors.

Consequently then, our original approach revealed the actual BLV infected herds fast and efficiently, by detecting 14.1 times more seroreactors on epidemiological parameters and 12.9 more on clinical parameters than undirected screening did.

Taken together, tests run on some 180 000 of Austria's 2.7 million cattle have shown a very low incidence of BLV. Efforts made and results achieved till now convincingly show that BLV can successfully be eradicated from individual herds. Nationwide eradication will be easy to achieve in a short time, if reactors are slaughtered earlier after the result of the serodiagnosis becomes known and if reluctant owners of BLV infected herds can be motivated to introduce an eradication programme.

INTRODUCTION

Following the detection of ID seroreactors with glycoprotein antigen of BLV (Miller et al.) in 1976 in Austria, we proposed a concept for nationwide detection and eradication of enzootic bovine leukosis from livestock (Bürki, 1978). It was, to start with, a screening programme on approximately 6 cows older than 4 years in each one of some 800 herds distributed all over the country and representing all breeds.

It was to be supplemented with ID testing of all animals over 6 months old in herds with (a) case(s) of lymphosarcomatosis or elevated leukocyte counts. Under a 3 year grant accredited to us by the Austrian Ministry of Health and Environmental Protection all herd owners of seroreactors were invited to submit on a voluntary basis to a test-and-slaughter programme, which should end with the official freedom from BLV infection of their entire herds.

Experiences gained and results achieved in this project should hopefully serve towards the future eradication of enzootic bovine leukosis from the entire Austrian livestock. Being traditionally one of the world's largest exporters of breeding cattle Austria should soon be able to attest official freedom from BLV infection, as it has for a long time from tuberculosis and brucellosis.

RESULTS ACHIEVED IN 2½ YEARS

Detection of BLV infected herds and animals

The screening performed on cattle over 4 years old was revealed as being highly efficient and inexpensive, being performed on residual sera left over from the national brucellosis control programme, which biannually covers half of Austria's cattle population. Efficiency of old animal testing soon became manifest in detecting actual BLV infected herds. With growing experience, it was also possible to qualify entire herds as free from BLV infection, at least under Austrian conditions, where in most herds line breeding is common (see discussion).

As evident from Table 1, ID screening according to our concept was performed on 4 135 cows from 757 larger herds from all over Austria (with only minor numbers from Tyrol and Styria). BLV dissemination proved to be very low with a total of 100 seroreactors (2.4%) plus 8 (0.2%) doubtful animals detected. They belonged to 46 herds which represented 6.1% of all herds screened. In these infected herds, however, BLV had spread to a remarkable extent among old livestock, manifested by 39.7% seropositive plus 3.2% doubtful cows.

TABLE 1

BLV RESULTS OF ID SCREENING OF '6 OLDEST ANIMALS' IN 757 LARGER HERDS

No. of animals tested	ID results		
	+	?	-
4 135	100	8	4 027
100%	2.4%	0.2%	97.4%

Additional informative ID testing was performed on 522 sera from 37 herds with (a) case(s) of lymphosarcomatosis or elevated leukocyte counts (Table 2). With 2.2% positive seroreactors and 0.2% doubtful, this approach showed a lower incidence of BLV infection because here all animals down to 6 months of age were serotested.

The summaries in Tables 1 and 2 revealed BLV seroreactors in 7 out of 9 Bundesländer (with Burgenland and Vienna exempted) and in all 5 Austrian cattle breeds, although nowhere in high density.

TABLE 2

BLV RESULTS OF ID TESTING OF 37 HERDS WITH CASES(S) OF LYMPHOSARCOMATOSIS OR ELEVATED LEUKOCYTE COUNTS

No. of animals tested (> 6 months)	ID results		
	+	?	-
522	12	1	539
100%	2.2%	0.2%	97.6%

Eradication of BLV infected cattle

Our own, the authorities', as well as cattle owners' confidence in the dependability of ID testing has been established by successfully retesting at intervals selected herds prior to starting the slaughtering of seroreactors. During this period, such animals were shown to remain seroreactors, and horizontal spread became manifest in additional seropositive younger livestock.

In consequence, herd owners submitting to the project had to slaughter their seroreactors within a 3 month period. By proceeding in this manner, BLV eradication in some herds was completed in a single step, this being proved by 2 entirely negative consecutive herd tests. In other herds, seroreactors were found in two consecutive herd tests, but thereafter BLV was stamped out. Lastly and rarely, a temporarily sanitised herd again showed a reactor among its young offspring and required further tests.

This latter observation prompts me to resume briefly the question, as to what extent a calf born to a seroreactor is likely to perpetuate BLV infection, although this question has been dealt with at former conferences. We made observations in one and the same herd, and specifically on two reactor cows, whose offspring we could follow up long enough, so that all possibilities could materialise:

- a calf may be born seropositive and remain positive,

- a calf may be born seropositive and turn negative,
- a calf may be seronegative for a limited time and then turn seropositive.

Our husbandry practices did not allow a calf to suckle its dam nor make physical contact with her later. As well, seropositive calves, kept amidst a large number of fellow calves, did not infect these others. This again raises the question of heredity of disposition to BLV, and prompts us to state that we should no longer encourage herd-owners, willing to eradicate BLV, to nurse calves of seroreactors with milk of negative foster-dams, but instead to fatten and slaughter such calves.

Table 3 summarises the gradual progress made within 2 years in 32 herds of BLV eradication based on the slaughter of ID reactors. These herds were recruited from the Bundesländer Salzburg, Carinthia, Lower Austria, and Vorarlberg. Starting with 783 head of cattle, these herds had an average of 24.5 animals over 6 months of age. To begin with, in their first serotest, they comprised 81 (10.3%) positive plus 11 (1.4%) doubtful animals. The fraction of incriminated animals then gradually diminished to 3.6% among 668 animals in the second test, and to 2.5% among 438 animals in the third test. The smaller total number of animals in the second test was mainly on account of actually smaller herds, as breeders waited for their own safe offspring to replace slaughtered reactors. The numbers of the third herd test declined due to the voluntary basis of our project: not all herds, whose sanitation had already become evident, were submitted to the additional final examination. This is statistically unfortunate because, had all herds completed investigation, we guess that in the third test there would have remained only about 1.5% reactors.

The voluntary campaign against BLV in Austria has displayed another drawback, evident from Table 4. This Table includes 22 tested herds whose owners were unwilling to eradicate BLV, primarily because of the low level of compensation offered in our project. Their herds averaged 40.6 cattle over

TABLE 3

BLV GRADUAL PROGRESS MADE WITH ERADICATION OF ID REACTORS FROM 32 HERDS, WHEN EXAMINED AT HALF YEAR INTERVALS

Bundesland (State)		ID results of individual animals 1st test n	%	2nd test n	%	3rd test n	%	4th test
Salzburg	+	51	11.8	10	2.5	10	3.2	0
	?	5	1.2	0	0	0	0	0
	-	378	87.0	398	97.5	301	96.8	14
	total	434		408		311		14
Carinthia	+	15	9.4	3	4.2	0		
	?	1	0.6	1	1.4	0		
	-	145	90.0	68	94.4	24		
	total	161		72		24		
Lower Austria	+	7	6.1	6	5.7	0		0
	?	4	3.5	0	0	0		0
	-	103	90.4	99	94.3	66		29
	total	114		105		66		29
Vorarlberg	+	8	10.8	4	4.8	1	2.7	
	?	1	1.4	0	0	0	0	
	-	65	87.8	79	95.2	36	97.3	
	total	74		83		37		
Total of table	+	81	10.3	23	3.4	11	2.5	0
	?	11	1.4	1	0.2	0	0	0
	-	691	88.3	644	96.4	427	97.5	43
	total	783[1]		668		438		43

1 Average herd numbers 24.5 animals over 6 months old.

TABLE 4

BLV ID REACTOR RATES OF 22 ENTIRELY TESTED HERDS WHOSE OWNERS WERE UNWILLING TO ERADICATE INFECTION

Bundesland (State)	ID results						total
	+		?		-		
	n	%	n	%	n	%	
Carinthia	147	35.3	4	1	265	63.7	416
Upper Austria	13	21.3	1	1.6	47	77.1	61
Tyrol	18	17.7	1	0.9	83	81.4	102
Salzburg	23	13.9	0	0	142	86.1	165
Styria	4	6.6	1	1.6	56	91.8	61
Vorarlberg	4	4.5	0	0	85	95.5	89
Total of table	....						894[1]

1 Average herd numbers 40.6 animals over 6 months old.

6 months of age, and, with reactors rates of 40 - 60% in extreme cases, averaged mostly higher infestation rates than in herds whose owners had decided for eradication. High cost and effort were not the only factors responsible for participation in our project; as the ciphers in Table 4 suggest, the owner's disinterest was also a major factor involved.

Other efforts for control of BLV in Austria

In the Bundesländer Tyrol and Salzburg, important cattle breeders had begun systematic leukocyte counts to remain competitive on international markets. This approach turned out, however, to be entirely unsatisfactory. Large numbers of herds and animals showed elevated leukocyte counts which the Coulter Counter was unable to recognise since apparently this is a physiological condition in mountain cattle. We claim a physiological elevation because negative ID testing in almost all cases ruled out BLV.

As a consequence, Tyrol and Salzburg, later to be followed by other Bundesländer, switched over to systematic ID screening instead of leukocyte counting. By linking the BLV survey with existing brucellosis serology, this will end within two years with ID tests performed on all Austrian cattle over 2 years old.

Table 5 contains data procured by Austria's State Laboratories in 1979 and kindly computed for this paper by Dr. G. Haunzwickl of the Austrian Ministry of Health and Environmental Protection. In 1979, 304 seroreactors were determined in this manner from the 174 463 animals tested, thus there were 0.17% seroreactors.

TABLE 5

BLV EXTENT OF SURVEY CONDUCTED AND PERCENTAGE OF ID REACTORS DETECTED BY STATE LABORATORIES IN 1979 IN 7 BUNDESLÄNDER OF AUSTRIA

Bundesland (State)	Number of animals > 2 years tested	ID reactors determined n	%
Carinthia	10 506	71	0.68
Lower Austria	17 405	15	0.09
Salzburg	8 975	45	0.50
Styria	26 068	65	0.25
Tyrol	9 261	4	0.04
Upper Austria	77 285	100	0.13
Vorarlberg	24 963	4	0.02
Total	174 463	304	0.17

Firstly, this confirms the extremely low infestation of Austrian livestock with BLV, which we have already pointed out at the 1978 Symposium (Bürki, 1978). Secondly, it reveals the effectiveness of our own approach to detect BLV revealing 14.1 times more reactors in our 'old-animal screening programme' (Table 1) and 12.9 times more reactors when taking lymphosarcomatosis or elevated leukocyte counts as guide-marks (Table 2).

The low reactor rates found have encouraged certain Bundesländer to raise financial compensation given for slaughtered seroreactors so as to speed up BLV eradication within their boundaries.

DISCUSSION

At the 1978 Symposium, Mammerickx et al. (1978) and Straub (1978) reported preliminary results of test-and-slaughter programmes performed on a few selected herds. Our data presented here very nearly approximate their data, showing that such an eradication policy is suitable for field application. Recently Forschner et al. (1979) indicated its suitability for sanitising hundreds of thousands of cattle, but put emphasis on standardisation and dependability of ID testing. So although there is no exactly parallel programme described, we still want to point out a few experiences pertinent to our work.

It turned out to be quite difficult to persuade authorities as well as cattle owners about the need to investigate and eradicate BLV, both conceptually and financially. Prior to 1976, no one had serologically or virologically worked on BLV in Austria, so our prime task was to convince people of its existence. The next step was to demonstrate the reliability and reproducibility of ID testing with glycoprotein antigen. Its great value was initially underestimated even by ourselves, taking into consideration efforts and reports in literature on other aetiologic test procedures. For some time we subjected sera with critical ID readings to immunofluorescence-inhibition tests (Ferrer et al., 1975), first using leukocyte-cultures of a donor cow, later Dr. Ressang's (1974) cocultivated FBL J 5 cell line as substrates.

With growing experience we realised that a carefully performed and read ID used alone is fully satisfactory for dependable detection and eradication of BLV, requiring no additional test procedure. As Table 3 shows, we started off with 1.4 to 3.5% of doubtful ID readings. These have dwindled down to practically zero in herds subjected to our project. We would of course judge an occasional single serum, with no herd background, as doubtful. But in project herds our readings may be conclusive.

This conclusiveness is based on our own experience gained in our follow-up controls as well as recent data in literature, ascertaining actual infection of doubtful ID reactors by ID post-testing (Forschner et al., 1979) or parallel ELISA testing (Behrens et al., 1979). Let me again point out what I recommended in 1978 (Bürki, 1978) that testing 3 diagnostical sera on a rosette with 6 peripheral basins allows far more accurate judging of weak results than by testing 4 (Commission of the European Communities, 1978). When summoned to perform controls on critical sera in our State Laboratories, which test 4 diagnostical sera per rosette, our decision-taking proved to be frankly superior.

Since such weak reactors, as Forschner et al. (1979) observed, apparently constitute the true shedders, their correct declaration as positive reactors will speed up and hence economise any eradication programme. To formulate it differently, simple as ID tests are to perform and read, scrutiny is a must and pays.

CONCLUSIONS

Our approach to detect and eradicate BLV on a nationwide scale has essentially proved to be effective and inexpensive. Primarily directed for positive findings, it turned out to be as informative regarding BLV exclusion, at least under Austrian conditions of husbandry, where closed herds with unsupervised breeding are common.

To the best of our knowledge we would have missed a single herd of some 30 000, tested by ourselves and State Laboratories, if we had restricted ID testing to cattle of 4 years or older. In this single herd, a 2 year old seroreactor had been introduced recently and has not yet spread BLV to his previously negative herd mates.

The drawbacks of our project (Bürki, 1978) are its voluntary status, its late removal of seroreactors and its small financial compensation paid for slaughtered animals. Comparison of Tables 3 and 4 clearly reveals that owners of smaller herds with fewer seroreactors were willing to join our project, while larger ones with higher infection rates refused to do so. So Austria, which might benefit from its exceedingly low infection rate, is unlikely to become the first country to eradicate BLV on a nationwide scale.

Fortunately, some Bundesländer, representing the principal export cattle producers, have recently become able to pay additional compensation. This should speed up overall eradication of BLV there.

In our 1978 presentation the question was raised on how long negative certificates should be valid, recommending 1 year for the entire herd and 6 weeks respectively for individual export or import certificates (Bürki, 1978). Although these periods will have to be agreed upon by state and interstate legislation, perhaps this forum of specialists could supply some pertinent information on this matter.

ACKNOWLEDGMENTS

We thank Dr. A.A. Ressang for kindly supplying us with his cocultured FBL J 5 cells, Dr. G. Haunzwickl for computing ID results state-wide for us, Dr. K. Möstl and Miss Eva Horvath for their excellent administrative and technical assistance.

REFERENCES

Behrens, F., Ziegelmaier, R., Toth, T., von Keyserlingk, M. and Forschner, E., 1979. Rinderleukose-Diagnostik: ELISA-ein neues Verfahren. Berl. Münch. Tierärztl. Wschr. 92, 429-432.

Bürki, F., 1978. A concept for nationwide detection and sanitation of bovine leukosis in Austrian cattle. Ann. Rech. Vét: 9, 909-913.

Commission of the European Communities, 1978. Summary record of the 2nd meeting for enzootic bovine leukosis. Brussels, 28 February, 1220/VI/78-E.

Ferrer, J.F., Piper, C.E., Abt, D.A., Marshak, R.R. and Bhatt, D.M., 1976. Natural mode of transmission of the bovine C type leukemia virus (BLV). Comparative Leukemia Research 1975, Bibl. Haemat. Nr. 43, 235-237 (Karger Basel).

Forschner, E., Ewald, P., von Keyserlingk-Eberius, M. and Seidler, M.J., 1979. Enzootische Rinderleukose: Der ID-Test und seine Standardisierung. Dtsch. Tierärztl. Wschr.: 86, 430-433.

Mammerickx, M., Cormann, A., Burny, A., Dekegel, D. and Portetelle, D., 1978. Eradication of enzootic bovine leukosis based on the detection of the disease by the GP immunodiffusion test. Ann. Rech. Vét., 9, 885-894.

Miller, J.M. and Van der Maaten, M.J., 1976. Serologic detection of bovine leukemia virus infection. Vet. Microbiol. 1, Straub O.C. (ed.) Elsevier Publishing Company Amsterdam and CEC, Luxembourg, 195-202.

Ressang, A.A., Mastenbroek, N., Quak, J., van Griensven, L.J.L.D., Calafat, J., Hilgers, J., Hageman, Ph., Souissi, T. and Sietske, S., 1974. Studies on bovine leukemia. I. Establishment of type C virus producing cell lines. Zbl. Vet. Med. B 21, 602-617.

DISCUSSION

B.S. Samagh *(Canada)*

When you speak of an eradication programme, it is not compulsory, so the owners of the animals can choose whether or not to become part of the programme. Is that right?

F. Bürki *(Austria)*

Yes, they have to sign a declaration that they will kill reactors within three months after the diagnosis becomes known. Unfortunately, the compensation they are paid is the lowest paid anywhere in Europe as far as I know. This is why they do not join the scheme. However, those who do join are then required to go through all the procedures until their herds are officially free which is the case after two entirely negative tests. We do not require five. However, for my own satisfaction this winter I will re-test the first twelve herds that have been classified as officially free. We are restricted in our country to taking samples only at certain times of the year because of the weather. In summer the herds are out on pasture and in the middle of winter they are often inaccessible because of heavy snow. So we have to take samples when the season dictates.

A.A. Ressang *(Netherlands)*

I agree entirely with Dr. Bürki when he says that the AGID test is a very simple test, very simple to perform, but that really it requires some training. The most important factor is the man who is doing it. Nevertheless, I always recommend a second test because these tests can complement each other.

Now, I have two questions: how do you handle your doubtful cases, and what exactly do you mean by 'lymphosarcoma'? Are you referring to EBL or to an animal with tumours?

F. Bürki

An animal with tumours, found at slaughter or, very occasionally, when skin or subcutaneous lymphnodes are enlarged, you see it clinically. But normally you find it at slaughter. There is no aetiology to it.

A.A. Ressang

I think we have some confusion over terminology; we should clarify our definitions of exactly what we mean by 'lymphosarcoma'. 'EBL' and so on.

F. Bürki

With regard to your first question, in doubtful cases we set up a second test; we dilute the reference serum while the diagnostic serum remains undiluted.

We dilute the serum 1 in 2 and 1 in 4 and we set it up with different concentrations of the reference serum. Then it may happen that we have here a faint line of identity which would not appear when you use the reference serum as it is supplied by the commercial houses.

We must be aware that by nature equivalence is the basis of precipitation and formerly, when it was done in tubes, any precipitation has been made in at least four dilutions. When the reaction is weak we dilute the reference serum. When the reaction is strong we dilute the diagnostic serum, 1 in 2, or even 1 in 5. 1 in 5 rarely gives us anything but it helps us to build up a diagnosis.

G.H. Theilen *(USA)*

In 1968 there was an international conference at the University of Pennsylvania. The proceedings of that conference were published in the Journal of the National Cancer Institute in 1968, and they contain clear definitions of terminology. I think it would be valuable to distribute this publication to members of this group.

M.J. Burridge *(USA)*

That article is: 'International Committee on Bovine Leukosis, Criteria for the determination of normal and leukotic state in cattle', published in the Journal of the National Cancer Institute, 1968, Vol. 41, p. 243.

R. Hoff-Jørgensen *(Denmark)*

May I go back to the discussion of ID test because, as you may know, we have decided on a common reference serum. That reference serum is going to be used to standardise the antigen so that the concentration of antigen is capable of taking off weak positives. Then, if you have the problem of very strong positives, you will see the shortening of the control line and you know you have to dilute.

F. Bürki

We buy the antigen from two commercial suppliers and we test every batch which arrives in concentrations 1 in 1, 1 in 2 and 1 in 4, the new batch with the old. Sometimes we make some corrections because it can happen that a very small dilution of the antigen gives us better results than if we use it as it is supplied.

C. Olson *(USA)*

You have two lines to judge rather than just one; it saves you repeating the whole test.

F. Bürki

Right, and since you have two guide lines to help you make a decision you feel much more certain than with one single one.

USE OF THE RADIOIMMUNOASSAY IN A PROGRAMME AIMED AT THE ERADICATION OF THE BOVINE LEUKAEMIA VIRUS (BLV) INFECTION FROM A HIGH-INCIDENCE HERD

J.F. Ferrer
School of Veterinary Medicine, University of Pennsylvania, New Bolton Center, Kennett Square, PA 19348, USA.

ABSTRACT

The present results indicate that BLV-free cattle can be accurately identified on the basis of negative results in two radioimmunoassays (RIAs) conducted at a 2 - 3 month interval after the age of 6 months, provided that in the interim exposure of BLV infected cattle is avoided or minimised.

Raising in isolation calves that were identified as BLV-free by this method has proven thus far to be an effective procedure for the eradication of BLV infection from a herd in which virtually all adult cattle are infected. On the other hand, this eradication programme would have failed if the agar gel immunodiffusion test had been used instead of the RIA for the initial identification of the BLV-free calves.

All 25 calves in this study were fed colostrum and milk from their infected dams. Therefore, the fact that all but one of these calves remained BLV-free for at least 2 - 2½ years, provides further evidence that milk-borne transmission of BLV is infrequent, if it occurs at all.

O.C. Straub (ed.), Fourth International Symposium on Bovine Leukosis

INTRODUCTION

The knowledge gained in recent years on the main mode of transmission of BLV and the development of reliable methods for the identification of BLV infected cattle have provided solid bases for the design of eradication and control programmes.

Studies at the University of Pennsylvania have shown that BLV is transmitted mainly by contact and that this probably occurs with the participation of insect vectors (Piper et al., 1975, 1979; Ferrer et al., 1976; Bech-Nielsen et al., 1978). Thus, it should be possible to eradicate BLV infection from a herd by either removing the infected animals or by isolating the non-infected cattle from the infected cattle. The second approach requires the implementation of measures to avoid transmission of the virus by vectors or fomites.

We have also shown that approximately 80% of the calves born to BLV infected dams are BLV negative at birth (Ferrer et al., 1976; Piper et al., 1979). Thus, in an eradication programme it should be possible to retain most of the calves born to infected dams.

The success and efficiency of an eradication programme depends largely on the sensitivity and reliability of the test used for the identification of the BLV-free cattle. The agar gel immunodiffusion test using a virion glycoprotein antigen (IDgp test) is probably the simplest and more popular procedure for the serological diagnosis of BLV infection. However, this test is considerably less sensitive than the radioimmunoassay (RIA), particularly for the detection of BLV infected cattle in early stages of infection (Lévy et al., 1977; Devare and Stephenson, 1977; Gupta and Ferrer, 1978).

This report describes the use of the RIA in a programme aimed at the eradication of BLV infection from a herd in which virtually all adult cattle are infected with BLV. From the results obtained thus far, it appears that complete eradication can be achieved by raising in isolation the calves that are negative in two RIAs conducted at 2 - 3 month intervals following the disappearance of the maternal antibodies.

MATERIALS AND METHODS

The BF herd

This is a dairy herd of Jersey cattle maintained at the University of Pennsylvania. To date, 76 histologically confirmed cases of lymphosarcoma have been observed in a population at risk of approximately 350 BG cattle. After 3 years of age all, or nearly all, the BF cattle are infected with BLV. In contrast, at birth and before the first colostral meal less than 20% of the BF calves are positive. In other words, more than 80% of the calves born to BLV infected BF cows are BLV negative at birth. Immediately after the ingestion of colostrum, all calves show passively-acquired maternal antibodies to BLV which disappear by the age of 6 months or earlier. As in most commercial herds, the BF calves are separated from the adult herd after weaning and kept separate until they reach puberty. The incidence of BLV infection increases only moderately until this age. Subsequently, however, after the BF heifers are returned to the herd and come in contact with the adult infected cows, the incidence of BLV infection increases rapidly so that by 3 years of age virtually all cattle are positive (Ferrer et al., 1976; Piper et al., 1979).

Serological tests

The RIA, using the virion gp antigen, was conducted as described by Devare and Stephenson (1977). The IDgp test was carried out in 0.7% noble special agar (Miller and Van der Maaten, 1977), using an antigen obtained by a procedure described in a previous publication (Gupta and Ferrer, 1978). This IDgp test is more sensitive than the IDgp test (Leukassay B) which is commercially available from Pitman-Moore, Inc. (Washington Crossing, NJ) (Ferrer, 1979).

Direct detection of BLV

The presence of BLV in blood leukocytes was examined by the competitive RIA (McDonald and Ferrer, 1976) and/or the syncytia infectivity assay (Ferrer and Diglio, 1976; Ferrer and Cabradilla, 1978). The preparations of the leukocyte extracts tested in the competitive RIA have been described (Kenyon et al., 1981).

Design

Since virtually all the cattle in the BF herd are BLV positive by the age of 3 years, the only possible approach for eradication in this herd is to identify the calves that are BLV-free and raise them in isolation. Since there is always a lag period of at least 3 weeks between infection and the development of detectable antibody titres, a single negative result even in the most sensitive serological test is not sufficient evidence to exclude BLV infection. Thus, repeated testing at 2 - 3 month intervals is always required. This is particularly true in the case of young cattle since in general these animals have a greater probability than adult cattle of being in early stages of infection.

After the ingestion of colostrum and until the age of 3 - 5 months, all calves born to BLV infected dams have passively acquired maternal antibodies against BLV (Ferrer et al., 1976; Piper et al., 1979; Ferrer and Piper, 1978). Thus, neither the RIA nor any other serological test can be applied to establish the diagnosis of BLV infection in this age period.

Obtaining a serum sample from a calf before the ingestion of colostrum is usually impractical. Therefore, in this study the testing procedure evaluated for the identification of BLV-free calves consisted of two series of RIAs at 2 - 3 month intervals, beginning at the age of 6 - 8 months.

Twenty-five calves that had been raised on colostrum and milk from their infected dams and gave negative results in these two series of RIAs were included. Ten of these calves were raised in a facility consisting of an open barn and an outside lounging area which was approximately 300 m away from the barns and pastures holding BLV infected cows. The personnel that attended this isolation facility had no contact with BLV infected animals. Vehicles, farm machinery, and utensils used in the barns holding the infected animals were not allowed in the isolation facility unless they were previously thoroughly cleaned and disinfected.

The remaining 15 calves were isolated under less stringent conditions in a similar facility that was only 50 m from the barn and pastures holding the BLV infected cows. These calves were attended by the herdsmen in charge of the infected herd. No precautions were taken to avoid the transportation of materials contaminated by excretions from infected cattle to this facility by personnel, farm machinery, utensils, etc.

All animals were tested at regular intervals (usually 2 - 3 months) for the presence of BLV antibodies, applying the RIA, as well as for the presence of BLV, applying the competitive RIA and/or the syncytia infectivity assay.

At the last evaluation the animals maintained in complete isolation were 23 - 25 months old; the animals raised in partial isolation were 25 - 29 months old.

RESULTS

The 25 calves that were negative in the RIA at 6 - 8 and 9 - 11 months of age had maternal antibodies against BLV during the first 3 - 5 months of life. Twenty-four of these calves were continuously negative for BLV until the age of 2½ years. At this age 90% or more of the non-isolated cattle in the BF herd were BLV positive. The remaining calf became positive at the age of 1½ years and was removed from the holding facility immediately after the RIA result was known. Since this calf belonged to the group raised in partial isolation, it is likely that it became infected horizontally after the initial testing procedure. On the other hand, the possibility should be considered that the calf became infected earlier and escaped detection by this procedure.

The original group of calves that were negative in the RIA at the age of 6 - 8 months and were maintained in partial isolation, included another calf that became positive in the RIA at 11 months of age. This calf was also removed immediately from the facility.

The RIA has been used to test precolostral serum samples from more than 40 BF calves that were negative in the RIA at the age of 6 - 8 months. All these precolostral samples were also negative. Thus, if in this eradication trial the calves had been classified initially as BLV-free on the basis of negative results in the RIA at birth before the ingestion of colostrum and at the age of 6 - 8 months, only one additional animal would have been found positive during the isolation period.

During the period in which the 25 calves included in this study were identified, there were in the herd several calves that were RIA positive at the age of 6 - 8 months. Five of these calves were negative in the IDgp test at this age and 2 - 3 months later. The presence of BLV was demonstrated in these 5 calves by the competitive RIA and/or the SIA. Therefore, it is evident that if the IDgp test had been used instead of the RIA for the initial identification of the BLV-free calves, 5 infected animals would have been introduced in the isolation facilities.

CONCLUSIONS

The present results show that BLV-free cattle can be accurately identified on the basis of negative results in two RIAs conducted at a 2 - 3 month interval after the age of 6 months, provided, of course, that during this interval exposure to BLV infected cattle is avoided or minimised.

Raising in isolation calves that were negative in the RIA at 6 - 8 and 9 - 11 months of age has proven thus far to be a highly effective procedure for the eradication of BLV infection from a herd in which virtually all adult cattle are infected.

In our experience all BF calves that were negative in the RIA at 6 - 8 months of age were also negative in the RIA before the ingestion of colostrum and only one became positive at the age of 9 - 11 months. Therefore, it appears that if in this eradication programme the calves had been selected initially on the basis of negative results in RIAs conducted in a precolostral serum sample and on a sample collected at the age of 6 - 8 months, only one additional animal would have been found positive during the period of observation. In contrast, the eradication programme would have failed if the initial classification of the calves had been made on the basis of two negative IDgp tests at a 2 - 3 month interval. Indeed, the data show that in this case 5 BLV infected calves would have been raised together with the isolated group of BLV-free calves. Most likely the infected calves would have spread the virus in this group.

The IDgp test has been used in eradication trials conducted by European workers (Bause et al., 1978; Mammerickx et al., 1978; Straub, 1978). In most of these trials, 3 or more series of tests performed over relatively long periods of time (often more than 1 year) were required to identify and remove all reactors. In one of three eradication trials conducted in the United States by Van der Maaten and Miller (1979), 27 IDgp negative cattle were segregated from the seropositive animals. When the seronegative group was retested 7 months later, 3 reactors were identified and removed. A third IDgp test conducted 5 months later revealed still another reactor. Thus, the removal of seropositive animals after repeated tests over one year has failed to eradicate BLV infection from the herd.

An even less satisfactory result was obtained in the attempt to eradicate BLV from the young animals in this herd. Of 8 IDgp negative heifers that were segregated from the seropositive animals, 6 reacted in the IDgp test 6 months later. In the second trial reported by Van der Maaten and Miller, 10 IDgp reactors were detected among 46 cows and removed immediately. When the remaining 36 cows and 2 recent additions were tested 4 months later, as many as 10 new reactors were identified. Although these reactors were also removed immediately, 2 months later another seropositive animal was identified. The conclusion that these trials were successful seems unwarranted. No evidence was reported to show that at the end of the trials the herds were indeed free of BLV. The last evaluation was made on the basis of a single test in which all the animals in the herd were negative. However, as it was mentioned earlier, a single negative result, even if the most sensitive test is used, is not sufficient evidence to exclude BLV infection.

The conditions under which the seropositive and seronegative cattle were separated could have been responsible for the relative inefficiency of these eradication trials. A more important factor was probably the limited sensitivity of the IDgp test. Indeed, this test fails to identify many infected animals that are positive in the RIA, particularly cattle in early stages of infection (Lévy et al., 1977; Devare and Stephenson, 1977; Gupta and Ferrer, 1978).

Clearly, the less sensitive the diagnostic test used, the longer it will take to identify and remove the infected animals that may continue to spread the virus in the herd, and the more expensive the eradication programme will be. The use of a sensitive and reliable test such as the RIA will, therefore, significantly shorten the time required to complete the eradication programme and reduce its cost.

All the calves in this study were raised on colostrum and milk from their infected dams. Therefore, the fact that only one of the 25 calves became BLV positive during the 2 - 2½ years of isolation extends previous evidence (Ferrer and Piper, 1978; Piper et al., 1979) suggesting that milk-borne transmission of BLV, if it occurs at all, is infrequent, or at least much less frequent than contact transmission. On the other hand, we have shown that BLV and/or BLV infected cells are present in the milk of most infected cows (Kenyon et al., 1981). The resistance of calves to milk-borne infection with BLV can be attributed mainly to the antiviral antibodies that all calves nursed on infected dams acquire through colostrum and have in their serum for at least 3 - 5 months (Ferrer et al., 1976; Ferrer and Piper, 1978; Piper et al., 1979). Most likely, these antibodies neutralise the virus and/or virus infected cells present in colostrum, and protect the calves against infection by milk and contact during the first months of life.

Heating at 56°C for 30 min completely destroys the infectivity of BLV without significantly affecting the activity of the virus neutralising antibodies (Diglio and Ferrer, 1976; Ferrer and Diglio, 1976). Therefore, the administration of heat-inactivated colostrum from BLV infected dams could be a safer and equally effective way of protecting calves against BLV infection during the first months of life.

The possibility should be considered that in some cattle infected prenatally or in early life, BLV remains in a covert state and becomes expressed only after the animals reach adulthood. Thus, for a final evaluation the present eradication trial will be continued until most cattle are at least 3 years old, an age at which virtually all BF cattle are BLV positive.

REFERENCES

Bause, I., Maas-Inderwiesen, H., Mitscherlich, E. et al., 1978. Results of an epidemiological survey of enzootic bovine leukosis in the northern part of Lower Saxony; based on serological diagnosis with agar gel immunodiffusion. Proc. of the Third International Conference on Bovine Leukosis, Paris, France, 1978. Ann. Rech. Vet., 9: 765-769.

Bech-Nielsen, S., Piper, C.E. and Ferrer, J.F., 1976. Natural mode of transmission of the bovine C-type virus (BLV). Proc. of the Seventh International Symposium of Comparative Leukemia Research. Copenhagen, Denmark, 1975. Bibl. Haematol., 43: 235-237.

Devare, S.C. and Stephenson, J.R., 1977. Radioimmunoassays for the major internal antigen (p24) and envelope glycoprotein (gp 51) of bovine leukemia virus. In: Ressang A.A. (Ed.), The serological diagnosis of enzootic bovine leukosis. CEC; directorate-general, Scientific and Technical Information and Information Management, Bâtiment Jean Monnet, Luxembourg, pp. 43-52.

Ferrer, J.F. and Piper, C.E., 1978. An evaluation of the role of milk in the natural transmission of the bovine leukemia virus. Ann. Rech. Vet., 9: 803-807.

Ferrer, J.F., Piper, C.E., Abt, D.A. et al., 1976. Natural mode of transmission of the bovine C-type virus (BLV). Proc. of the Seventh International Symposium of Comparative Leukemia Research, Copenhagen, Denmark, 1975. Bibl. Haematol., 43: 235-237.

Ferrer, J.F., 1979. Proc. Bovine Leukosis Symposium, College Park, Md., pp. 77-92.

Gupta, P. and Ferrer, J.F., 1978. A critical comparison of the virus neutralization, radioimmunoprecipitation and immunodiffusion tests for the serological diagnosis of BLV infection. Proc. of the third International Conference on Bovine Leukosis, Paris, France, 1978. Ann. Rech. Vet., 9: 683-688.

Kenyon, S.J., Gupta, P. and Ferrer, J.F., 1981. Presence of the bovine leukemia virus (BLV) in milk of naturally infected cattle. Proc. 4th International Symposium on Bovine Leukosis, Bologna, Italy, November 1980 (this publication).

Levy, D., Deshayes, L., Parodi, A.L. et al., 1977. Bovine leukemia virus specific antibodies among French cattle, II. Radioimmunoassay with the major structural protein (BLV p24) Int. J. Cancer, 20: 543-550.

Mammerickx, M., Cormann, A., Burny, A., Dekegel, D. and Portetelle, D., 1978. Eradication of enzootic bovine leukosis based on detection of the disease by the GP immunodiffusion test. Ann. Rech. Vét. 9, 885-894.

McDonald, H.D. and Ferrer, J.F., 1976. Detection, quantitation and characterization of the major internal antigen of the bovine leukemia virus by radioimmunoassay. J. Natl. Cancer Inst., 57: 875-882.

Miller, J.M. and Van der Maaten, M.J., 1977. Use of glycoprotein antigen in the immunodiffusion test for bovine leukemia virus antibodies. Eur. J. Cancer., 13: 1369-1375.

Piper, C.D., Abt., D.A., Ferrer, J.F. et al., 1975. Seroepidemiological evidence of the horizontal transmission of the bovine C-type virus. Cancer Res., 35: 2714-2716.

Piper, C.E., Ferrer, J.F., Abt., D.A. et al., 1979. Prenatal and postnatal transmission of the bovine leukemia virus. J. Natl. Cancer Inst., 62: 165-168.

Straub, O.C., 1978. Preliminary results of a new sanitation programme for the eradication of enzootic bovine leukosis. Ann. Rech. Vét. 9, 895-898.

DISCUSSION

D.H. Roberts *(UK)*

Suppose a farmer accidentally fed a calf with colostrum with antibody to BLV, which might contain the virus BLV, at what age would you consider it would up safe if you still had a negative test, with any test used?

J.F. Ferrer *(USA)*

In our experiment, if the calves were fed colostrum and milk from a BLV infected dam, and were negative according to radioimmunoassay at six and eight to twelve months of age, only one of them converted to positive up to the age of 24 to 28 months. I don't know if this answers your question.

D.H. Roberts

So at what age would you add a calf to an EBL free herd, using your system of testing?

J.F. Ferrer

At one and a half years. I would add that a safer way to protect the calves from infection would be to give them colostrum from BLV infected dams which has been heat inactivated. If you heat inactivate, you will destroy the infectivity of the virus but you will not destroy the virus neutralising antibodies.

D.H. Roberts

Yes, but it is better not to buy from an infected herd at all, if you have the choice.

J.F. Ferrer

But then the calf is not protected. It does not have antibodies.

SESSION X

1. Prophylaxis
2. Pathology, Histology, Ultrahistology
3. Miscellaneous

Chairmen : A.L. Parodi and G. Vacirca

VACCINATION AGAINST BOVINE LEUKAEMIA VIRUS INFECTION

G.H. Theilen[1], Janice M. Miller[4], Joanne Higgins[1], R.N. Ruppanner[2] and W. Garrett[3]

[1]Department of Surgery, Section of Clinical Oncology

[2]Department of Epidemiology and Preventive Medicine

[3]Department of Animal Science

School of Veterinary Medicine, University of California, Davis, CA 95616, USA

[4]USDA, APHIS National Veterinary Service Laboratory, Ames, Iowa 50010, USA.

ABSTRACT

Bovine leukaemia virus (BLV) is widespread in many countries, especially in the United States. Test and slaughter programmes have proved successful in some countries but would be very costly if not economically prohibitive in countries with widespread BLV infection rates. In countries where BLV is widespread, vaccination would be more economical. This is a report of a study using non-viral immunogens as a vaccine source.

BL-3 lymphoid cell suspension culture was initiated from tissue of a 4 month old calf with lymphosarcoma and used as source of vaccine. BL-3 cells were harvested fresh by centrifugation at 1 200 RPM, washed 3 times in phosphate buffered saline (PBS) and then resuspended in 2.0 ml of PBS at a concentration of 1 x 10^7 cells. Cattle were vaccinated once with BL-3 cells alone and twice with 10% suspension of aluminium hydroxide adjuvant pH 7.2. To test immunogenicity 12 6 month old calves were divided into three groups. Five were vaccinated and challenged with BLV, 3 were vaccinated and not challenged with BLV but left in contact with other cattle, 4 were not vaccinated (controls) and challenged with BLV. BLV status of pre- and post-vaccination and post-challenged cattle was determined by syncytial assay for virus infection and antibody responses were determined by immuno-diffusion test for glycoprotein and radioimmune assay for p24 BLV protein.

Technical Assistance of Mr. Doug DeBoer and Dr. Stephen Paul is greatly appreciated.

O.C. Straub (ed.), Fourth International Symposium on Bovine Leukosis

Of the 4 vaccinated cattle negative for BLV before vaccination none developed BLV infection on challenge with 2.5 x 10^5 BLV infected lymphocytes. Two of the 3 non-vaccinated cattle negative before BLV challenge became infected following change. Three cattle vaccinated and not challenged with BLV but in contact with other cattle remained negative for BLV infection.

This vaccination trial indicates there is a protective component in BL-3 cells that prevents BLV infection. BL-3 cells used as an immunogen has the advantage over other BLV vaccines by not inducing BLV antibody in vaccinated cattle thereby making it easy to determine whether BLV infection has occurred.

INTRODUCTION

Neoplasms of the haemolymphatic system comprise a complex of diseases that have been described in most animal species and man. Cell types are categorised as primitive, non-lymphoid mononuclear, mixed mononuclear, lymphocytic, myelopoietic and miscellaneous types (Rappaport, 1966). Pathologic grading of malignant lymphomas is determined by degree of differentiation of cells and diffuseness or nodularity of the malignant process. Immunologic classification considers whether the cells are B, T or null cells (Lukes and Collins, 1974). Bovine leukaemia (Leukosis) almost always arises from lymphoid cells and the resulting leukaemia is lymphatic and the solid tumour phase is a lymphosarcoma also referred to as leukosis (Theilen and Madewell, 1979). Cell types may be primitive, mature or a mixture, and organ involvement may be nodular or diffuse. Immunologically the malignant cells may arise from either B or T cells but most frequent origin is from B cells (Garcia de Lima and Mitscherlich, 1973). In one report, the 'calf' form had an absence of both B and T cells (Takashima et al., 1977). The most consistent karyotype is either 57, 58, 59 or 63 - 65 chromosomes but no constant pattern exists between individuals, although within the same animal, chromosomal patterns remain the same, indicating a possible unifocal origin of neoplasia (Hare et al., 1967).

On the basis of seroepidemiology and transmission experiments the causal agent of bovine leukaemia is established as a RNA virus belonging to the retroviridae family (Van der Maaten, 1979). The bovine leukaemia virus (BLV) is widespread in many countries. It infrequently causes tumours in infected cattle but readily produces neoplasms within 9 to 18 month incubation period in experimentally inoculated sheep (Olson et al., 1972).

Because of the great economic loss to cattlemen from the tumorous phase (lymphosarcoma), various nations in the European Economic Community (EEC) have established a 'test and slaughter' programme to eradicate enzootic bovine leukosis (EBL). Purchase of cattle or semen from infected herds is prohibited by law in EC countries having official control programmes, which has been a great monetary loss for United States cattlemen. Test and slaughter is costly, for instance in 1978 the British Government spent about 4½ million dollars in testing for BLV infection and then paying an indemnity for 455 slaughtered cattle (editorial in Vet. Rec., 1979). The British government is attempting to keep EBL from spreading because it may have only recently been introduced into the British Isles. In many countries, such as the United States, EBL is widespread and endemic in many herds, making a test and slaughter programme so costly that its economic impact would be prohibitive for control of EBL.

It seems a more efficient way, in countries with widespread infection, to prevent spread of EBL through use of effective vaccines. Effective vaccines should also protect cattle or sheep against subsequent development of tumours. This is a report of a vaccination trial using whole live transformed lymphoid cells (BL-3) grown in suspension culture. The BL-3 cells are non-BLV 'producers'.

MATERIALS AND METHODS

Cell culture

Source of vaccine was BL-3 lymphoid suspension cultures established at the University of California (Kniazeff et al., 1968). The BL-3 line was derived from bone marrow and thymus cells obtained from a 4 month old Hereford male with the 'calf' form of lymphosarcoma according to techniques previously published (Theilen et al., 1968). BL-3 cells grow well in suspension in either Eagles minimum essential medium, Leibovitz L-15 medium, or RPMI 1640. Cells are passaged by 1 to 2 or 1 to 3 splitting and transferred to new flasks or roller bottles every 2 to 3 days in a concentration approximately 1 x 10^6 cells/ml. Cell concentrations above 5 x 10^6 are undesirable for maximum growth. Long term storage is accomplished in 10%

dimethylsulfoxide containing 15% foetal calf serum at a cell concentration of about 1 x 10^7 cells/ml. Morphologically the BL-3 line is a typical lymphoid cell culture similar in appearance to BL-1 and BL-2 lymphoid cell cultures (Theilen et al., 1968). It contains cells with a hypodiploid (54 - 59) karyotype and a second population of cells with normal diploid chromosomal number of 60. All cells contain male XY chromosomes and are of B cell origin (Paul et al., 1980). Injected into nude mice, BL-3 will induce lymphosarcoma (Irvin et al., 1975). Using the syncytial assay (SYN) for detection of BLV infection and radioimmune assay for p24 antibody, the BL-3 cell line was determined to be a non-virus 'producer'.

Animals

Twelve six month old Hereford crossbred beef cattle were selected from a group of 87 for vaccination trial. All cattle were on a nutrition feeding experiment being conducted concomitantly at the University of California at Davis. Housing was in outdoor pens and those selected for the vaccination trial were divided into 3 groups being located in 4 different pens. Four to 6 other animals not in the vaccination trial were in direct physical contact with the study group animals. Those in group I were vaccinated and challenged with BLV (Nos. 808, 818, 832, 836 and 878). Those in group II were vaccinated and not challenged with BLV (Nos. 814, 823 and 860). Those in group III were not vaccinated and challenged with BLV (Nos. 822, 834, 342 and 868).

Preparation of vaccine

Cattle were vaccinated at 2 week intervals for 3 times by dividing the vaccine dosage 1 : 1 and injecting 1 ml subcutaneously and 1 ml intramuscularly. BL-3 cells were harvested by centrifugation at 1 200, RPM washed 3 times in phosphate buffered saline (PBS), and then resuspended in 2.0 ml of PBS at a concentration of 1 x 10^7 cells as a vaccination dosage. The cells used for vaccination were held at 4°C until used within 1 to 3 hours. Vaccine used the second and third times contained

0.2 ml of Alhydrogel (aluminium hydroxide) adjuvant pH 7.2 in addition to the same amount of BL-3 cells suspended in PBS.

Vaccination trial

Two serological tests were used to evaluate pre- and post-vaccination and post-BLV challenge for antibody response to the BLV antigen. The agar gel immunodiffusion (AGID) test for antibody to BLV glycoprotein antigen and the radioimmunoassay (RIA) for antibody to p24 antigen have been reported previously (Miller and Van der Maaten, 1977; Devare et al., 1977). Vaccinates and controls were also tested for pre-vaccination, post-vaccination, and post-BLV challenge for BLV infection using the syncytium assay (SYN) reported elsewhere (Ferrer and Diglio, 1976).

Evaluation for antibody and BLV infection was determined at 2 to 3 week intervals twice before vaccination, 3 times before BLV challenge and 4 times after BLV challenge. Group I (vaccinated cattle) and Group III (control cattle) were challenged with 2.5×10^5 peripheral blood lymphocytes from a persistently infected animal. The lymphocytes were isolated from blood by Ficoll-hypaque flotation (Muscoplat et al., 1974).

RESULTS

The vaccination results summarised in Table 1 demonstrated that BLV pre-vaccination infection and antibody against p24 and glycoprotein was present in 2 animals, 832 in Group I and 842 in Group III. The other cattle were negative at time of vaccination. The pre-vaccination positive animals remained persistently infected throughout the 18 weeks of the vaccination trial. The other 10 animals were negative on all tests before vaccination. At 16 weeks post-vaccination and 9 weeks after BLV challenge no vaccinated animals (Groups I and II) negative at time of vaccination were positive for BLV infection nor did they have an antibody response although 2 of 3 unvaccinated negative animals (834 and 868) became positive 5 weeks after

TABLE 1

PRESENCE OF ANTIBODY AND BLV INFECTION IN VACCINATION TRIAL CATTLE BEFORE AND AFTER VACCINATION AND BLV CHALLENGE

Group of animal numbers	Pre-vaccination			16 weeks post-vaccination and 11 weeks post-challenge		
	ID[1]	RIA[2]	SYN[3]	ID[1]	RIA[2]	SYN[3]
Group I: Vaccinated-challenged						
808	-	-	-	-	-	-
818	-	-	-	+/-	-	-
832	+	+	+	+	+	+
836	-	-	-	+/-	-	-
878	-	-	-	-	-	-
Group II: Vaccinated-not challenged						
814	-	-	-	-	-	-
823	-	-	-	-	-	-
860	-	-	-	-	-	-
Group III: Not vaccinated-challenged						
822	-	-	-	-	-	-
834	-	-	-	+	+	+
842	+	+	+	+	+	+
868	-	-	-	+	+	+

[1]ID = Immunodiffusion to measure antibodies to BLV glycoprotein

[2]RIA = Radioimmunoassay p24 inhibition

[3]SYN = Virus syncytium assay

challenge. One unvaccinated animal (822) remained negative after BLV challenge. The control cattle (834 and 868) developed antibody against glycoprotein identified by the ID test more slowly than against p24 protein although the delay was rot more than 4 weeks (Table 2). Detection of infection was followed in one to two weeks by strong antibody response in 834 and 868.

TABLE 2

RESULTS OF ANTIBODY RESPONSE AND BLV INFECTION IN GROUP III ANIMALS BEFORE AND AFTER BLV CHALLENGE

Time interval in weeks		Animals											
		834			868			822			842		
		ID	RIA	SYN	ID	RIA	SYN	ID	RIA	SYN	ID	RIA	SYN
Pre-vaccination	O	-	-	-	-	-	-	-	-	-	+	+	+
Vaccination(1)	2	-	-	-	-	-	-	-	-	-	+	+	+
(2)	4	-	ND	-	-	ND	-	-	ND	-	+	ND	+
(3)	6	-	-	-	-	-	-	-	-	-	+	+	+
Challenge	9	-	-	-	-	-	-	-	-	-	+	+	+
Post-challenge													
(3)	12	-	-	-	-	-	-	-	-	-	+	+	+
(5)	14	-		+		+	+	-	-	-	+	+	+
(7)	16		+	+		+	+	-	-	-	+	+	+
(9)	18	+	+	+	+	+	+	-	-	-	+	+	+

ID = Immunodiffusion to measure antibodies to BLV glycoprotein

RIA = Radioimmunoassay p24 inhibition

SYN = Virus syncytium assay

CONCLUSIONS

Following challenge with BLV, 4 of 4 vaccinated calves negative at time of first vaccination remained negative during the 18 week period of study, giving evidence of immune protection against BLV infection. Evidence for this conclusion was absence of viraemia as indicated by negative syncytial assay (SYN) results and lack of antibody production against structural BLV proteins detected by radioimmune assay (RIA) and immunodiffusion (ID) tests. Conversely, 2 of the 3 non-vaccinated cattle negative before vaccination developed a persistent viraemia beginning 5 weeks after challenge and strong RIA and ID antibody responses from 5 to 9 weeks after BLV challenge. Cattle vaccinated but not challenged did not develop a viraemia indicating they were protected against possible contact exposure. Two animals positive at the beginning of the vaccination trial remained positive throughout the 18 weeks of the trial. The persistently viraemic animal in vaccination Group I was vaccinated and the vaccination did not alter the viraemia.

Reasons why one non-vaccinated animal did not become infected after BLV challenge are not clear. Perhaps the animal was improperly exposed to BLV or it might have had an unusual natural resistance to BLV infection. It is unlikely that the challenging dose was inactivated because from the same source of challenging infected lymphocytes two unvaccinated animals became infected.

Multiple vaccination with addition of aluminium hydroxide (AH) adjuvant on second and third vaccinations were deemed necessary to increase antigenicity of the vaccine. In an unrelated BLV vaccination trial, one of us (JHM) determined that AH adjuvant and multiple vaccination increased the antigenicity of the antigen in the vaccine (Miller and Van der Maaten, 1978). Virus neutralisation assays were not done in this trial although it would have given additional information of whether antibody was produced that was directed toward whole virus inactivation.

From the studies reported herein, it is difficult to determine whether protection against BLV was directed toward humoral antibody which inactivated virus before cellular invasion, or whether it was cell mediated that prevented virus infection of host lymphocytes, or a combination of both.

BL-3 cells did not induce a viraemia or antibody response directed against structural BLV proteins (p24 and glycoprotein). Protection against virus infection upon BLV challenge, however, was evident. This indicated that BL-3 cellular antigen(s) provided protection against BLV virus infection. The nature of the cellular antigen(s) has not been elucidated although presumably they are not related to BLV structural proteins. Animals with the 'calf' form of lymphosarcoma are usually negative for BLV, the type of lymphosarcoma from which BL-3 was derived (Onuma and Olson, 1976). In addition, BLV has not been cultured from the 'thymic', 'skin' and some adult animals with lymphosarcoma. These types of lymphosarcoma are found sporadically and the aetiology is undetermined while the enzootic type of lymphosarcoma is associated with BLV infection. It is intriguing to speculate that the protective antigenic component(s) of the BL-3 cell are tumour associated transplantation antigens (TATA) located on the cell surface. It is also possible that protective component(s) are located internally in the BL-3 cell. If this hypothesis is correct, BL-3 antigenic component(s), TATA, provide an immune surveillance in vaccinated cattle whereby receptor sites on host lymphocytes are altered preventing initial virus infection. Results of our study support the idea that BLV infection did not occur in host lymphocytes or otherwise antibodies should have been detected in vaccinated cattle after BLV challenge. Future studies are designed to discover what is the protective component(s) in BL-3 and whether that component(s) is(are) preserved by cellular inactivation. Future studies will also be designed to discover whether BL-3 cells contain footprints of BLV by doing molecular hydridisation studies.

Clearly this is a report of a BLV vaccination trial that is preliminary in nature; however, results are encouraging and provide a basis for future studies. The BL-3 vaccine has distinct advantages over other BLV vaccines because it does not induce antibody responses confused with BLV infections (Miller and Van der Maaten, 1978).

Vaccinated and unvaccinated sheep are presently being studied to determine the oncogenic potential of BL-3 cells in this species. It is unlikely that BL-3 cells are oncogenic in homologous or heterologous hosts although this question needs testing because genetic information for oncogenesis is present in BL-3 cells that lead to lymphosarcoma in athymic nude mice (Irvin et al., 1975). Lymphosarcoma induction in athymic nude mice is presumably a cell transplantation in immune deficient animals whereas in immunologic intact cattle or heterospecies, transplantation antigens would prevent growth of BL-3 cells.

REFERENCES

Devare, S.G., Chander, S., Samagh, B.S. and Stephenson, J.R., 1977. Evaluation of radioimmunoprecipitation for the detection of bovine leukemia virus infection in domestic cattle. J. Immunol. 119: 277-282.

Ferrer, J.F. and Diglio, C.A., 1976. Development of an *in vitro* infectivity assay for the C-type bovine leukemia virus. Cancer Res. 36: 1068-1073.

Garcia de Lima, E. and Mitscherlich, E., 1973. Untersuchungen über die Zahl der B-und T-Lymphocyten im strömenden Blut von gesunden, leukoseverdächtigen und leukosekranken Rinden der Deutschen Schwarzbunten. Zbl. Vet. Med. B 20: 665-684.

Hare, W.C.D., Yang, T.J. and McFeely, R.A., 1967. A survey of chromosome findings in 47 cases of bovine lymphosarcoma (leukemia). J. Nat. Cancer Inst. 38: 383-392.

Irvin, A.D., Brown, C.G.D. and Kanhai, G.K., 1975. Comparative growth of bovine lymphosarcoma cells and lymphoid cells infected with *Theileria parva* in athymic (nude) mice. Nature 255: 713-714.

Kniazeff, A., Owens, R.B. and Theilen, G.H. Establishment of BL-3 lymphoid cell suspension culture. Unpublished data, June 1968.

Lukes, R.J. and Collins, R.D., 1974. Immunologic characterization of human malignant lymphomas. Cancer 34: 1488-1503.

Miller, J.M. and Van der Maaten, M.J., 1977. Use of glycoprotein antigen in the immunodiffusion test for bovine leukemia virus antibodies. Euro. J. Cancer 13: 1369-1375.

Miller, J.M. and Van der Maaten, M.J., 1978. Evaluation of an inactivated bovine leukemia virus preparation as an immunogen in cattle. Ann. Rech. Vet. 4: 871-877.

Muscoplat, C.C., Alhaj, I., Johnson, D.W., Pomeroy, K.A., Olson, J.M., Larson, V.L., Stevens, J.B. and Sorensen, D.K., 1974. Characteristics of lymphocyte responses to phytomitogens: Comparison of responses of lymphocytes from normal and lymphocytotic cows. Am. J. Vet. Res. 35: 1053-1055.

News and reports, 1979. Animal disease outbreaks in 1978. Vet. Rec. 104: 401.

Onuma, M. and Olson, C., 1976. Bovine leukemia virus antigen in bovine lymphosarcoma cell cultures. Bovine leukosis: Various methods of molecular virology, Commission of the European Communities Eur. 5685, Ed. A. Burny, pp. 95-118 (ECSC, EEC, EAEC, Luxembourg).

Olson, C., Miller, L.D., Miller, J.M. and Hoss, H.E., 1972. Transmission of lymphosarcoma from cattle to sheep. J. Natl. Cancer Inst. 49: 1463-1467.

Paul, P., Theilen, G.H. and Taylor, N., 1980. Morphologic characterisation and cytogenetic analysis of continuous cell suspension culture, BL-3. Unpublished data.

Rappaport, H., 1966. Tumors of the hematopoietic system. In: Atlas of Tumor Pathology, Section III, Fascicle 8. Washington DC Armed Forces Institute of Pathology, p. 13.

Takashima, I., Olson, C., Driscoll, D.M. and Baumgartener, L.E., 1977. B-lymphocytes and T-lymphocytes in three types of bovine lymphosarcoma. J. Nat. Cancer Inst. 59: 1205-1209.

Theilen, G.H. and Madewell, B.R., 1979. Bovine leukemia disease complex (malignant lymphoma, leukosis, lymphosarcoma). In: Veterinary Cancer Medicine, Ed. G.H. Theilen and B.R. Madewell, pp. 252-272, Lea and Febiger, Philadelphia.

Theilen, G.H., Rush, J.D., Nelson-Rees, W.A., Dungworth, D.L., Munn, R.J. and Switzer, J.W., 1968. Bovine leukemia: establishment and morphologic characterization of continuous cell suspension culture, BL-1. J. Nat. Cancer Inst. 40: 737-749.

Van der Maaten, M.J., 1979. Review of recent international developments regarding bovine leukosis. Proceedings of Bovine Leukosis Symposium. Ed. by Joint Committee, pp. 173-176, May 22-23, University of Maryland, College Park, Maryland.

DISCUSSION

B.S. Samagh *(Canada)*

Did you know that at the University of Guelph similar work is done?

G.H. Theilen *(USA)*

No, I did not know that.

M.J. Van der Maaten *(USA)*

I tried to infect that cell line with BLV, and I could not infect it either.

ATTEMPT FOR A NEW CYTOLOGICAL AND CYTOIMMUNOLOGICAL CLASSIFICATION OF BOVINE MALIGNANT LYMPHOMA (BML) (LYMPHOSARCOMA)

A.-L. Parodi[1], Martine Mialot[1], F. Crespeau[1], D. Lévy[2], H. Salmon[3], G. Noguès[4] and R. Gérard-Marchand[5]

[1]Laboratoire d'Anatomie-Pathologique ENVA, F-94704 Alfort Cedex

[2]Unité INSERM 152 - Hôpital Cochin, F-75014 Paris

[3]Laboratoire d'Immunologie et de Virologie, INRA, F-78 Thiverval-Grignon

[4]CERMA, F-75996 Paris Armées

[5]Service d'Anatomie-Pathologique, Institut G. Roussy, F-94000 Villejuif

France.

ABSTRACT

According to the principles of the KIEL classification of human malignant lymphomas (ML), a classification of bovine ML is proposed. This classification is based upon cytological, cytoenzymological and immuno-chemical methods. It was applied to 43 bovine ML - juvenile and adult. The results lead to the conclusion that the criteria used for the human ML are applicable to their bovine counterpart. Most of the cases observed, both in adults and calves, were B-lymphocyte derived. Cytoenzymological markers, known as T-lymphocyte specific in human, were detected in three juvenile cases. Investigation into the presence of BLV antibodies in the sera of the animals failed to establish a correlation between sporadic or enzootic forms of bovine leukosis and the cytological types of the tumours.

O.C. Straub (ed.), Fourth International Symposium on Bovine Leukosis

INTRODUCTION

Four clinical and pathological forms of bovine lymphosarcoma, a neoplasm of lymphoid tissue, are differentiated: the common adult type or adult lymphosarcoma (ALS), the adult skin lymphosarcoma (SLS), the calf or juvenile lymphosarcoma (JLS) and the thymic form (TLS)(International Committee on Bovine Leukosis, 1968). Only the ALS or enzootic form is known to be enzootic and associated with bovine leukaemia virus (BLV). The other, or sporadic, forms are non-associated with BLV (Lévy et al., 1976).

During the last ten years, new cytological and functional concepts of the lymphoid system have arisen, establishing the basis of the relationship between the various lymphoid cells in normal lymphoid tissue (Lennert, 1978).

These new concepts led to some new classifications of human lymphosarcomas or malignant lymphomas (ML) (Lukes et al., 1974; Gérard-Marchand et al., 1974; Lennert et al., 1975).

Using the basis of these classifications, essentially the so-called KIEL classification (Gérard-Marchand et al., 1974) and the cytological criteria used in human ML (Lennert, 1978), we attempted to classify cases of bovine malignant lymphoma (BML).

MATERIALS AND METHODS

Tumour cases

Our study was performed on 43 cases of BML, including 19 ALS, one SLS, 20 JLS and 3 TLS. Those developed in animals less than 2 years old were considered as juvenile BML. Only cases with large thymic tumours, associated generally with lymph node localisations, were initially classed as TLS but, in addition, after *post mortem* examination, we included 7 other cases with mild thymic infiltration - all of them were less than 2 years old.

Histopathology and cytopathology

Various lymph node and visceral tumour samples were cut off, in each case, in order to obtain imprints and paraffin blocks.

Imprints and thin sections were stained, using various methods, as seen in Table 1.

In order to detect intracytoplasmic immunoglobulins (C-IgG), a peroxidase-antiperoxidase soluble complex technique was performed (Bellet et al., 1979) using a rabbit anti-bovine immunoglobulin G serum (Cappel Laboratories Inc.).

The two cytoenzymological techniques used (acid-phosphatase and β glucuronidase) (Goldberg et al., 1962), were performed referring to the specific enzymatic activities observed in human T-lymphocytes (Lennert, 1978).

Detection of anti-BLV antibodies

The agar gel immunodiffusion test (AGID), using a commercial antigen (Seromed) and the radioimmunoassay (RIA) as described previously (Lévy et al., 1977) were performed in each case before euthanasia.

RESULTS

The classification of the 43 cases, according to the cytological criteria used in human ML in the KIEL classification, is reported in Table 2. The most prevalent types are the immunoblastic (19 cases) and centroblastic or centroblastic/centrocytic types (17 cases). The lymphoblastic types are more rare (4 cases), and two of them were of the convoluted cell type described in human lymphoblastic ML by Lukes et al. (1975). No lymphocytic type was observed. Two pleomorphic cell cases without similarities to any forms of human ML, were tentatively considered to be histiocytic types.

TABLE 1

HISTOLOGICAL AND CYTOLOGICAL METHODS FOR DIAGNOSING MALIGNANT LYMPHOMA

PARAFFIN SECTIONS
a) After AFA[1] fixation:
- Hemalun - eosin - saffron
- Giemsa
- Methyl - green - pyronin
- Silver staining (optional)
b) After Bouin (or AFA)[1] fixation:
- Immunoperoxidase (PAP) method, with anti-bovine IgG rabbit immunoserum
IMPRINTS
a) Without fixation:
- May - Grünwald - Giemsa
b) After formalin-acetone fixation:
- Acid - phosphatase (Katayama method)
- β Glucuronidase

[1] Alcohol-formalin-acetic acid

All these tumours were of the diffuse type.

None of these cytological types was over-represented in juvenile or adult forms. The lymphoplasmacytoid case was observed in the SLS.

The three clinical TLS were of the immunoblastic type in two cases and of the centroblastic/centrocytic type in one case.

Using macroscopic milk thymic infiltration, confirmed by histological examination, the following types were observed in the other seven cases: centroblastic/centrocytic (1), centroblastic (2), immunoblastic (1), immunoblastic with plasmablastic differentiation (1), immunoblastic/centroblastic (1), lymphoblastic (1).

TABLE 2

CYTOLOGICAL CLASSIFICATION OF 43 CASES OF BOVINE LEUKOSIS

Lymphocytic	0
Lymphoplasmacytoid	1
Centrocytic	0
Centroblastic/Centrocytic	9
Centroblastic	8
Immunoblastic:	
Pure immunoblastic	11
Immunoblastic with plasmablastic differentiation	4
Immunoblastic/Centroblastic	4
Lymphoblastic	4
Histiocytic	2

No prevalence of cytological type with BLV infection was observed. Two juvenile cases (one year and 18 months old) were BLV positives. Conversely, five adult cases were BLV negative. Clinical TLS and SLS were BLV negative (Figure 1).

There was evidence of intracytoplasmic IgG in 12 cases out of the 41 confirmed lymphoid tumours. The types in which C-IgG appeared most frequently were the immunoblastic type with plasmablastic differentiation (3/4) and the immunoblastic/ centroblastic type (2/4) (Table 3). The lymphoplasmacytoid type was also positive. The prevalence of C-IgG was low in the pure immunoblastic type (3/11) and the centroblastic (2/8) and centroblastic/centrocytic types (1/9). No lymphoblastic ML was C-IgG positive.

A focal intracytoplasmic enzymatic activity (acid-phosphatase and β glucuronidase) was observed in three cases: one immunoblastic from TLS, and two lymphoblastic with convoluted cell type, both in juvenile cases, one of them with thymic infiltration, the other one without thymic involvement.

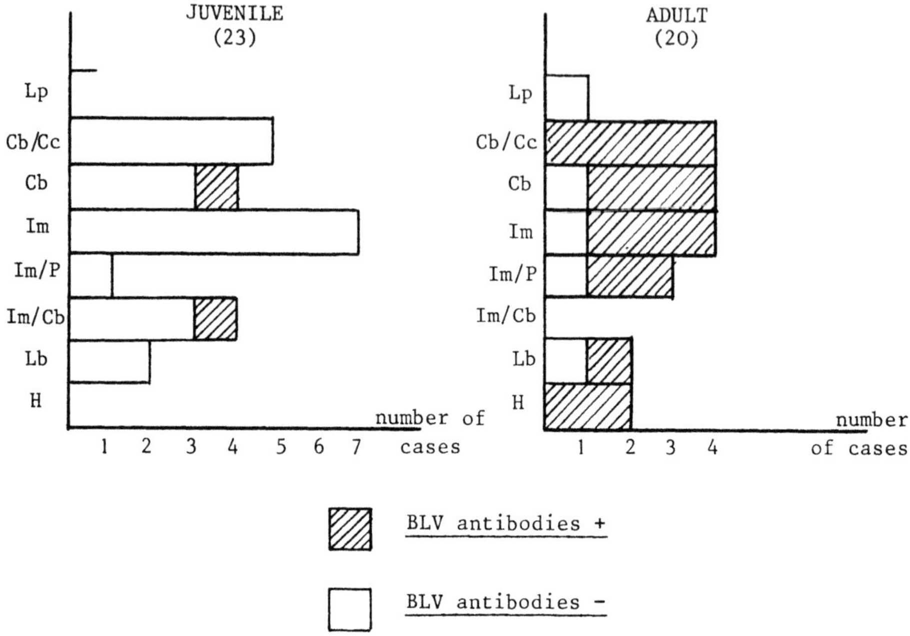

Fig. 1. Classification of 43 cases of adult and juvenile bovine lymphosarcomas according to their cytological types and presence of BLV antibodies

DISCUSSION

The basic, cytological criteria of this classification of BLM were transposed from those of human ML.

According to these cytomorphological criteria, most of the BLM cases seem to be derived from the B-lymphocyte sub-line. That is the case with the lymphoplasmacytoid (1), centroblastic/ centrocytic (9), centroblastic (8), immunoblastic with plasmablastic differentiation (4) and immunoblastic/centroblastic (4) types. The pure immunoblastic and the lymphoblastic types could be derived both from the T and the B-lymphocyte sub-lines. However, the presence of C-IgG, considered as specific to the B-lymphocyte, may support the adherence of the tumoral cells to this sub-line. In three pure immunoblastic cases, the tumour cells contained intracytoplasmic IgG. None of the lymphoblastic cases contained tumour cells with C-IgG.

TABLE 3

CLASSIFICATION OF 43 CASES OF BOVINE LYMPHOSARCOMA ACCORDING TO THEIR CYTOLOGICAL, CYTOENZYMOLOGICAL AND IMMUNOCHEMICAL CHARACTERISTICS

Clinical type	Gross pathology	Cytological type	Enzymological activities	Cytoplasmic IgG	Total
JUVENILE (23)	Thymic (3)	Cb/Cc	O/1	O	1
		Im	1/1	O	2
	Multicentric (20)	Cb/Cc	O/1	O	4
		Cb	O/4	O	4
		Im	O/4	3	5
		Im/P	-	1	1
		Im/Cb	O/4	2	4
		Lb	2/2	O	2
	Cutaneous (1)	Lp	O/1	1	1
ADULT (20)	Multicentric (19)	Cb/Cc	O/3	1	4
		Cb	O/3	2	4
		Im	O/2	O	4
		Im/P	O/2	2	3
		Lb	O/1	O	2
		H	O/1	2	2

The prevalence of B-lymphocyte derived tumour cells in adult BML has been observed previously using other criteria (Takashima et al., 1977; Onuma et al., 1979). JLS was considered not to be B-lymphocyte derived, the tumoral cells lacking specific markers.

It appears from our observations that B-lymphocyte derived ML was also identified in JLS, including cases with thymic involvement. This situation, which differs from those found in previous studies where different markers were used, does not seem to be a pathological impossibility because in all of the cases with thymic involvement, many other lymphoid organs, including lymph nodes, were simultaneously tumoral. The tumour cells could arise from these extra thymic localisations and, further, invade the thymus. These factors lead us to consider classical TLS as a clinical type of BML, but not as an obligatory T-lymphocyte derived ML.

The cytological analogies between human and bovine ML led us to the hypothesis that the focal intracytoplasmic acid phosphatase and β glucuronidase activities could be markers of T-lymphocyte derived tumour cells. Two of our cases with these markers belong to the lymphoblastic types with convoluted-cells, known to be T cell derived in humans. The third belongs to the immunoblastic type which can also be T-lymphocyte derived. None of them contained positive C-IgG cells.

Conversely, no case considered as B-lymphocyte derived, according to the cytomorphological criteria and/or the presence of C-IgG, had these enzymatic activities.

However, the use of other lymphocyte markers is necessary to demonstrate that these enzymatic positive cells are T-lymphocyte derived.

No correlation was observed between any cytological types and the presence, or absence, of BLV infection. However, the two JLS with evidence of BLV infection were considered as

B-lymphocyte derived: one was a centroblastic type, C-IgG negative, the other was an immunoblastic/centroblastic type C-IgG positive. No case considered as possibly T-lymphocyte derived (all JLS) was BLV associated. This finding seems to be in agreement with other observations (Paul et al., 1977).

In conclusion, the transposition to BML based on the criteria used in the KIEL classification for human ML led us to establish that:

(a) Most of the various cytological and functional types described in human ML can be found in BML. A good correlation exists between the immunochemical marker represented by the presence of C-IgG and the cytological types known to be B-lymphocyte derived. According to these cytological and functional criteria most of the BLM are B-lymphocyte derived. A good correlation seems to exist between the localised intracytoplasmic acid phosphatase and β glucuronidase activities and certain cytological types considered in humans as T-lymphocyte derived; namely the convoluted cells, lymphoblastic type. However, more specific functional markers are necessary to confirm this analogy.

Owing to the fact that B-lymphocyte derived ML can develop with thymic involvement, TLS seems to be no more than a clinical type of JLS.

(b) No correlation exists between a prevalent cytological type and the presence or absence of BLV infection. However, no ML tentatively considered as T-lymphocyte derived was associated with BLV infection.

ACKNOWLEDGMENTS

We thank Mrs. Chantal Pinelli for her excellent technical assistance.

This work was supported by a grant n°80 - 7 - 044C from the Délégation Générale à la Recherche Scientifique et Technique and, in part, by a grant from la Direction de la Qualité, Service Vétérinaire.

REFERENCES

Bellet, D., Caillaud, J.M. and Arrang, J.M., 1979. Marqueurs biologiques en cancérologie. Journées de Biologie Clinique Necker. Institut Pasteur, 13-17.

Gérard-Marchand, R., Hamlin, I., Lennert, K., Rilke, F., Stanfeld, A.G. and Van Unnik, J.A.M., 1974. Classification of non-Hodgkin's lymphomas. (Letter to the Editor) Lancet: 406-408.

Goldberg, A.F. and Barka, T., 1962. Acid phosphatase activity in human blood cells. Nature (London), 195: 297.

Lennert, K., Stein, H. and Kasserling, E., 1975. Cytological and functional criteria for the classification of malignant lymphomata. Brit. J. Cancer, 31, suppl. II: 29-43.

Lennert, K., 1978. Malignant lymphomas other than Hodgkin's disease. Springer Verlag, Berlin.

Lévy, D., Deshayes, L., Guillemain, B., Irgens, K. and Parodi, A.-L., 1976. Studies on BLV infection: a serological survey on French cattle. In: Bovine Leukosis: Various methods of molecular virology. A. Burny (Ed.), CEC publication, Luxembourg, pp. 199-208.

Lévy, D., Deshayes, L. Parodi, A.-L., Lévy, J.P., Stephenson, J.R., Devare, J.G. and Gilden, R.V., 1977. Bovine leukemia virus specific antibodies among French cattle. II: Radioimmunoassay with the major structural protein (BLV p24). Int. J. Cancer, 20: 543-550.

Lukes, R.J. and Collins, R.D., 1974. Immunologic characterization of human malignant lymphomas. Cancer, 34: 1438-1503.

Lukes, R.J. and Collins, R.D., 1975. New approaches to the classification of the lymphoma. Brit. J. Cancer, 31, suppl. II: 1-28.

Onuma, M., Honma, T., Mikami, T., Ichijo, S. and Konishi, T., 1979. Studies on the sporadic and enzootic forms of bovine leukosis. J. Comp. Path., 89: 159-167.

Paul, P.S., Pomeroy, K.A., Castro, A.E., Johnson, D.W., Muscoplat, C.C. and Sørensen, D.K., 1977. Detection of bovine leukemia virus in B-lymphocyte by the syncytia induction assay. J. Nat. Cancer Inst., 59: 1269-1272.

Takashima, I., Olson, C., Driscoll, D.M. and Baumgartener, L.E., 1977. B- and T-lymphocytes in three types of bovine lymphosarcoma. J. Nat. Cancer Inst., 59: 1205-1209.

X. : An international committee on bovine leukosis: Criteria for the determination fo the normal and leukotic state in cattle. J. Nat. Cancer Inst., 41: 243-263, 1968.

DISCUSSION

A.A. Ressang *(Netherlands)*

This is a practical question which should be of interest to all of us. On the grounds of the histological picture, could you distinguish between the juvenile form and the EBL form?

A.-L. Parodi *(France)*

This was one of the aims of the study but we do not have a prevalent type in juveniles, in the same form.

STUDIES ON A RANDOM SERIES OF CASES OF BOVINE LEUKOSIS

L.M. Markson, D.H. Roberts and R. Bradley

Central Veterinary Laboratory,
New Haw, Weybridge, Surrey, UK.

ABSTRACT

A random series of 19 clinical field cases of bovine leukosis from England and Wales was studied clinically, haematologically, serologically, virologically and by use of the electron microscope to count nuclear pockets in circulating lymphocytes. Additionally calves were inoculated with whole blood and a tissue lymphocyte suspension from the first six cases and subsequently studied periodically by the same methods. Herds of origin of the field cases were examined for clinical evidence of leukosis, for evidence of leukaemia and for serum antibody to bovine leukosis virus (BLV). No evidence was found to suggest that 18 of these field cases were other than sporadic and non-infectious: neither BLV nor specific antibody to it was demonstrated; no increase in lymphocytic nuclear pockets was seen; the transmission tests were negative. The nineteenth case was of the enzootic form of the disease, recently discovered in Britain. BLV was isolated from the animal, antibody to BLV was demonstrated in its serum and in the serum of other cattle in the herd of origin and a significant increase was found in the proportion of circulating lymphocytes containing nuclear pockets. It would appear that sporadic bovine leukosis and enzootic bovine leukosis are aetiologically separate entities. The IgM and IgG concentration in serum from 12 of the sporadic cases and from 6 cattle seropositive for antibody to BLV was within normal limits. Lymphocytes from 6 sporadic cases could not be identified as either T or B cells. A common tumour-associated antigen was not detected in 10 of the sporadic cases and a single enzootic case, which supports the opinion that sporadic bovine leukosis does not have a single viral origin.

O.C. Straub (ed.), Fourth International Symposium on Bovine Leukosis

INTRODUCTION

An interim account of this project was presented at the Third International Symposium on Bovine Leukosis which took place in October 1978 at Alfort (Markson et al., 1978). Since then the project has been completed and is now reported in full.

Until two years ago there had been no evidence that enzootic bovine leukosis (EBL) existed in Great Britain (Markson, 1977). A project was therefore set up to study the British forms of bovine leukosis (BL) and compare them with EBL as seen in other countries. In this way they could be studied in isolation from EBL; alternatively, evidence for the existence of EBL in indigenous British cattle might be discovered.

PROJECT PLAN

Field Cases

Live cases of BL were sought in England and Wales, transported to the Central Veterinary Laboratory and, after clinical examination, studied as follows:

(i) Haematology. Haematological parameters - RBC, Hb, PCV, WBC (total and differential) - were assayed by standard techniques. The EC leukosis key (Mammerickx et al., 1978) was used to evaluate the lymphocyte counts.

(ii) Serology. Serum samples were examined for antibody to bovine leukosis virus (BLV) by an indirect fluorescent antibody test according to the method of Ressang et al. (1974). More recently an agar gel immunodiffusion test has been introduced using the Leukassay B kit of Pitman-Moore Inc., Washington Crossing, New Jersey, USA.

(iii) Lymphocytic nuclear pockets (LNP). The ultrastructure of circulating lymphocytes was studied with particular reference to LNP, using the method of Weber and his colleagues (1969). As interpreted by these authors, when fewer than 1% of 200 lymphocytes had LNP, the diagnosis was read as negative, 1 to 2% as suspicious and over 2% as positive.

(iv) Morbid anatomy. The animals were killed and the gross and microscopic pathological abnormalities assessed.

(v) Virology. Lymphocyte cultures were set up from peripheral blood, lymph nodes, spleen and thymus, and the cells examined by electron microscopy for the presence of C-type particles. Attempts were also made to isolate BLV using the cocultivation technique described by Ressang et al. (1974). Additionally the herd of origin of the field cases was examined clinically, haematologically and serologically as above.

Transmission Experiments

Before inoculation 30 healthy calves a few days old were bled to provide material for haematological, serological, virological and ultrastructural examination as above. Material from each of the first six leukosis cases to be received was inoculated into a separate group of five calves; 50 ml of citrated whole blood were administered intravenously; 20 ml of a crude 10% suspension of lymphomatous tissues in beef infusion broth with antibiotics were injected by the intraperitoneal route. After inoculation they were observed clinically and bled periodically for similar examination.

RESULTS

In the 3½ years which the project lasted, 19 cases of leukosis were received: 12 were juvenile multicentric cases, 3 were thymic, 2 cutaneous, 1 adult multicentric and 1 was a case of EBL; 9 were aleukaemic (including 1 of the cutaneous cases, the 3 thymic and 5 of the juvenile multicentric cases). One of the 2 cutaneous cases died on the journey and was therefore unsuitable for detailed investigation; but the veterinary surgeon who submitted it had provided haematological data which indicated a lymphocyte count of 18 800/mm^3. The EBL case, a Canadian Holstein cow, had come to light in the course of a retrospective serological survey of imported cattle.

BLV was recovered from circulating lymphocytes and various lymphnodes of the only single EBL case in the series. In lymphocyte cultures from the other cattle in the series no BLV was demonstrated nor any C-type particle. The heifer with cutaneous leukosis, which was used in one of the transmission experiments, was pregnant with a live foetus of 160 - 165 days gestation in which BLV was not demonstrated.

Nuclear pockets were found in 7.5% of lymphocytes in samples of blood from the cow with EBL. Otherwise no significant difference was found between the number of lymphocytes containing NP in the leukaemic and aleukaemic animals respectively: in each of them it comprised < 1%.

Access to the herd of origin of these cases of leukosis could not be enforced with the result that only 13 herds were investigated. No more clinical cases of leukosis were found in any of them, not even in the herd in which the BLV infected cow had been identified. Of 129 serum samples obtained from the latter herd, 11 were positive for antibody to BLV. All the serological tests from the 12 other herds were negative. Only 39 sequestrenated blood samples could be obtained from the BLV infected herd: 2 of these had a positive lymphocyte count, 4 were in the doubtful range and the rest were haematologically negative. In blood samples from the remaining 12 herds, such positive lymphocyte counts as were detected were just within the positive range and, on subsequent retesting, were found to be negative.

The first 6 leukosis cases which survived to be killed were used to set up the transmission experiments: 3 juvenile multicentric, 1 adult multicentric, 1 thymic and 1 cutaneous, all sporadic cases in which neither BLV nor antibody to it had been detected. Three calves, which died of intercurrent disease when quite young, were negative for evidence of BLV infection by the criteria determined for the project. The remainder were kept on experiment for 3 years and then killed. During this period, despite repeated testing, no antibody to BLV was detected in serum samples from the inoculated animals, no evidence of an abnormal number of lymphocytes with NP was found in any blood sample and the few instances of a lymphocyte count within the positive range of the EC key were shown by subsequent testing to have been transient.

During the long course of this project, as new staff and new techniques became available, additional parameters were assayed in several of the field cases of SBL studied and investigated. Thus Dr. D.A. Higgins, while he was at the CVL, attempted to identify the lymphocytes in 6 cases of SBL, using the method described by Higgins and Stack (1977). Fewer than 5% could be identified as T or B cells: the neoplastic cell type was apparently a 'null' (non-T and non-B) lymphocyte as in some cases of human leukaemia. Onuma and Olson (1977) found tumour-associated antigens on the membrane and in the cytoplasm of lymph node cells and circulating lymphocytes from clinical cases of EBL. Following the procedure they described, antiserum against neoplastic cells from a case of SBL was prepared in a calf. Lymphocyte suspensions from 10 cases of SBL were examined for common antigens using an indirect fluorescent antibody test with this antiserum and serum from an animal positive to serological tests for BLV antibody: a common antigen was not detected. The concentration of IgM and IgG in the serum of 12 of the SBL cases and of 6 cattle seropositive for BLV antibody was assayed using a quantitative immunodiffusion kit (Miles Laboratories, Inc.): all the results obtained were within the normal limits.

DISCUSSION

Anderson et al. (1969) examined all tumours in cattle, sheep and pigs passing through 100 slaughterhouses in Great Britain during a period of 12 months. Lymphosarcoma in its different manifestations was the most common malignant neoplasm in all 3 species. Seventy five cases, all single incidents, were diagnosed in 1.3 million bovine carcasses which were reckoned to be about one third of the annual national total, thus giving a national prevalence in slaughtered cattle of about 225. Adding live cases which end up in knackeries or diagnostic laboratories suggests an annual incidence of about 300 cases of bovine leukosis of which only a minority would be seen clinically. Thus British veterinary surgeons in general practice must have had little if any experience of the disease, which would partly account for our difficulty in obtaining live cases and would also explain the 4 non-leukotic cattle mistakenly offered to us as leukosis cases.

Our project was set up at a time when there was no evidence that EBL existed in England (Markson, 1977). Recently, however, serological, virological and haematological evidence of EBL has been found in imported cattle, in some of their progeny and in indigenous cattle with which these affected animals were subsequently reared (Chasey et al., 1978; Loxam et al., 1978). Although more such infected herds have been identified since then, clinical disease in infected cattle has been a very rare occurrence. One such case is included in the series reported here; but it came too late to be included in the limited transmission experiments planned. Another case was identified after the death of a Holstein cow from perforation of a lymphosarcomatous abomasum with consequent fatal haemorrhage. More recently Grimshaw et al. (1980) have confirmed a case of EBL in an Aberdeen Angus x Friesian cow. The origin of the animal is obscure, but the thought that the Friesian parent may in fact have been a Holstein is tempting. Be that as it may, the number of cases of proven EBL is far too few, only one live case having been available to us, for a detailed comparison with our 18 cases of SBL. Nevertheless, it is common knowledge now that EBL is a contagious disease of adult cattle caused by a retrovirus which provokes an antibody response now demonstrable by a wide range of serological tests. The single case in our series was seropositive by the agar gel immunodiffusion test for antibody to BLV, as were 11 other cattle in the herd of origin. Two of 39 sequestrenated blood samples obtained from the herd had a lymphocytic leukaemia within the positive range of the EC criteria, as did the leukotic cow. The latter's exophthalmia was associated with retro-ocular lymphosarcoma which is a feature peculiar to EBL. The 18 other cases in our series were all single cases and exemplified all the recognised types of SBL except for the rare 'atypical' or unicentric leukosis. No serological or virological evidence of infection with BLV was demonstrated either in the leukotic animals or in the herd of origin. They have all therefore been identified as cases of sporadic bovine leukosis. Several attempts at transmission were negative in all respects, although the inoculated animals were kept for 3 years during which they were examined repeatedly for evidence of transmission or of infection by BLV. Thus the evidence here appears to confirm that there is no aetiological relationship between EBL and the different forms of SBL.

Weber et al. (1969) suggested a positive correlation between the prevalence of nuclear pockets in circulating lymphocytes and the ability of cells from such a population to produce C-type viral particles. Weber et al. (1973) subsequently suggested that "LNP evaluations in cattle may be a significant aid in the early diagnosis of bovine lymphocytic leukaemia". Bloch et al. (1975) disagreed with this opinion, maintaining that a correlation between lymphocytosis and an increase to over 2% in the proportion of lymphocytes containing NP could be found even in cattle free of EBL. One case of EBL hardly provides sufficient evidence to support or refute a hypothesis. Nevertheless it is a fact that our single case of EBL had NP in 7.5% of the circulating lymphocytes examined - a proportion well within the EBL positive range of Weber et al. (1973) - whereas the LNP count in the remainder of our cases, leukaemic and aleukaemic alike, was invariably < 1%. However, perhaps the LNP count should now be considered to have only academic value in view of the variety of sensitive serological tests now available to identify the presence of specific antibody in cattle infected with BLV.

According to Muscoplat and his colleagues (1974) the percentage of B lymphocytes in normal cattle varies from 18 to 28%, whereas in leukaemic, BLV infected cattle the proportion of B lymphocytes could be as high as 68%. In 6 of our SBL cases examined by Higgins very few lymphocytes (< 5%) were identified as either T or B cells. The neoplastic cells were considered to be 'null' (non-T, non-B) lymphocytes such as are seen in some cases of human leukaemia.

Our failure to demonstrate a common tumour-associated antigen in 10 cases of SBL and our single case of EBL supports the opinion that SBL is neither related to EBL nor does it have a single viral origin.

Trainin et al. (1973) found both EBL and SBL to be characterised by a deficiency of serum IgM; the concentration of IgM and IgG in serum from 12 of our SBL cases and 6 clinically normal cattle seropositive for BLV antibody showed no such deviation from normality.

ACKNOWLEDGMENTS

The authors are most grateful to the many colleagues - too many to mention individually - throughout the State Veterinary Service who, by their co-operation and efforts, have made possible the execution of this project. Exception must be made, however, to thank J. Bailey, D.A. Stagg, G. Wibberley and Mary Quinn who carried the burden of the laboratory work. The project was carried out under contract to and with financial assistance from the Commission of the European Communities.

REFERENCES

Anderson, L.J., Sandison, A.T. and Jarrett, W.F.H., 1969. A British Abattoir Survey of Tumours in Cattle, Sheep and Pigs. Vet. Rec. 84, 547-551.

Bloch, B., Bendixen, H.J. and Lund, E., 1975. The Possible Utilization of Nuclear Pockets on Lymphocytes in the Diagnosis of Enzootic Bovine Leucosis. Acta Path. Microbiol. Scand., Sect. A, 83, 511-518.

Chasey, D., Wibberley, G., Markson, L.M. and Roberts, D.H., 1978. Demonstration of Enzootic Bovine Leukosis Virus in Great Britain. Vet. Rec. 103, 449-450.

Grimshaw, W.T.R., Wiseman, A., Petrie, L., Selman, I.E., Gibbs, H.A. and Thompson, H., 1980. A Confirmed Clinical Case of Enzootic Bovine Leukosis in Britain. Vet. Rec. 107, 110.

Higgins, D.A. and Stack, M.J., 1977. Bovine Lymphocytes: Enhanced E-rosette Formation after Storage or Gradient Centrifugation. Clin. Exp. Immunol. 29, 304-310.

Loxam, J.G., Edwards, W.A. and Watson, W.A., 1978. Enzootic Bovine Leukosis in Great Britain. Vet. Rec. 103, 270-271.

Mammerickx, M., Lorenz, R.J., Straub, O.C., Donnelly, W.J.C., Flensburg, J.C., Gentile, G., Markson, L.M., Ressang, A.A. and Taylor, S.M., 1978. Bovine Haematology III. Comparative Breed Studies on the Leukocyte Parameters of Several European Cattle Breeds as Determined in the Common Reference Laboratory. Zbl. Vet. Med. B, 25, 257-267.

Markson, L.M., 1977. Bovine Leukosis in Great Britain. Bovine Leukosis: Various Methods of Molecular Virology, Ed. A. Burny, pp. 381-386 (CEC, Brussels)

Markson, L.M., Roberts, D.H. and Bradley, R., 1978. Studies on Bovine Leukosis as it is seen in England and Wales. Ann. Rech. Vet. 9, 899-902.

Muscoplat, C.C., Johnson, D.W., Pomeroy, K.A., Olson, J.M., Larson, V.L., Stevens, J.B. and Sorensen, D.K., 1974. Lymphocyte Surface Immunoglobulin: Frequency in Normal and Lymphocytotic Cattle. Am. J. Vet. Res. 35, 593-595.

Onuma, M. and Olson, C., 1977. Tumor-associated Antigen in Bovine and Ovine Lymphosarcoma. Cancer Res. 37, 3249-3256.

Ressang, A.A., Mastenbroek, N., Quak, J., van Griensven, L.J.L.D., Calafat, J., Hilgers, J., Hageman, P.C., Souissi, T. and Swens, S., 1974. Studies on Bovine Leukemia. I. Establishment of Type C Virus Producing Cell Lines. Zbl. Vet. Med. B, 21, 601-617.

Trainin, Z., Mairom, R., Klopfer, U. and Meidan, G., 1973. Levels of IgM and IgG in the Sera of Normal and Leukaemic Calves. J. Comp. Path. 83, 87-90.

Weber, A., Andrews, J., Dickinson, B., Larson, V., Hammer, R., Dirks, V., Sorensen, D. and Frommes, S., 1969. Occurrence of Nuclear Pockets in Lymphocytes of Normal, Persistent Lymphocytotic and Leukemic Adult Cattle. J. Nat. Cancer Inst. 43, 1307-1315.

Weber, A., Fahning, M., Hammer, R.H. and Jessen, C., 1973. Relationship between Nuclear Pockets in Bovine Peripheral Blood Lymphocytes and C-type Virus Particles in Cultures of These Cells. J. Nat. Cancer Inst. 51, 81-88.

ULTRASTRUCTURAL RESEARCH ON BOVINE CUTANEOUS LEUKOSIS

P. Simoni and S. Cinotti
Istituto di Patologia Generale e Anatomia Patologica Veterinaria
Istituto di Patologia Speciale e Clinica Medica Veterinaria
Università di Bologna
I-40126, Bologna, Italy.

ABSTRACT

Four cases of bovine cutaneous leukosis have been studied. At the peak of clinical manifestation the leukotic nodules appear histologically and ultrastructurally constituted by prolymphocytes bridled by a loose network of fibroblasts and collagen fibres. Later the external clinical manifestation tends to disappear. At this time the nodules have reduced volume and appear mainly constituted of loose connective tissue in which few leukotic cells are dispersed.

O.C. Straub (ed.), Fourth International Symposium on Bovine Leukosis

INTRODUCTION

In Italy few cases of bovine cutaneous leukosis have been studied until now (Gentile, 1967; Caporale et al., 1970; Gentile, 1971; Rizzi and Stanzani, 1973; Persechino and Roperto, 1978). None of this research nor that conducted elsewhere (Lesbouyries et al., 1935; Dungworth et al., 1964; Bendixen and Friis, 1965; Clegg and Moss, 1965; Marshak et al., 1966; Horvath et al., 1976) have been carried out with the aid of electron microscopy. This paper describes the ultrastructural characteristics of the cutaneous lesions of four affected animals.

MATERIALS AND METHODS

All samples of the cutaneous nodules were fixed in formalin. In one case we made a surgical biopsy of some cutaneous nodules 15 days before slaughtering, at the peak of clinical manifestation. In this case the bioptical material was fixed in formalin and in glutaraldehyde as well. A second drawing of samples was made when the animal was slaughtered because it was in agony. At slaughtering a certain remission of cutaneous symptoms was observed. All the tissue blocks were post-fixed in OsO_4 and, after dehydration, embedded in araldite. After preparation all tissue blocks were subjected to light and electron microscopic observation.

RESULTS

At the peak of clinical manifestation the lesions were nodular, covering the entire body. Certain nodules were surgically excised. When sectioned they appeared white to pink with a fatty consistence. Histologically (Figure 1) the neoplastic cells of all animals appeared to infiltrate the derma often bridled by a loose network of fibroblasts and collagen fibres, orientated in a prevalently perpendicular manner to the cutaneous surface. Under the electron microscope most of the neoplastic cells resembled immature lymphocytes (Figure 2), i.e. containing little heterochromatin and large, often numerous,

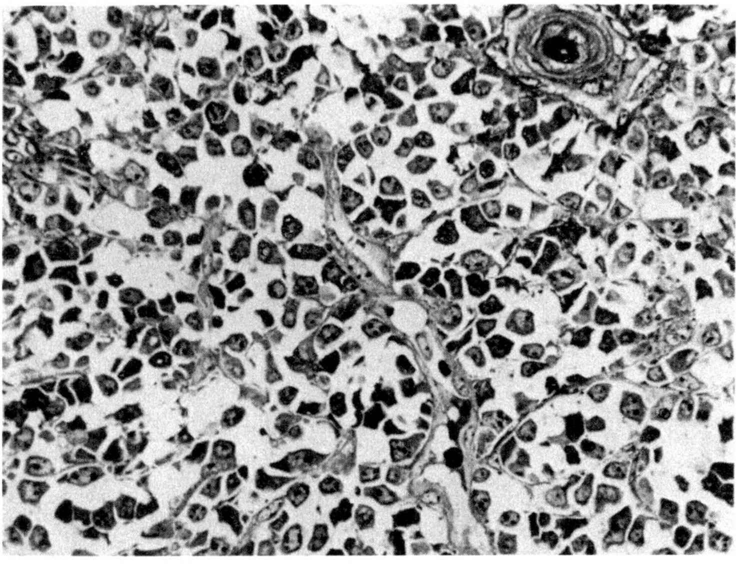
Fig. 1.

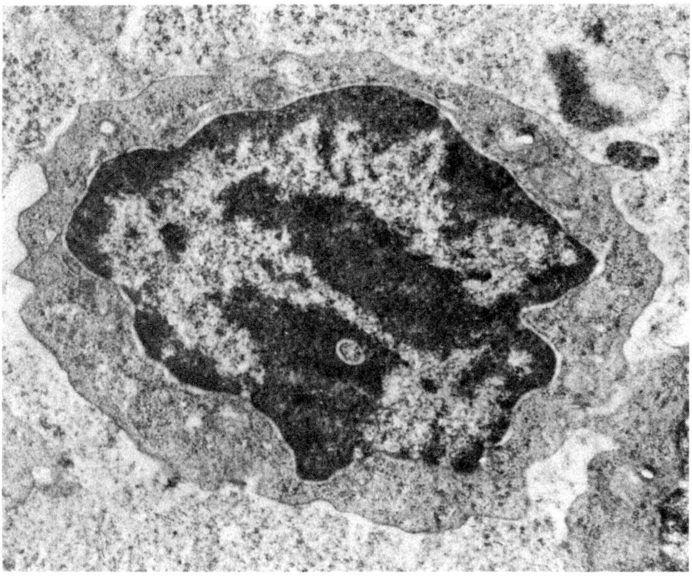
Fig. 2.

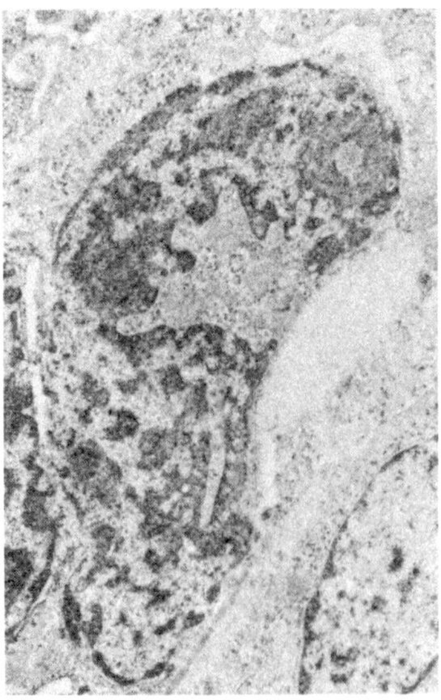
Fig. 3.

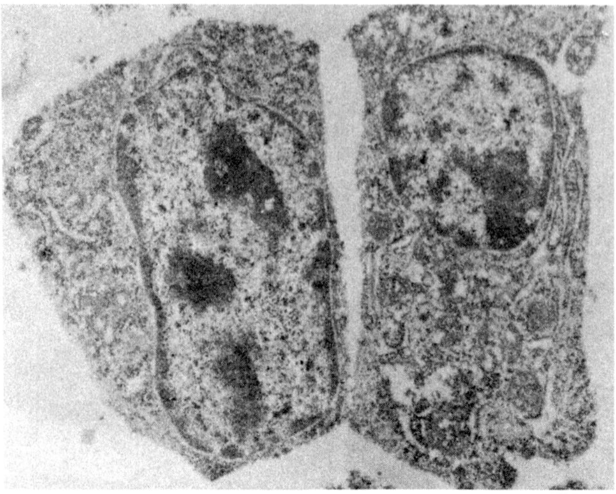
Fig. 4.

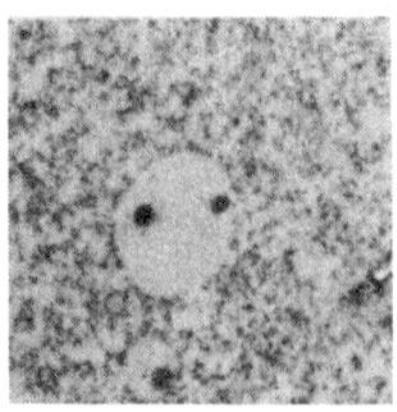
Fig. 5.

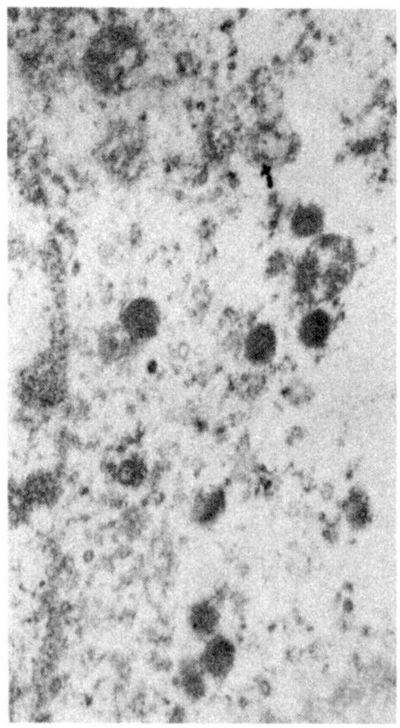
Fig. 6.

reticular nucleoli disposed for the most part along the nuclear membrane. The surface of the nuclear membrane of some cells was irregular (Figure 3) with frequent nuclear pores. The cytoplasm contained numerous mitochondria (Figure 3) and sometimes showed signs of cellular damage such as sequestration of cytoplasmic organelles and secondary lysosomes. In some cells the rough endoplasmic reticulum was unusually developed (Figure 4). In the cytoplasm of some cells we observed vacuoles of the endoplasmic reticulum which contained a few viral-like particles (Figures 5 and 6). Some structures resembling the 'budding' from the cytoplasmic membrane of some retroviruses were also present. When the external clinical manifestation was disappearing the histological sections showed absence of leukaemic tissue that was partly replaced by loose connective tissue. A few small groups of immature lymphatic cells were observed dispersed in the connectival matrix.

CONCLUSIONS

On the basis of histological and ultrastructural observations we can conclude that our animals were affected by prolymphocytic leukosis. As regards the aetiology of the bovine cutaneous leukosis we have inadequate findings to assume that a virus may be involved. In fact the 'viral-like particles' we observed might be degenerating proteic and/or lipidic structures of necrotising cells. Moreover, immunodiffusion tests for BLV were negative.

REFERENCES

Bendixen, J.J. and Friis, N.F., 1965. Hautleukose bei Rindern in Dänemark. Wien Tierärztl. Mschr. 52, 496-505.

Caporale, G., Rossi, G.A. and Caporale, V., 1970. Osservazioni su un caso di leucosi cutanea sporadica del bovino. Atti Soc. Ital. Buiatria. 2, 702-720.

Clegg, F.G. and Moss, B., 1965. Skin leukosis in a heifer: an unusual clinical history. Vet. Rec. 77, 271-272.

Dungworth, D.L., Theilen, G.H. and Lengyel, J., 1964. Bovine lymphosarcoma in cattle. II. The thymic form. Path. Vet. 1, 323-350.

Gentile, G., 1967. La leucosi cutanea del bovino. Atti Soc. Ital. Sci. Vet. 21, 569.

Gentile, G., 1971. La leucosi cutanea del bovino. Clinica Vet. 94, 295-304.

Horvath, Z., Tury, E. and Sellyei, M., 1976. An atypical case of bovine skin leukosis in Hungary. Magyar Allatorvosok Lapya. 31, 305-310.

Lesbouyries, G., Berthelon, M. and Marlot, T., 1935. Lymphosarcomatose chez une génisse. Bull. Acad. Vét. 8, 359-364.

Marshak, R.R., Hare, C.D., Dutcher, R.M., Schwartzman, R.M., Switzer, J.W. and Hubben, K., 1966. Observations on a heifer with cutaneous lymphosarcoma. Cancer. 19, 724-734.

Persechino, A. and Roperto, F., 1978. Osservazioni su di un caso di leucosi cutanea del bovino. Acta Med. Vet. 24, 47-66.

Rizzi, P. and Stanzani, F., 1973. Su un caso di leucosi cutanea sporadica del bovino. Atti Soc. Ital. Buiatria. 5, 455-464.

BOVINE LEUKOSIS: SHEEP AS AN EXPERIMENTAL MODEL FOR HAEMATOLOGICAL, MACROSCOPIC AND MICROSCOPIC ALTERATIONS

L.R. Neira, F. Lozano A. and O. Mariño
Laboratorio de Investigaciones Médicas Veterinarias
Instituto Colombiano Agropecuario ICA,
Bogotá, Colombia. Apartado Aéreo 29743.

ABSTRACT

Three groups of 5 lambs were inoculated intraperitoneally with peripheral blood leukocytes, cultured lymphocytes, and macerated neoplastic lymphnodes respectively. Inoculums were obtained from a 6 year old Holstein-Friesian cow that was diagnosed as having enzootic bovine leukaemia. Changes associated with ovine lymphosarcomas were observed in lambs inoculated with 1.4 x 10^8 *leukocytes. Serum antibodies against bovine lymphosarcoma virus (BLV) were detected at four weeks post inoculation (p.i.) and simultaneously increases in the peripheral lymphocyte counts were observed until week 32 PI, together with the presence of immature and neoplastic cells. Gross alterations were minimal, however increases in the size of retropharyngeal, mediastinal and mesenteric lymph nodes were observed in lambs in group I. Neoplastic lymphoid proliferations were observed microscopically in the lymph nodes, liver and heart in the lambs from group I.*

O.C. Straub (ed.), Fourth International Symposium on Bovine Leukosis

INTRODUCTION

Bovine lymphosarcoma is a neoplastic disease which causes large economical losses especially on dairy farms. In Colombia bovine lymphosarcoma has been recognised for many years, but according to recent studies an increase in the incidence of this disease has occurred in milk producing areas. Ovines can suffer from the disease under natural or experimental conditions, and for that reason, lambs can be used as a model to study bovine lymphosarcoma.

MATERIALS AND METHODS

Twenty 1 - 15 day old lambs were used in this experiment (5 were Corriedale and 15 native x Romney Marsh). A 6 year old Holstein-Friesian cow with enzootic bovine leukaemia was used as a donor.

Inoculum 1

One hundred and fifty ml of peripheral blood was collected with 100 iu of heparin/ml and leukocytes were obtained by centrifugation at 160 g for 5 minutes after the erythrocytes were lysed with distilled water. Five lambs (nos. 8212, 8243, 8248, 8622 and 8638) were used in group I and were inoculated intraperitoneally with 1.4×10^8 peripheral blood leukocytes.

Inoculum 2

Twenty ml of blood was collected to obtain peripheral blood lymphocytes (Boyum, 1968). These lymphocytes were cultured in RPMI 1640 culture medium supplemented with 10% bovine foetal calf serum and phytohaemagglutinin-M. Lambs in group II were inoculated intraperitoneally with 2.6×10^8 cultured lymphocytes.

Inoculum 3

Small pieces of neoplastic lymph nodes were macerated with 20 ml of phosphate buffered saline, 100 mg of streptomycin and 100 iu of penicillin were also added. Five lambs in group III were inoculated intraperitoneally with 0.5 g of this preparation. Five lambs in the control group IV were inoculated intraperitoneally with 3 ml of sterile saline and were kept under the same conditions of management as groups I, II and III.

All the lambs were fed during the 6 weeks with a mixture of heated cows' milk (70%), water (27%) and sugar (3%). After the seventh week p.i. the lambs received pasture only. All the lambs were bled prior to inoculation and fortnightly thereafter 5 ml of blood was collected with EDTA to determine the haemoglobin concentration and packed cell volume, together with the total and differential white blood cell counts. Ten ml of blood was collected to obtain serum to determine the total serum protein levels. Bovine leukosis virus (BLV) antibody titres were measured using the agar gel immunodiffusion test (Miller and Olson, 1972). All the lambs that died during the experiment were examined *post mortem* and tissue samples of cerebrum, cerebellum, spinal cord, sciatic nerve, lung, tongue, oesophagus, abomasum, small and large intestine, liver, kidney, urinary bladder, uterus, heart, aorta and spleen were taken together with the following lymphnodes: retropharyngeal, prescapular, mediastinal, mesenteric, prefemoral and popliteal. Tissue sections were fixed in 10% buffered neutral formalin. Paraffin embedded tissues were sectioned at 4 μm and then stained with haemotoxylin-eosin.

RESULTS

The lambs numbered 1, 2 and 5 from group II died during the first month from malnutrition. During the second month lamb no. 8242 from group I, 6 from group III and 11 and 12 from group IV died as a result of bloat. Lambs nos. 7 and 10 from group III died from pneumonia. The packed cell volumes decreased in groups II, III and IV, but there was a greater decrease in group I (Table 1). Haemoglobin concentration also decreased in groups II, III and IV while this fall was moderate in group I (Table 2). Total white blood cell counts increased from week 6 until week 20 p.i., however, this increase was more marked in the lambs in group I, although the total leukocyte counts were within the normal limits for the ovine species. Absolute peripheral lymphocyte counts were similar in the lambs in groups II, III and IV whereas the lambs in group I showed marked increases from week 2 p.i. until week 32 p.i., as compared with group IV (Table 3).

TABLE 1

MEAN PACKED CELL VOLUMES OF BLV INFECTED LAMBS. THE LAMBS IN GROUPS I, II, III AND IV WERE INOCULATED IP[1] WITH PERIPHERAL BLOOD LEUKOCYTES, CULTURED LYMPHOCYTES, MACERATED NEOPLASTIC LYMPHNODES AND STERILE SALINE RESPECTIVELY.

Weeks PI[2]	Group I X[3]	Group II X	Group III X	Group IV X
0	42.0	44.0	40.6	42.6
2	40.0	43.0	40.4	39.0
4	38.5	37.0	39.3	41.3
6	38.5	38.0	37.0	40.3
8	36.5	40.0	38.0	40.5
10	37.5	40.0	36.0	37.3
12	38.0	38.0	34.0	35.5
14	36.0	37.0	35.0	33.8
16	33.5	34.0	33.0	34.0
18	32.3	34.0	34.0	33.0
20	28.3	34.0	33.0	34.7
22	28.7	34.0	33.0	33.0
24	28.0	33.0	34.0	33.0
26	29.3	-[4]	35.0	32.3
28	29.0		34.0	33.0
30	29.0		33.0	34.0
32	27.0		34.0	33.0

[1] Intraperitoneally
[2] Post-inoculation
[3] Mean
[4] The lambs in group II died from causes different from those of the experiment

Lymphoblast, prolymphocytes and anaplastic cells in the peripheral blood were seen between the 6th and 8th week p.i. in lambs in group I. No abnormal or atypical cells were seen in lambs in groups II, III and IV. No significant changes in the absolute blood neutrophil, eosinophil, monocyte and basophil counts were seen in the experiment. The total serum protein concentration was similar in the lambs in groups II, III, IV but a slight decrease was observed in lambs in group I. From 4 weeks p.i. lambs nos.8212 and 8248 in group I showed specific serum antibodies against BLV, 2 weeks later specific antibodies were detected in lambs nos. 8622 and 8633 that belonged to the same group. Specific serum antibodies were not detected in lambs in groups II, III and IV. Lambs nos. 8212, 8248 and 8638 in group I

TABLE 2

MEAN HAEMOGLOBIN CONCENTRATION (g/100 ml) OF BLV INFECTED LAMBS. THE LAMBS IN GROUPS I, II, III AND IV WERE INOCULATED INTRAPERITONEALLY WITH PERIPHERAL BLOOD LEUKOCYTES, CULTURED LYMPHOCYTES, MACERATED NEOPLASTIC LYMPHNODES AND STERILE SALINE, RESPECTIVELY.

Weeks PI[1]	Group I $\bar{X}$[2]	Group II $\bar{X}$	Group III $\bar{X}$	Group IV $\bar{X}$
0	13.4	13.8	12.7	13.5
2	12.7	13.2	12.5	12.2
4	12.0	11.2	11.7	12.5
6	11.0	12.2	11.6	12.9
8	11.7	13.0	11.7	12.8
10	12.0	13.0	11.5	12.2
12	11.0	12.2	10.9	11.0
14	10.4	12.0	11.2	10.6
16	9.4	10.4	10.3	10.7
18	9.5	10.4	10.4	10.6
20	9.0	10.8	10.3	11.2
22	9.2	10.3	10.3	10.2
24	9.0	10.2	10.6	10.4
26	8.0	-[3]	10.8	9.7
28	8.9		10.6	10.0
30	8.9		10.5	10.0
32	8.1		10.5	10.0

[1] Post-inoculation
[2] Mean
[3] The lambs in group II died from causes different from those of the experiment

were examined *post mortem* at 32 weeks p.i. and showed slight subcutaneous oedema and small amounts of ascitic and hydrothoraxic fluid.

TABLE 3

MEAN LYMPHOCYTE COUNTS (x 10^3/ml) OF BLV INFECTED LAMBS. THE LAMBS IN GROUPS I, II, III AND IV WERE INOCULATED IP[1] WITH PERIPHERAL BLOOD LEUKOCYTES. CULTURED LYMPHOCYTES, MACERATED NEOPLASTIC LYMPHNODES AND STERILE SALINE, RESPECTIVELY.

Weeks PI[2]	Group I $\bar{X}$[3]	Group II $\bar{X}$	Group III $\bar{X}$	Group IV $\bar{X}$
0	4.50	4.89	3.51	4.41
2	4.66	4.12	4.02	4.14
4	5.39	4.13	4.04	4.46
6	6.02	5.48	4.95	4.77
8	6.98	5.64	5.74	5.15
10	8.52	5.97	5.59	5.61
12	8.35	6.15	5.69	5.38
14	8.48	6.19	5.85	5.75
16	8.25	6.26	5.04	5.48
18	8.47	5.46	5.49	5.21
20	8.23	4.96	4.52	4.91
22	8.39	4.97	4.53	4.95
24	8.07	4.76	5.54	4.72
26	7.80	-[4]	5.93	4.61
28	7.86		5.50	4.53
30	7.69		5.40	4.51
32	7.77		5.21	4.63

[1] Intraperitoneally
[2] Post-inoculation
[3] Mean
[4] The lambs in group II died from causes different from those of the experiment

Retropharyngeal, prescapular, mediastinal and mesenteric lymphnodes were 2 - 3 times their normal size and the cut surfaces had a white-grey colour, some of them contained nodular formations and no clear demarcation between cortical and medullar zones was observed. Microscopically, lambs 8212, 8248 and 8638 in group I showed lesions in the liver, heart, spleen and lymph nodes. Moderate lymphocytic infiltration was observed in the portal areas of the liver; also immature and neoplastic lymphoid cells were seen in the same area. Slight diffuse lymphocytic infiltration was observed in the heart, together with immature and neoplastic lymphoid cells. Sarcosysts were also evident. Slight reticular cell hyperplasia and haemosiderosis were seen in the spleens. Oedemas, congestion and neoplastic lymphoid proliferation were seen in the retropharyngeal prescapular, mediastinal, mesenteric, prefemoral and popliteal lymphnodes. Neoplastic proliferation was more evident in the cortical zones and these areas had a monotonous, uniform appearance. Subcapsular and marginal sinuses were invaded by neoplastic cells. No clear differentiation was observed in the germinal centres and the primary lymph nodules.

CONCLUSIONS

Ovine lymphosarcoma was reproduced by intraperitoneal inoculation with peripheral blood leukocytes from a cow with enzootic bovine leukaemia. The disease was neither reproduced by the intraperitoneal inoculation with cultured peripheral blood lymphocytes nor by the intraperitoneal inoculation with macerated neoplastic lymph nodes obtained from the same cow. The failure to reproduce the disease may have been due to low virus viability or low infectivity. In the neoplastic stage of the disease the high levels of antibodies may not allow the virus to be released from infected cells. Mitogens as phytohaemagglutinins could also prevent the replication or release of BLV in tissue cultures. Specific serum antibodies against BLV appeared simultaneously with the increase in the peripheral lymphocyte counts and persisted during the experiment. Persistent lymphocytosis was observed and associated with the presence of lymphoblasts, prolymphocytes and neoplastic cells. The presence of specific serum antibodies means that the animals are, or were, infected with BLV and does not indicate whether the animals are showing signs of the disease or are carriers. Haematologic studies show 3 possibilities:

a) seropositive animals without haematological changes

b) seropositive animals with persistent lymphocytosis

c) seropositive animals with persistent lymphocytosis together with immature and neoplastic lymphoid cells.

The histological findings observed in the lymphnodes, liver and heart were characteristic of the changes associated with ovine lymphosarcoma.

REFERENCES

Boyum, A., 1968. Separation of leukocytes from blood and bone marrow. Scandinavian Journal of Clinical and Laboratory Investigation, 21: 109.

Miller, J.M. and Olson, C., 1972. Precipitating antibody to an internal antigen of the C-type virus associated with bovine lymphosarcoma. Journal of the National Cancer Institute, 49: 1459-1461.

DISCUSSION

J.F. Ferrer *(USA)*

How many haematological examinations do you do before you consider an animal has persistent lymphocytosis?

A. Fernando Lozano *(Colombia)*

Three.

J.F. Ferrer

So, therefore you consider you have persistent lymphocytosis when you have three elevated lymphocyte counts?

A. Fernando Lozano

Yes.

PRELIMINARY STUDIES ON IMPACT OF BOVINE LEUKAEMIA VIRUS INFECTION ON DAIRY PRODUCTIVITY*

M.J. Burridge, M.C. Thurmond, D.M. Puhr,
C.J. Wilcox and N.A. Simerl

Department of Preventive Medicine,
College of Veterinary Medicine,

Dairy Science Department, Institute
of Food and Agricultural Sciences,

University of Florida, Gainesville, Florida 32610, USA.

ABSTRACT

A preliminary study was undertaken to investigate the economic impact of bovine leukaemia virus (BLV) infection on milk production in a Florida dairy herd. Relationships between BLV infection status (as determined by reaction to the agar gel immunodiffusion test with a glycoprotein antigen) and 4 production variables (total milk yield, daily milk yield, fat percentage in milk, and length of lactation) were examined statistically. Cows were separated into sire-lactation groups for data analysis to minimise any genetic or age influences. There was no evidence of any difference between BLV positive and BLV negative cattle with regard to the production variables studied.

*Supported by United States Department of Agriculture cooperative agreement 58-519B-0-872.

O.C. Straub (ed.), Fourth International Symposium on Bovine Leukosis

INTRODUCTION

There is evidence from recent work in Israel that leukaemic cattle produce antibodies of reduced immunocompetence (Trainin et al., 1968, 1973, 1976; Klopfer and Trainin, 1970; Trainin and Klopfer, 1971; Ungar-Waron et al., 1978), suggesting that bovine leukaemia virus (BLV) might be an immunosuppressive agent. It is already known that other animal retroviruses such as the feline leukaemia virus can produce immunosuppression in the infected host (Essex, 1980). Consequently, there is a possibility that BLV might decrease an infected animal's resistance to disease, thus having an economic impact on bovine productivity. This paper describes the preliminary results of a study designed to investigate the impact of BLV infection on milk production in a Florida dairy herd.

MATERIALS AND METHODS

Cattle

The cattle studied were the milking cows in the University of Florida Dairy Research Unit herd between 1975 and 1979. This herd is heavily infected with BLV, having an annual BLV antibody prevalence of over 75% in adult cattle (Burridge et al., 1979). The cows were either of the Holstein or Jersey breed, with Holstein predominating. Every one of the 200-plus animals was bled between August and October each year for serum collection. The following production data were collected from each cow by lactation: total milk yield in pounds, fat percentage, and length of lactation in days. Furthermore, the sire of each cow was identified and recorded.

Serology

Each serum sample was tested for BLV antibodies using the agar gel immunodiffusion test with a glycoprotein antigen (Leukassay-B, Pitman-Moore Inc., Washington Crossing, New Jersey), according to the method of Burridge et al. (1979). Each positive reaction to the test was interpreted to indicate past infection with BLV. This test was chosen for the present study because of its simplicity and because of its high relative sensitivity and relative specificity when compared with established tests for the serodiagnosis of BLV infection (Miller and Van der Maaten, 1976, 1977; Olson et al., 1976).

Data analysis

Relationships between BLV antibody status and 4 variables (total milk yield, daily milk yield, fat percentage in milk, and length of lactation) were examined statistically using the t-test procedure of the Statistical Analysis System (SAS User's Guide, 1979). The cows were separated into sire-lactation groups for data analysis so that the animals in each group all had the same sire and the same lactation number. This analytical method minimised any genetic or age influences when the production variables of BLV positive and BLV negative cows were compared.

RESULTS

The mean total milk yield, mean daily milk yield, mean fat percentage, and mean length of lactation are compared between BLV positive and BLV negative cows within 6 sire-lactation groups in Table 1. There was no indication of any difference between BLV positive and BLV negative cattle with regard to the production variables studied.

TABLE 1

COMPARISON OF PRODUCTIVITY OF BOVINE LEUKAEMIA VIRUS (BLV) POSITIVE AND BLV NEGATIVE COWS IN A FLORIDA DAIRY HERD

Sire registration no.*	Lactation no.	BLV-antibody status	No. of cows	Mean total milk yield in lbs.	Mean daily milk yield in lbs.	Mean fat %	Mean length of lactation in days
		-	5	9186	36.2	3.41	261.2
1432733	1			(P=0.588)**	(P=0.714)	(P=0.474)	(P=0.381)
		+	8	10109	34.3	3.19	286.9
		-	11	9915	35.7	3.13	260.3
1515207	1			(P=0.557)	(P=0.979)	(P=0.836)	(P=0.193)
		+	10	10759	35.8	3.10	299.7
		-	7	10760	40.2	3.59	266.9
1515207	2			(P=0.630)	(P=0.546)	(P=0.287)	(P=0.369)
		+	20	9854	42.0	3.35	231.9
		-	3	14327	50.0	3.32	288.0
1515207	3			(P=0.318)	(P=0.445)	(P=0.670)	(P=0.369)
		+	12	11412	47.1	3.43	238.2
		-	4	8278	36.1	3.28	224.8
1516360	1			(P=0.544)	(P=0.565)	(P=0.431)	(P=0.600)
		+	10	9650	38.4	3.13	248.9
		-	3	5967	26.8	4.42	228.0
605836	2			(P=0.950)	(P=0.052)	(P=0.718)	(P=0.374)
		+	5	6060	21.6	4.60	281.6

* Sire number 605836 was a Jersey; all others were Holsteins.

** P value for t-test.

CONCLUSIONS

Four production variables were examined: total and daily milk yield as measures of milk production, fat percentage as a measure of milk quality, and length of lactation as a quantitative measure of disease problems such as mastitis and abortion. There was no evidence that BLV infection had any significant effect on any of these variables.

Only one previous study (Langston et al., 1978) has investigated the effect of BLV infection on dairy productivity. It found no difference in productivity between BLV positive and BLV negative cows. However, that study was not controlled for genetic factors. Consideration of genetic influences in such studies is essential since available data indicate that both milk production variables (Wilcox, 1974) and susceptibility to BLV infection (Burridge et al., 1979) are traits of appreciable heritability.

Optimally, study of the economic impact of BLV infection on dairy productivity should involve within-cow comparisons, comparing production variables in a lactation before infection with those in a later lactation after infection. Such an experimental design would be controlled for genetic influences, and the data could be adjusted for age before analysis. Unfortunately this approach could not be followed in our study since the majority of cows became infected before completion of their first lactation (Burridge et al., 1979).

REFERENCES

Burridge, M.J., Wilcox, C.J. and Hennemann, J.M., 1979. Influence of genetic factors on the susceptibility of cattle to bovine leukemia virus infection. Europ. J. Cancer 15: 1395-1400.

Essex, M., 1980. Feline leukemia and sarcoma viruses. In: Viral Oncology, ed. G. Klein. Raven Press, New York, pp. 205-229.

Klopfer, U. and Trainin, Z., 1970. Haematological findings and IgM levels in a leukotic cow. Refuah Vet. 27: 60-63.

Langston, A., Ferdinand, G.A.A., Ruppanner, R., Theilen, G.H., Drlica, S. and Behymer, D., 1978. Comparison of production variables of bovine leukemia virus antibody-negative and antibody-positive cows in two California dairy herds. Am. J. vet. Res. 39: 1093-1098.

Miller, J.M. and Van der Maaten, M.J., 1976. Serologic detection of bovine leukemia virus infection. Vet. Microbiol. 1: 195-202, Straub, O.C. (ed.). Elsevier Publishing Company Amsterdam and CEC, Luxembourg.

Miller, J.M. and Van der Maaten, M.J., 1977. Use of glycoprotein antigen in the immunodiffusion test for bovine leukemia virus antibodies. Europ. J. Cancer 13: 1369-1375.

Olson, C., Baumgartener, L.E., Miller, J.M. and Van der Maaten, M.J., 1976. A comparison of tests on reference serums for BLV antibody. Vet. Microbiol. 1: 275-278, Straub, O.C. (ed.). Elsevier Publishing Company Amsterdam and CEC, Luxembourg.

SAS User's Guide, 1979. SAS Institute Inc., Raleigh, North Carolina.

Trainin, Z., Nobel, T.A., Klopfer, U. and Neumann, F., 1968. Absence of gamma macroglobulin (IgM) in the sera of leukotic cattle and the diagnosis of bovine leukosis. Refuah Vet. 25: 185-187.

Trainin, Z. and Klopfer, U., 1971. Immunofluorescent studies of lymph nodes and spleens of leukotic cattle for cells producing IgM and IgG. Cancer Res. 31: 1968-1971.

Trainin, Z., Mairom, R., Klopfer, U. and Meidan, G., 1973. Levels of IgM and IgG in the sera of normal and leukaemic calves. J. Comp. Pathol. 83: 87190.

Trainin, Z., Ungar-Waron, H., Meirom, R., Barnea, A. and Sela, M., 1976. IgG and IgM antibodies in normal and leukaemic cattle. J. Comp. Pathol. 86: 571-580.

Ungar-Waron, H., Avraham, R., Gluckmann, A. and Trainin Z., 1978. Reduced immunocompetence of antibodies produced in leukemic cattle. Ann. Rech. Vét. 9: 815-819.

Wilcox, C.J., 1974. Breedings for milk production. In: Animal Agriculture, H.H. Cole and M. Ronning (eds.). W.H. Freeman & Co., San Francisco, p.280.

STUDIES ON BOVINE LEUKOSIS VIII. THE SEROLOGIC RESPONSE OF LEUKOTIC CATTLE TO INJECTIONS WITH AUJESZKY'S DISEASE AND BORDETELLA VACCINES, TETANUS TOXOID AND PORCINE ERYTHROCYTES. THE CUTANEOUS REACTION FOLLOWING ADMINISTRATION OF *Mycobacterium microti* AND THE EFFECT OF POKEWEED AND PHYTOHAEMAGGLUTININ STIMULATION ON LEUKOTIC LYMPHOCYTES

A.A. Ressang, W. Rumawas, P.R. Rondhuis,
J. Haagsma and S. Bercovich

Central Veterinary Institute ,
P.O. Box 6007, 3002 AA Rotterdam, The Netherlands.

ABSTRACT

The serological reactions to parenteral administrations of Aujeszky's disease vaccine, bordetella vaccine, porcine erythrocytes and tetanus toxoid in leukotic and non-leukotic cattle were examined and compared. No significant difference in the humoral immune response was observed. Both groups of experimental animals were also given Mycobacterium microti by the intravenous route. The delayed type hypersensitivity skin reaction was significantly more clear in the leukotic group. Leukocytes from the leukotic and non-leukotic animals were cultured, stimulated with pokeweed and thereupon their thymidin uptake determined. The stimulation indices were equal. Leukocytes from leukotic animals stimulated with phytohaem-agglutinin had lower indices.

Thus it seemed that suppression of the humoral immunological system did not occur in clinically healthy cattle affected with enzootic bovine leukosis. In contrast, the cellular immunological apparatus was significantly activated in this disease.

Cross-reacting antibodies to pig erythrocytes, bordetella vaccine and tetanus toxoid, were found.

Paper published in full in: Zbl. Vet. Med., Reihe B, 27, 576-587 (1980)

O.C. Straub (ed.), Fourth International Symposium on Bovine Leukosis

CLOSING REMARKS

J. Connell *(CEC)*

In closing this seminar, I thank Professor Gentile and Professor Straub most sincerely for their enormous efforts in preparing such a successful meeting. Furthermore, I do assure you it is an honour for the Commission to be able to gather together so many eminent scientists on such an important topic. The outcome of this meeting, the 4th CEC International Symposium on Bovine Leukosis, will add greatly to the work which has appeared from earlier research supported from Brussels and in the member states of the European Community. Certainly, on the subject of bovine leukosis, considerable progress has been made by the Commission and scientists in this lecture room. On behalf of the CEC Division which co-ordinates agricultural research (VI F 4) and the CEC Division which deals with legislation relating to veterinary matters (VI B 4), Mr. J. Caffrey and I thank you all for your participation and contributions to the proceedings which will be published for a much wider international audience interested in your conclusions.

LIST OF PARTICIPANTS

AUSTRIA

Prof. Dr. F. Bürki	Institut für Virologie Tierärztliche Hochschule Wien Linke Bahngasse 11 A-1030 Vienna

BELGIUM

Prof. A. Burny	Université de Bruxelles Département de Biologie Moléculaire 67 rue des Chevaux B-1650 Rhode Saint-Genèse
Dr. J.P. Caffrey	Commission of the European Communities DG VI 200 rue de la Loi B-1049 Brussels
Dr. J. Connell	Commission of the European Communities DG VI 200 rue de la Loi B-1049 Brussels
Dr. R. Kettmann	Université de Bruxelles Département de Biologie Moléculaire 67 rue des Chevaux B-1640 Rhode Saint-Genèse
Dr. M. Mammerickx	Institut National de Recherches Vétérinaires 99 Groeselenberg B-1180 Brussels
Dr. D. Portetelle	Université Libre de Bruxelles Département de Biologie Moléculaire 67 rue des Chevaux B-1640 Rhode Saint-Genèse

CANADA

Dr. B.S. Samagh	Animal Diseases Research Institute 801 Fallowfield Road Box 11300, Station H Nepean, Ontario K2H 8P9
Dr. P. Seguin	Canadian Embassy 35 Montaigne 75008 Paris France

COLOMBIA

Dr. A. Fernando Lozano	Apartado Aéreo 29743 Bogotá

ČSSR

Dr. B. Hofírek — Vysoká škola veterinární
Palackého 1-3
612 42 Brno

DENMARK

Dr. J.C. Flensburg — Veterinaerdirektoratet
Frederiksgade 21
DK-1265 Copenhagen K

Dr. R. Hoff-Jørgensen — Statens Veterinaere Serum Laboratorium
Bülowsvej 27
DK-1870 Copenhagen V

FEDERAL REPUBLIC OF GERMANY

Dr. F. Behrens — Behringwerke AG
Postfach 1140
D-3550 Marburg/Lahn

Prof. Dr. O.-R. Kaaden — Institut für Virologie der Tierärztliche Hochschule
Bischofsholer Damm 15
D-3000 Hannover 1

Dr. R.J. Lorenz — Bundesforschungsanstalt für Viruskrankheiten der Tiere
Postfach 1149
D-7400 Tübingen

Prof. Dr. M. Mussgay — Bundesforschungsanatalt für Viruskrankheiten der Tiere
Postfach 1149
D-7400 Tübingen

Dr. E. Schaal — Direktor des Staatlichen Veterinäruntersuchungsamtes
Zur Taubeneiche 10-12
D-5760 Arnsberg 2

Prof. Dr. F.-W. Schmidt — Tierärztliches Institut der Universität Göttingen
Geiststrasse 7
D-3400 Göttingen

Prof. Dr. O.C. Straub — Bundesforschungsanstalt für Viruskrankheiten der Tiere
Postfach 1149
D-7400 Tübingen

FRANCE

Dr. Thérèse Astier — Institut National de la Santé et de la Recherche Médicale
U-117
Fondation Bergonié
229 cours de l'Argonne
33076 Bordeaux Cedex

Dr. T. Gauthier — L'Institut RONCHESE
Zone Industrielle de Libourne
F-33501 Libourne

Dr. L. Deshayes — Laboratoire Immunologie et Virologie des Tumeurs
Groupe INSERM U-152
Hôpital Cochin
27 rue du Faubourg Saint-Jacques
F-75674 Paris Cedex 14

Dr. B. Guillemain — Institut National de la Santé et de la Recherche Médicale
U-117
Fondation Bergonié
229 cours de l'Argonne
F-33076 Bordeaux Cedex

Dr. D. Lévy — Laboratoire Immunologie et Virologie des Tumeurs
INSERM U-152
Hôpital Cochin
27 rue du Faubourg Saint-Jacques
F-75014 Paris Cedex 14

Dr. R. Mamoun — Institut National de la Santé et de la Recherche Médicale
U-117
Fondation Bergonié
229 cours de l'Argonne
F-33076 Bordeaux Cedex

Dr. Mialot — Département de Pathologie
Ecole National Vétérinaire
7 Avenue de Général de Gaulle
F-94704 Maisons-Alfort

Prof. Dr. A.L. Parodi — Département de Pathologie
Ecole Nationale Vétérinaire
7 Avenue de Général de Gaulle
F-94704 Maisons-Alfort

GERMAN DEMOCRATIC REPUBLIC

Dr. R. Schön — Zentralinstitut für Molekularbiologie
Lindengerweg 70
DDR-1115 Berlin - Buch

GREECE

Dr. I.A. Dimitriadis — Bas. Sofias 65
Ag. Paraskeyi
Athens

HUNGARY

Prof. Dr. Z. Horvâth — Veterinäruniversität
Landler J u.2
H-1400 Budapest

IRELAND

Dr. P.J. Kavanagh — Veterinary Research Laboratory
Abbotstown
Castleknock
Co. Dublin

ISRAEL

Prof. Dr. Y. Becker — Department of Molecular Biology
Hebrew University
Hadassah Medical School
P.O. Box 1172
Jerusalem

ITALY

Dr. F. Biancifiori — Istituto Zooprofilattico Sperimentale
Umbria E Marche
Via Salvemini 1
I-06100 Perugia

Dr. V. Caporale — Istituto Zooprofilattico Sperimentale
Teramo

Prof. Dr. C. Cavrini — Direzione Generale Servici Veterinari
Ministero della Sanita
I-EUR-Rome

Prof. Dr. G. Gentile — Il Direttore
Clinica Medica Veterinaria
Viale Q. Filopanti 5
I-40126 Bologna

Prof. Dr. A. Mantovani — Facoltà di Medicina Veterinaria
Via S. Giacomo 9/2
I-40126 Bologna

Prof. Dr. P.S. Marcato — Istituto di Patologia Generale
Facoltà di Medicina Veterinaria
Via Belmeloro 10
I-40126 Bologna

Dr. G. Poli	Istituto di Microbiologia e Immunologia Veterinaria Facoltà di Medicina Veterinaria Via Caloria 10 I-20100 Milan
Dr. D. Rutili	Istituto Zooprofilattico Sperimentale Via S. Constanza 14 I-06100 Perugia
Dr. M. Severini	Istituto di Ispezione degli Alimenti O.A. Facoltà di Medicina Veterinaria Via S. Constanza 14 I-06100 Perugia
Dr. P. Simoni	Istituto di Patologia Generale Facoltà di Medicina Veterinaria Via Belmeloro 10 I-40126 Bologna
Prof. Dr. S. Tura	Cattedra di Ematologia Policlinico S. Orsola Via Massarenli I-40126 Bologna
Prof. Dr. G. Vacirca	Clinica Medica Veterinaria Via Celoria 10 I-20100 Milan

JAPAN

Dr. M. Onuma	Faculty of Veterinary Medicine Hokkaido University Sapporo 060

SWEDEN

Prof. Dr. G. Hugoson	National Veterinary Institute Department of Epizootiology S-750 07 Uppsala
Prof. Dr. Z. Dinter	Department of Virology The Royal Veterinary College Biomedicum Box 585 S-751 23 Uppsala

SWITZERLAND

Dr. H.W. Holy	Technicon International Division SA 12-14 chemin Rieu CH-1208 Geneva
Mrs. V. Reicher	Technicon International Division SA 12-14 chemin Rieu CH-1208 Geneva

THE NETHERLANDS

Dr. G. de Vries	Stichting Gezondheidszorg voor Dieren Bachmanstraat 48 The Hague
Mr. J. Quak	Centraal Diersgeneeskundig Instituut P.O. Box 6007 Prof. Poelslaan 35 NL-3028 EP Rotterdam
Prof. Dr. A.A Ressang	Centraal Diergeneeskundig Instituut P.O. Box 6007 Prof. Poelslaan 35 NL-3028 EP Rotterdam

UNITED KINGDOM

Mr. S.E.W. Hallam	Janssen Services 33a High Street Chislehurst Kent BR7 5AE
Dr. M.H. Lucas	Ministry of Agriculture, Fisheries and Food Central Veterinary Laboratory New Haw Weybridge Surrey KT15 3NB
Mr. L.M. Markson	Central Veterinary Laboratory New Haw Weybridge Surrey KT15 3NB
Dr. D.H. Roberts	Ministry of Agriculture, Fisheries and Food Central Veterinary Laboratory New Haw Weybridge Surrey KT15 3NB
Mrs. M.J. Robins	Janssen Services 33a High Street Chislehurst Kent BR7 5AE
Dr. W.A. Watson	Ministry of Agriculture, Fisheries and Food Hook Rise South Tolworth Surbiton Surrey

USA

Dr. M.J. Burridge	Associate Professor of Epidemiology College of Veterinary Medicine Department of Preventive Medicine Box J-136 University of Florida Gainesville Florida 32610
Prof. Dr. J.F. Ferrer	University of Pennsylvania School of Veterinary Medicine Kennett Square New Bolton Center RD 1 Pennsylvania 19348
Prof. Dr. C. Olson	Department of Veterinary Science University of Wisconsin 1655 Linden Drive Madison Wisconsin 53706
Prof. Dr. G.H. Theilen	University of California School of Veterinary Medicine Davis California 95616
Dr. M.C. Thurmond	College of Veterinary Medicine Department of Preventive Medicine Box J-136 University of Florida Gainesville Florida 32610
Dr. M.J. Van der Maaten	US Department of Agriculture National Animal Disease Center P.O. Box 70 Ames Iowa 50010

VENEZUELA

Dr. C. Marin Aponte	Instituto de Investigaçiones Veterinarias Apdo. 70 Maracay 300 Caracas

YUGOSLAVIA

Prof. Dr. I. Jazbec	Tierärztliche Fakultät Cesta v Mestnilog 47 YU-61000 Ljubljana

Manuscript prepared by JANSSEN SERVICES,
33a High Street, Chislehurst, Kent BR7 5AE, UK.

GPSR Compliance

The European Union's (EU) General Product Safety Regulation (GPSR) is a set of rules that requires consumer products to be safe and our obligations to ensure this.

If you have any concerns about our products, you can contact us on ProductSafety@springernature.com

In case Publisher is established outside the EU, the EU authorized representative is:

Springer Nature Customer Service Center GmbH
Europaplatz 3
69115 Heidelberg, Germany

Batch number: 10620157

Printed by Printforce, the Netherlands